NAVIGATING THE MAZE OF RESEARCH

4TH EDITION

Enhancing Nursing and Midwifery Practice

Australian and New Zealand edition

NAVIGATING THE MAZE OF RESEARCH

4TH EDITION

Enhancing Nursing and Midwifery Practice

Australian and New Zealand edition

SALLY BORBASI RN, PHD

Honorary Professor of Nursing, Faculty of Health Sciences,
Australian Catholic University, McAuley Campus,
Brisbane, Queensland, Australia

DEBRA JACKSON FACN, PHD

Professor of Nursing, Faculty of Health & Life Sciences,
Oxford Brookes University, UK
Professor, Nursing Research, Oxford University Hospitals
NHS Trust, UK
Professor of Nursing, University of New England,
Armidale, New South Wales, Australia

ELSEVIER

ELSEVIER

Elsevier Australia. ACN 001 002 357
(a division of Reed International Books Australia Pty Ltd)
Tower 1, 475 Victoria Avenue, Chatswood, NSW 2067

Navigating the Maze of Nursing Research: An interactive adventure
Copyright © 2001 by Mosby, Inc.
ISBN: 978-0-323-00947-8

This adaptation of Navigating the Maze of Nursing Research: An interactive adventure, 1e, by Rae Langford, was undertaken by Elsevier Australia and is published by arrangement with Elsevier Inc.

Navigating the Maze of Research: Enhancing Nursing and Midwifery Practice; 4th edition
Copyright © 2016 Elsevier Australia. 3rd edition © 2012; 2nd edition © 2008; 1st edition © 2004 Elsevier Australia.
ISBN: 978-0-7295-4213-5

National Library of Australia Cataloguing-in-Publication entry

---

Borbasi, Sally, author.

Navigating the maze of research : enhancing nursing and midwifery practice / Sally Borbasi & Debra Jackson.

4th edition.

9780729542135 (paperback)

Nursing–Research–Australia.
Midwifery–Australia.
Nursing–Australia.

Jackson, Debra, author.

610.73072

Senior Content Strategist: Melinda McEvoy
Content Development Specialist: Tamsin Curtis
Project Manager: Devendran Kannan
Edited by Rosemary McDonald
Proofread by Forsyth Publishing Services
Index by Robert Swanson
Typeset by Toppan Best-set Premedia Limited
Cover and internal design by Georgette Hall
Printed in China by CTPS

CONTENTS

ACKNOWLEDGMENTS

As colleagues who have witnessed huge progress in the evolution of nursing and midwifery scholarship during past decades, we take delight in conveying our appreciation to all our readers for seeking out this up-to-the minute interactive learning resource to promote understanding of a topic fundamental to both professions. We couldn't have produced this exemplary text without the assistance of some very talented people, whom we would like to acknowledge. So we say a big thank you to all of our contributors for their excellent work in this edition while not forgetting to acknowledge those contributors who appeared in earlier editions. We also want to thank the peer reviewers for their thoughtful and helpful critique and a big thank you to Melinda McEvoy, Senior Content Strategist, Tamsin Curtis, Content Development Specialist and Devendran Kannan, Project Manager, for their support and encouragement, and finally to you, the reader. We congratulate you for wanting to better understand what research can bring to your professional practice. We hope you find this book an informative and engaging stimulus to your life of learning and we wish you all the very best for your future career in nursing or midwifery whether as a consumer of research or indeed as consumer *and* researcher.

Sally Borbasi

Debra Jackson

PUBLISHER'S NOTE

A range of exciting and instructive activities are provided on the accompanying Evolve website (http://evolve.elsevier.com/AU/Borbasi/maze/) to extend student learning and enhance understanding of critical concepts in each chapter. Elsevier Australia wishes to thank contributors for the development of this material.

FOREWORD

The need for this new edition of *Navigating the Maze of Research: Enhancing Nursing and Midwifery Practice* reflects the significant success of the work overall and is a measure of its utility, quality and relevance. This fourth edition bears all of the hallmarks of earlier editions of the work. Once again the highly regarded editors of, and expert contributors to, the work have continued to provide a highly accessible, engaging, pedagogically sound, comprehensive, contemporary and scholarly introduction to research in nursing and midwifery. As one would expect, the new edition has surpassed the high standard achieved in earlier versions. This edition provides the most up-to-date thinking behind research and research processes for nursing, midwifery and health with enhanced examples of application to clinical practice.

In this research text, Professors Sally Borbasi and Debra Jackson demonstrate the importance of developing research literacy, where clinical nurses and midwives develop a greater understanding of the evidence generated by research findings. They are then able to implement this evidence into practice. Nurse and midwife clinicians and students need to be able to understand and evaluate the available evidence related to their practice, in order to give the best possible care to their patients and clients. This introductory research textbook will certainly assist them to develop these skills. It will certainly excite both new and experienced practitioners to navigate the maze and to break down the barriers to understanding research, thus enhancing their practice.

Like earlier editions, this high-quality text will be a valuable asset to undergraduate students and academic staff in nursing and midwifery programs, particularly in nursing and/or midwifery inquiry and research methods components. It will continue to serve as an important vehicle for use in demystifying the complexities of research and in informing and inspiring students of research in nursing and midwifery.

We commend this text to students, teachers and clinicians engaged in learning and discovery in nursing and midwifery research.

John Daly PhD, RN, FACN, FAAN
Dean and Professor of Nursing, Faculty of Health
Head, WHO Collaborating Centre for Nursing, Midwifery & Health Development
University of Technology, Sydney, New South Wales, Australia

Michelle Campbell RN, BAppSc, MNS, DN
Professor and Executive Dean, Faculty of Health Sciences
Australian Catholic University

ABOUT THE AUTHORS

Sally Borbasi and Debra Jackson are both registered nurses, long-standing nursing academics and professors of nursing, although Sally has recently retired from full-time work and Debra has moved to take up an exciting position overseas. Sally and Debra met at the University of Sydney in the early 1990s.

FROM THE AUTHORS

Over the years we have worked across different states in Australia and have had the pleasure of teaching research and evidence-based practice to student groups at baccalaureate, masters and doctoral levels. We have also worked with baccalaureate, masters, doctoral and post doctoral levels and practising clinicians to make research less mystifying and more readily applicable to clinical practice. As teachers we have experimented with a number of differing pedagogies/learning practices to make research come alive for students and practitioners.

This learning package is in part a result of that experimentation, stemming as it did from the original edition of Rae Langford's book, published first in the USA. In this latest edition, the fourth of our collaboration on this title, we have reshaped and advanced the work of previous editions and added some significant content. Once again we have sought contributions from a range of highly experienced leading academics and scholars in nursing and midwifery. We are pleased ethics, Indigenous research and knowledge translation are more visible in this issue. Most of our contributors have been using this book with their students for many years and therefore had first-hand knowledge of how the material could be expanded and improved. Together, we have produced a cutting-edge collection of work to inform, challenge and stimulate. We believe we bring you a book that is even better geared to making you, the student, understand and navigate the maze we call research. We make research accessible!

Many of the quizzes and challenges included in this edition have been tested with undergraduate students, who have found them fun and challenging. Students have commented this approach makes research seem more real and relevant, and helps them to feel more confident in reading and making sense of research articles. Academics have given us positive feedback, claiming their students are increasingly discussing and applying research findings to clinical situations and classroom activities.

The goal of this book is to equip you as a student and beginning research consumer with the skills to enable you quickly to find, critically read and readily identify possible uses for relevant clinical research. The book aims to introduce you to the research process and provide insight into how research is conducted and why. Importantly, this book highlights that not all nurses or midwives will actually conduct or *do* research but that we all need to be able to *use* the findings from research in our daily practice. In order to do this, clinicians need to understand the foundations of basic research and be able to evaluate critically and, if appropriate, implement research findings. Knowledge is constantly 'moving' and this book provides the latest facts and tips about how you can keep on top of it and use it to your best advantage. The approach taken is interactive and multimodal, aimed at getting students actively involved in the learning process with provision of multiple opportunities to practise and integrate newly acquired skills. We hope you find this approach as useful as we and our students have. Happy navigating!

Sally Borbasi
Debra Jackson

TO THE READER

In order to promote your understanding of the comprehensive material provided in this book, we thought we would walk you through the chapters as a precursor to your own navigation. Let us start at the very beginning – **Section 1** sketches the research backdrop. This section introduces you to research as a strategy for generating knowledge and is devoted to honing your library, internet, reading, abstracting and research appreciation skills. The important distinction between actually conducting research yourself as opposed to informing your practice through other people's research is made. Using research in the provision of care is called evidence-based practice and its implementation is due mainly to a process described as 'knowledge translation'. In order to conduct or use research, students need to become research consumers. Research consumers are able to find and then read research articles, evaluate their relevance and apply the results/knowledge to their practice. **Chapter 1** sets the scene by introducing you to the concept of research as an important avenue for gaining disciplinary knowledge on which to base professional practice; to do this requires some understanding of what is called the 'research process'. In this chapter you will be introduced to fundamental concepts associated with the research process, particularly around the design and conduct of research studies. This is a really important chapter for laying the foundations to your understanding so make sure you read it well.

In order to practice from an evidence (research) base, clinicians need to understand the research literature and how to find it. **Chapter 2** navigates the 21st century library and its many assets providing insights for efficient and effective database searching (knowledge access) while also explaining the core features of a library and how they have changed rapidly in recent years and continue to change.

Chapter 3 explores the vast resources for furthering practice that are available on the internet. However, be warned not all knowledge is valid and reliable or trustworthy and the ability to discern the good from the bad is crucial to best practice for patient care. Here we introduce you to the importance of critiquing the information/literature you access through library databases and internet sources.

Chapter 4 covers important concepts for clinicians to know if they are to understand and appreciate the ethical principles that apply to research.

Section 2 of the book is further designed to give you the vocabulary necessary to read, understand and appraise research studies by introducing you to the main types of research design – quantitative, qualitative and mixed methods. We also introduce an important new paradigm that seeks to uncover Indigenous perspectives. As an introductory textbook **Chapters 5, 6, 7 and 8** explain basic concepts for beginners in the field. Over time, as you grapple more deeply with research fundamentals through further study, your ability to feel comfortable with the material will inevitably increase.

Having provided some hints and tips for evidence searching and explored some of the major research paradigms described in the literature, the next steps for understanding the machinations of research are presented in **Section 3**. Firstly, **Chapter 9** explores the notion of reading research and scholarship, and teaches you essential elements in appraising evidence/research using a systematic approach. In so doing, the text builds upon some of the basic concepts and principles learned in Section 1. This chapter should make clear the necessary steps in reviewing literature critically before contemplating its implementation.

Chapter 10 extends on the idea of evidence being considered worthy of implementation by looking at just how that might take place and why a lot of good/ 'best' evidence does not get carried over into practice but sits in journals on library databases. Once we have established that research is good research we need to think about how we get that research evidence into practice. How do we translate that knowledge to practice so that patients benefit? What are the barriers and facilitators to that end? **Chapter 11** comprises an example of the research process in action and is designed to bring much of what has been covered beforehand, together. Through a case study the researchers describe the steps they took in carrying out a piece of research and then discuss how the study was formally appraised as evidence. Finally, **Chapter 12** continues the theme of using research to make practice change and influence the system by looking to the future and discussing the importance of nurses and midwives translating knowledge into practice while providing examples of models that have been developed to fulfill this aim. The requirement for you to embrace a lifetime of learning is also raised in this section.

That brings us to the end of the book. One comment we would like to make is that in our experience, many students tend to approach research as a topic that doesn't seem to have much relevance for them. They will ask, why do I need to know this? However, they will soon discover their professional associations consider research so vital to the professions of midwifery and nursing that they expect all practitioners, regardless of educational preparation, to be research consumers. In this, the 21st century, you need to keep continually abreast of the knowledge that forms the basis of your practice and to do that you need to know the material we present in this book. In addition, you will need to update your knowledge and skills constantly as you move through your career. This is where this learning package (textbook and website) takes off! It is designed to enhance your skills in finding information fast and using that information effectively so that you can successfully read, understand, evaluate and apply research findings in your everyday clinical practice. It encourages you to examine what you do in the clinical area and to pose questions such as: 'Am I providing the best possible care?' 'Why am I doing this intervention?' 'Is this the best way to carry out this intervention?' It seeks to involve you as an active participant in this learning process. Student activities and critical thinking opportunities are featured throughout the text, along with interactive exercises and quizzes you will find on the Evolve website. The more you participate in the various activities, exercises and discussions about the identified research content, the more confident and competent you will become in using research as a tool to improve your practice and/or argue for change. Most importantly, this book represents an excellent starting point for you to become that lifelong learner you read about in **Chapters 10** and **12**.

By the final pages we hope you will have gained a much better understanding of research and why it is such an important avenue for the development of the nursing and midwifery disciplines. Understand too, that research as a form of knowledge making is subject to constantly shifting sands (associated with internal and external forces and perhaps a little bureaucracy) and so our peek into the future is designed to help you plan your own journey. Whatever you do, don't overlook the many special features of this book as they are especially designed to boost your learning! They are listed below. Used well, you may find you not only learn how to translate research effectively in your midwifery or nursing practice, but you also increase your ability to read and think critically, to analyse situations and to use and manage available resources better.

Okay that's enough from us! We invite you now to begin the first step in your journey to navigate the maze that is nursing or midwifery research. Bon Voyage: Enjoy the Ride!

Special features

- Student quotes: You can probably identify with other students' feelings about research.
- Abstracts: Just as a research article has an abstract – an introductory paragraph that summarises the article – so too does each chapter of the book.

- Learning objectives: These describe what you should be able to do after reading each chapter and working through the activities.
- Chapter outline: Each chapter contains a list of the major headings to give you an idea of the topics covered.
- Key terms: A list of the terms that are important to know is provided for each chapter.
- Student challenges: Try these activities to apply what you are reading and learning.
- Hints and other boxed information: Be sure to remember these useful tips and notes.
- Resource kits: These provide a list of materials to refer to for further information.
- Glossary: A list of all the key terms in the book is provided at the back of the book.
- Evolve website: This website, located at http://evolve.elsevier.com/AU/Borbasi/maze/, provides links to internet sites that correspond to activities in the text, and other websites relevant to nursing and midwifery research. Also included on Evolve are quizzes and student activities for each chapter, as well as teaching tips and PowerPoint slides for faculty members.

LIST OF CONTRIBUTORS

Sharon Andrew PhD, MSc(Hons), BAppSc, RN
Professor of Nursing, School of Nursing and Midwifery, Anglia Ruskin University, England

Wendy Cross BAppSc., MEd., PhD
Professor and Head, School of Nursing and Midwifery, Monash University, Victoria, Australia

Hannah G Dahlen RN, RM, BN(Hons), MCommN, PhD, FACM
Professor, School of Nursing and Midwifery, University of Western Sydney, New South Wales, Australia

Rebecca Disler MSc (KCL), PDAN (UMelb), BN (Latrobe), BSc (UMelb)
Senior Lecturer, Director of International Activities, Centre for Cardiovascular and Chronic Care, Faculty of Health, University of Technology Sydney, New South Wales, Australia

Leah East BN (Hons), PhD
Post Doctoral Fellow, School of Nursing and Midwifery, Faculty of Health, Deakin University, Victoria, Australia

Anne Gardner RN, BA, CritCareCert, MPH, PhD
Professor of Nursing, School of Nursing, Midwifery and Paramedicine, Australian Catholic University, Australian Capital Territory, Australia

Terri Gibson RN, Dip Applied Science (Nursing), BN (Education), MA Nursing Studies, PhD
Senior Lecturer & Program Director Postgraduate & International, School of Nursing and Midwifery, University of South Australia, South Australia, Australia

Elizabeth J. Halcomb RN, BN(Hons), GradCertICNurs, GradCertHE, PhD, FACN
Professor of Primary Health Care Nursing, School of Nursing, University of Wollongong, New South Wales, Australia

Louise D. Hickman RN, MPH, PhD
Director Postgraduate Nursing Studies, Faculty of Health, University of Technology, New South Wales, Australia

Anne T. Hofmeyer RN, PhD
Senior Lecturer, School of Nursing and Midwifery, University of South Australia, South Australia, Australia

Marie Hutchinson RN, RM, PhD
Associate Professor, School of Health and Human Sciences, Southern Cross University, New South Wales, Australia

Judy Mannix RN, BEd (Nsg), MN(Hons)
Director of Academic Programs – Postgraduate, School of Nursing and Midwifery, University of Western, Sydney, New South Wales, Australia

Jane Mills PhD, MN, MEd, BN, GradCertEdu, FACN
Professor, Director Centre for Nursing and Midwifery Research, College of Healthcare Sciences, James Cook University, Queensland, Australia

Kath Peters RN, BN (Hons), PhD
Associate Professor, School of Nursing & Midwifery, University of Western Sydney, New South Wales, Australia

Tamara Power RN, BN (Hons), PhD
Lecturer, Faculty of Health, University of Technology, Sydney, New South Wales, Australia

Lucie Ramjan RN, BN(Dist.), BN(Hons-1st Class), PhD
School of Nursing and Midwifery, University of Western Sydney, New South Wales, Australia

Bob Ribbons RN, ICCert, BAppSc (Nur), MEd (Computing)
Undergraduate Coordinator Bachelor of Nursing, Health Science and Biotechnology, Holmesglen, Victoria, Australia

Virginia A. Schmied BA, MA(Hons), PhD
Professor, School of Nursing and Midwifery, University of Western Sydney, New South Wales, Australia

Juanita Sherwood RN, Primary Teaching Dip Education, Post Grad Cert Collaborative Research, PhD
Professor and Academic Director, National Centre for Cultural Competence, Deputy Vice Chancellor (Indigenous Strategy and Services), University of Sydney, New South Wales, Australia
Adjunct Professor of Indigenous Health, Public Health, James Cook University, Queensland, Australia

Sally K. Tracy DMid, MA, BNurs, Grad Dip N, RGON, RM
Professor of Midwifery, Faculty of Nursing and Midwifery, The University of Sydney, New South Wales, Australia
Professor of Midwifery, Midwifery and Women's Health Research Unit, Royal Hospital for Women, New South Wales, Australia

Kim Usher RN, BA, DipAppSc, MNSt, PhD, FACN, FACMHN
Head of School, Health, University of New England, New South Wales, Australia

Denise Wilson RN, BA (SocSc), MA (Hons), PhD
Professor, Maori Health, School of Public Health & Psychosocial Studies; Director, Taupua Waiora Centre for Maori Health Research, Auckland University of Technology University, Auckland, New Zealand

LIST OF REVIEWERS

Lesley Andrew MSc, BSc (Hons), RN, RHV. (PhD candidate)
School of Exercise and Health Science, Faculty of Health, Engineering and Science, Edith Cowan University, Western Australia, Australia
Registered Nurse, Nursing and Midwifery Board of Australia; Fellow of the Higher Education Academy

Catherine Chung RN, MAdvNsgPrac (Emerg), Grad.Dip AdvNsgPrac (Emerg), Grad.Cert HPE, BN
Lecturer, Nursing & Midwifery, Federation University, Victoria, Australia; ANF, ACCCN, CENA, NTEU

Leigh Davis PhD, BN (Hons 1st), RN, RM
Casual Academic, University of Queensland; Sessional Tutor, Queensland University of Technology; Clinical Nurse and Midwife, Royal Brisbane and Women's Hospital, Queensland, Australia

Judith Finn PhD, MEdSt, GradDipPH, BSc, DipAppSc, RN, RM, ICCert, FACN, FAHA
Curtin University, Perth; Monash University, Melbourne, Victoria, Australia

Yvonne Hauck PhD
Professor of Midwifery, School of Nursing and Midwifery, Curtin University, Western Australia, Australia

Tracey Moroney RN, BN (Hons), PhD, Grad Cert Ed Studies (Higher Ed), MACN
Dean, School of Nursing, The University of Notre Dame, Sydney, Australia

Jane O'Donnell NZRN, BHSc, MN, GradCert Clinical ED
Fisher & Paykel Healthcare Ltd, East Tamaki, Auckland, New Zealand

Amanda Towell D Cur, M Cur, B Cur (Ed et Adm), DCH, RCCN, RN
Edith Cowan University, School of Nursing and Midwifery, Western Australia, Australia; Adjunct Researcher, Sir Charles Gairdner Hospital, Western Australia, Australia

Rachel Walker RN, BN, BA, MA (Research), PhD
Research Fellow, NHMRC Centre of Research Excellence in Nursing, Centre for Health Practice Innovation, Menzies Health Institute Queensland, Griffith University, Australia
Division of Surgery, Princess Alexandra Hospital Queensland, Australia

Jo Wu RN, DrHlthSc, FACN
Senior Research Fellow, School of Nursing, Midwifery and Paramedicine, Faculty of Health Sciences, Australian Catholic University, Queensland, Australia
Fellow of Australian College of Nursing (FACN); Visiting Fellow, School of Nursing, Queensland University of Technology; Honorary Research Fellow, Mater Research Institute-University of Queensland; Honorary Research Fellow, Royal Brisbane & Women's Hospital; Editorial Board member of International Nursing Review

SECTION 1

Finding it fast and reading it well

We live in a time when information on almost any topic is readily available. Information is produced every minute of every day. The 21st century requires learners to be able to find and access information quickly. Much of the information you will be interested in will be based on research. Unfortunately, many new learners fail to take advantage of the wealth of information and research available and have little idea about how to find and use it. Taking advantage of the information explosion and being able to access information is critical to success. This chapter will help you to be better prepared. The trick is not to be overwhelmed by the challenge but to identify your deficits and learn the skills you need to be successful. This section will introduce you to research as an important source of information/knowledge, to the need for research to be ethical, to the resources available in today's library and teach you how best to use the library and electronic resources to get the information you need.

CHAPTER 1

INTRODUCTION TO NURSING AND MIDWIFERY RESEARCH

Kim Usher and Jane Mills

CHAPTER OUTLINE

KEY TERMS

deductive reasoning
epistemology
evidence-based practice
inductive reasoning
interdisciplinary teamwork
intuition
knowledge translation
midwifery research
mixed methods research
nursing research
qualitative research
quantitative research
reasoning
research

LEARNING OBJECTIVES

After reading this chapter and following critical reflection the student will be able to:

1. Explore preconceived self-notions about research
2. Define the terms 'research', 'nursing research' and 'midwifery research'
3. Describe ways to acquire knowledge
4. Describe the historical development of nursing or midwifery research
5. Discuss why nursing or midwifery research is important
6. Define the term 'evidence-based practice'
7. Identify in any research paper the research question, the study design and the findings
8. Discuss the contribution research can make to inform and change practice.

STUDENT QUOTE

I expected to learn about research at university and I am delighted I have been able to link it to both my studies and clinical practice.

ABSTRACT

Research is one way to acquire knowledge in order to make sense of the world. Research offers a systematic method of confirming existing knowledge and building new knowledge in a profession or discipline. Nursing and **midwifery research** is a way to explore and discover new knowledge to refine and expand the body of knowledge that clinicians, managers and policy-makers draw upon to advance practice. Nurses and midwives use **research** findings and their professional experience with patients and clinical practice to provide quality care based on the best and most up-to-date available evidence; this is known as **evidence-based practice**. Research in nursing and midwifery was relatively late to develop compared with other disciplines, largely because nursing education was moved into the tertiary sector relatively recently, but research is increasingly important to sustain in a complex and rapidly changing healthcare landscape.

How do you feel about research?

Teachers of nursing and midwifery, when facing a new class, will often pose a series of questions to beginning research students:

- What image comes to mind when you hear the word 'research'?
- What are your feelings about studying research?
- Is research important to nursing and midwifery?
- Who should conduct research?
- How does research relate to evidence-based practice?

Students will have a notion of what research is but might be unsure about its application in the day-to-day practice of nursing and midwifery. Although students probably agree that research has a place in nursing and midwifery, they might think someone else should be doing or using it. Students might be excited and curious about studying research but somewhat anxious about getting started.

STUDENT CHALLENGE

Preconceived Notions

Consider each of these questions one at a time and record your answers.

1. What image comes to mind for the word 'research'? Paint a word picture or draw an image.
2. What characteristics does a researcher possess? List traits you think a researcher needs.
3. How do you feel about research? How do you feel about your study of research? Use 'feeling' words such as happy, sad, scared or anxious. Try to examine why you might be feeling this way.
4. Do you think research is important to nursing and midwifery? Why or why not?
5. Who do you think should do nursing or midwifery research?

6. Who should use the findings of nursing or midwifery research?
7. How does research relate to evidence-based practice? Can you 'do' evidence-based practice without understanding the basics of research?

Compare your answers with those of two or three of your peers. Discuss similarities and differences. What do your answers tell you? Did you learn anything that might be useful as you begin your study?

This chapter presents research as a resource for nurses and midwives to use in their practice and studies. Although nurses and midwives often begin performing research only after they embark on postgraduate studies, findings from research are an immediate and important source of information for students. The wise use of research findings in practice helps clinicians and patients choose the best available therapies and care. Research has increasing relevance to nursing and midwifery practice; students will also find that in their studies appropriate reference to research evidence is an essential requirement of academic writing.

One of the hallmarks of a profession is that its members (in this case nurses and midwives) know things that are of worth to others. For instance, a professional nurse should know the answer to a question such as: 'How will my leg ulcer heal when I live alone with no one to help me?'

In order to maintain public trust in both nursing and midwifery, it is the responsibility of members of each profession to update that knowledge bank regularly. It would be considered irresponsible of a nurse to undertake the care of a person with a leg ulcer if that nurse was not able to develop and apply knowledge of the best available evidence about supporting the patient, treating the ulcer, and sharing this information with the patient. The way knowledge is generated and tested is through a process called research.

Research is an important tool in the rapidly changing practice of nursing and midwifery.

Nurses and midwives have worked hard to establish a research tradition in order to generate their own evidence base. Nurse and midwife researchers seek to find answers to questions that can inform practices and therapies complementary to, but independent from, medicine. Unless, however, research evidence is read, appraised and used by clinicians to develop their own knowledge and point of care delivery, it is difficult to demonstrate the worth of clinical research in a meaningful way. Poor research utilisation in practice is a problem shared by all health professions and, as such, encouraging research utilisation has become a priority for evidence-based practice organisations. The process of getting evidence from research studies into practice is called **knowledge translation**. If nurses and midwives translate research findings to their own practice, the results will be the incorporation of evidence to the point of care (see Chapter 10 for further reading on this topic). Figure 1.1 illustrates how the domains of research, nurses and midwives' knowledge and evidence-based practice interrelate.

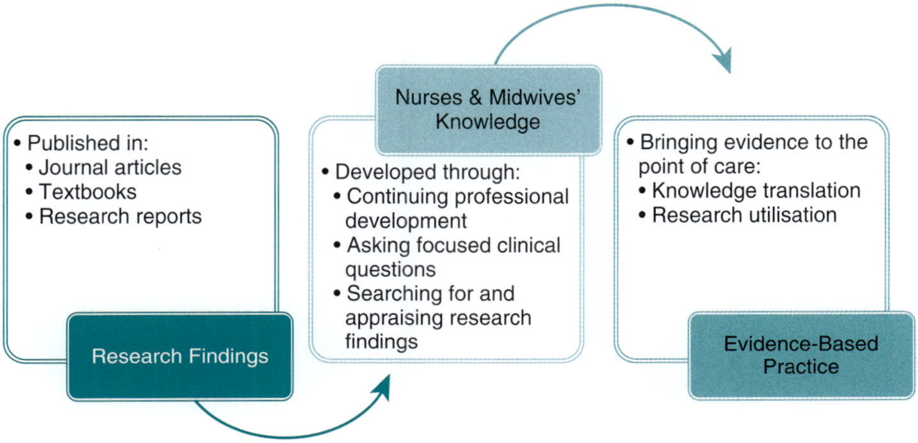

FIGURE 1.1
Linking the domains of research, knowledge and evidence-based practice

In order to develop your own knowledge about a particular area of interest with the aim of using or applying research findings, it is necessary to make judgments about the quality of the research and its relevance to a particular context or purpose. Knowing about the processes of research prepares people to determine the rigour of studies. Accessing research papers only from peer-reviewed journals may reassure some less-informed readers about the quality of these studies, as such journals only publish papers that have been critically reviewed and judged acceptable by a panel of experts. However, the review process in these journals is not perfect and, at some stage through an undergraduate degree, students will be expected to undertake the critique of research for themselves. This is why research is introduced at the undergraduate level – to provide the knowledge and skills to appraise research findings. This book is designed to help undergraduate nursing and midwifery students appreciate how research is conducted and how appraised research findings might be utilised in practice.

Before embarking on the study of research, readers are reminded that research is one source of knowledge amongst a number of different sources (Box 1.1). Understanding how people come to know things helps to develop knowledge wisely.

Box 1.1
Sources of knowledge

Tradition and custom
Authority and role models
Trial and error
Personal experience
Intuition
Reasoning
Research

What is knowledge?

Knowledge is the understanding of facts, truths or principles. It is the information used to conduct our personal and professional lives. The study of knowledge (or theorising knowledge) is called **epistemology**. People acquire knowledge in several ways and may use more than one of these methods at a time when working on a solution to a problem or the answer to a troubling question. All methods of acquiring knowledge are viable options and are valid at various times. Each offers a way to deal with the world and possesses strengths and weaknesses that can be used to advantage. The following sections discuss each method of knowledge acquisition in more depth.

STUDENT CHALLENGE

How Do We Know What We Know?

1. Either alone or with a small group of friends, brainstorm how you as a student nurse or midwife come to know what you know.
2. When you are finished, compare your findings to the list in Box 1.1.
3. Did you come up with other sources of knowledge that are not listed?
4. Can you think of examples of how you use each of these sources of knowledge in your daily life?

How do nurses and midwives know?

Tradition and custom

Knowledge derived from tradition is 'truth' that is passed from previous generations. It is often a reflection of culture or heritage. It involves those things known or done because 'this is the way it has always been'. These truths are usually accepted as given with little questioning. This can be advantageous because it offers a common cultural ground from which to communicate and make decisions. Many practices that evolve from this kind of knowledge are ritualistic in nature. The reason or rationale for such practice may have been lost or may have disappeared over the years.

An example of this is provided in the following story. Two friends were preparing dinner together. One of them took the roast, cut off each end and then placed it in the oven to brown.

The other asked, 'Why did you cut off the ends first?'

'I don't know,' said the first, 'It's the way my mother taught me.'

However, being curious, she called her mother and asked for an explanation. Her mother didn't know either, having learned to cook a roast by watching her mother. So the woman called her grandmother in search of an answer.

'Well,' the grandmother said, 'I used to cut the ends off the roast because the dish I cooked it in was too small to hold the whole thing.'

Large amounts of information and many practices in nursing and midwifery are based mainly on tradition. For example, nurses and midwives routinely take patient vital signs each shift and encourage daily baths and daily linen changes. Many nursing practices were originally instituted for good reasons. However, much like cutting off the end of the roast, the reason for the practice may no longer be appropriate. So it may be to patients' and professionals' advantage to re-examine those 'ritualistic' things done in nursing and midwifery that we 'know' by tradition – the practices carried out because 'that is the way it is customarily done'.

Authority

'Experts' are authorities who are relied upon to provide information to guide good decisions and teach the performance of certain functions. The first authority figures children encounter are parents. At school, children begin to rely on teachers and textbooks to expand their knowledge base. Adults also rely on the opinions of authorities that have expertise in areas they do not. This is a natural evolution, as it would be impossible for all people to be knowledgeable about all things.

When first embarking on a new profession, people look to authorities in the field to teach what they know. Novices imitate the example set by authority figures, who serve as role models. Students and novice clinicians can learn attitudes, knowledge and skills by selecting and using discipline academics or expert clinicians as role models.

When using knowledge gleaned from authority figures, or when imitating their behaviours, care must be taken to pick these role models wisely by asking questions such as the following: What makes this person an expert? What is his or her educational background and experience? How did he or she acquire this knowledge? Do I accept the word of my lecturers and tutors or practising clinicians without question? How well read and current are my nursing and midwifery academics? Are they involved in scholarly activity and research? Are their clinical skills current? What about the health professionals I see in the clinical area? Do they keep up with the latest discoveries in their specialty area? Do they show evidence of critical thinking in their clinical decision-making, or do they justify actions with 'That's the way we do it here'?

Textbooks and other information sources, including the internet, often assume an authority role in the life of a nursing or midwifery student. A lot of credibility is assigned generally to the written word. Many words are written in the modern nursing world – not all of them true – and these words must be tested by, for example, asking questions such as the following: Do you take every piece of information you read at face value? Do you know if you are learning the best information available? Do you regularly use nursing or midwifery journals as information sources?

Information in most textbooks can be three to five years old by the time it is published, which must be a consideration for students reading research. The following cautionary tale has been drawn from the authors' circle of professional associates. An academic co-authored a quick-reference handbook on diseases. Within one month of sending her work to the publisher, six major developments occurred that affected the content of the book. After she finished writing the book, the academic had to wait a year before the book was printed. The number of changes that occurred in that one-year period was enormous. By the time it was available to the public, her book was no longer current. Similarly, while the internet offers access to copious amounts of information, there is no control over the information available and no guarantee it is accurate. The high rate at which material is added to the internet makes it difficult for clinicians to sift through the information to determine what is relevant, and to assess the reliability of the information (Estabrooks et al 2003). To ensure that decisions are based on the best evidence, students and nurses need to be certain their sources are both reliable and accurate.

In addition, information must always be viewed with a critical eye. One might try asking is the information in line with other authorities in the same area? Is it backed up by sound rationale? Is it presented clearly and logically? Is it current?

Trial and error

The process of trial and error involves trying out a successive number of ideas to solve a problem until one works. The successful idea is adopted until it ceases to work, whereupon it is rejected and the process is started again. This method is often used when someone has a limited frame of reference on which to draw, when seemingly equal options are easily accessible, or when standard approaches have been exhausted. Trial and error tends to be a haphazard approach and, often, results cannot be reproduced a second time. For example, try to reproduce a meal thrown together with a little of this and a little of that – a particularly futile task.

In using trial and error, one might also end up using one option when another would work better. This occurs because the selected option solves the problem adequately, leaving the better option unexplored. By way of example, a teenager has produced a longed-for result on his computer and proudly shown the results of his handiwork to a more computer-literate friend. The friend proceeds to show the boy how to get the same result in one or two keystrokes. Using a system of trial and error might also entail a certain amount of risk. In nursing, for example, using trial and error to find the correct dose of medication for a patient is quite plainly irresponsible and inappropriate.

However, in some situations, trial and error can bring about surprising results. When one approaches an obstacle from a 'let's try this and see what happens' perspective, he or she is not bound by the restraints of logic. This type of exploration may provide solutions that might not have been discovered with a more logical approach.

Personal experience

Knowledge derived from the cumulative experiences of living is familiar and powerful. It comes from seeing, hearing, touching, tasting, feeling and doing something ourselves. It is first-hand knowledge: known because one has been there before and experienced the same thing before. Every person is intimately acquainted with using personal experience as a reliable method of knowing, and most people trust personal experience and value it highly in the decision-making process. The more experience gained in a situation, the greater the comfort and skill in future situations. As the number and variety of these experiences increase, so too is knowledge transferred, adapted and extended from previous situations to fit new situations. As the depth and breadth of experience grows, the operating knowledge base becomes increasingly complex. Personal experience is individual and is often hard to translate or explain to others, particularly to those people who have no similar experiences to draw upon. Students begin nursing or midwifery from a range of backgrounds. It is important to note past experiences outside healthcare, and the degree to which knowledge is drawn from them, as students become practitioners.

Patricia Benner (1984) describes five levels a nurse goes through in developing clinical expertise: novice, advanced beginner, competent, proficient and expert. Movement from one level to the next occurs with experience. Experience is only gained when previous knowledge is refined or challenged by clinical evidence. The novice nurse or midwife begins with knowledge, gained in large part from authoritative sources, and from the ability to use that knowledge and reason to solve problems. Experience is then added to the equation. Expertise develops over time as the nurse or midwife tests and refines this body of knowledge in real-world situations; thus, says Benner, experience is a necessary prerequisite for developing expertise.

Intuition

Intuition is a 'hunch' or 'gut feeling' about a situation that is not readily explained or easily backed up by logic or facts. It is an insight or understanding of the whole, seen apart from its component parts. Intuition is closely tied to personal experience. Extensive experience in a particular situation allows knowledge to be ingrained so that it becomes second nature. Acting on this deeply embedded knowledge often occurs automatically and quickly, appearing to be a flash of insight or an immediate recognition of the whole. For expert nurses and midwives it is often difficult even to recall or recount what produces this insight.

Intuition has long been discounted as an evidential source of knowledge because it is not easily examined or readily categorised by the research process. It also appears to occur apart from consideration of available facts and use of a **reasoning** process. So, in a society that holds logic at a premium, intuition is labelled as unreliable or as a 'lucky guess'.

Benner (1984) and Benner, Tanner and Chesla (2009) propose that intuition is a perceptual awareness. In their estimation, intuition is not a lack of knowledge or a 'lucky guess'; rather it is deep knowledge derived from long hours of clinical observation and experience. Intuition is about being attuned to very subtle shifts that may be important only in the case of a specific patient. Benner et al document several instances where expert nurses recognise impending warning signs of a life-threatening situation long before the objective signs revealed something was going wrong. This type of clinical knowledge needs greater study so it can be more clearly understood and taught.

Reasoning

Reasoning is a way of using the mind to work out puzzles and present ideas and plans. To reason is to think through an issue or a problem in an objective, systematic and logical way: to take stock of what appears to be happening, make associations between things, and determine the likely consequence of a range of responses. For example, a nurse or midwife might see a urine sample, notice it is much clearer than the day before, know the patient is taking antibiotics and determine the treatment for urinary tract infection is beginning to work. The clinician is thus making associations between pieces of information and a plausible conclusion. Following on from this, the nurse/midwife will use this reasoning to encourage the patient to continue to take the antibiotics until the course is finished. Giving a patient a reason for their treatment shows respect for them and for their intelligence.

Reasoning is used to formulate arguments and is therefore a skill perfected by politicians, lawyers and scientists. Political debates portrayed in the media demonstrate that when individuals want to undermine the position their opponent is taking, they will question the rationale behind the opponent's argument and try to find a flaw. Children also learn the art of reasoning quickly; for example, 'If I am able to play now, I could do my homework with less distraction later' is a more persuasive argument than 'I want to play now'.

Research

Research is a systematic process used to confirm and refine existing knowledge and to build new knowledge both inductively and deductively. **Inductive reasoning**, or where reasoning moves from the particular to the general, underlies qualitative research, while **deductive reasoning**, where two or more variables form the basis for assuming the existence of a relationship that can be tested, underpins quantitative research. Inductive research is useful when little is known about a particular area. Through the process of exploration, investigators using inductive methods of research construct concepts or theories that can explain what is going on in a particular context. Deductive research begins with a proposed theory about the effect of an intervention, which an investigator then tests and verifies before recommending it as evidence-based practice.

Quantitative research is used to describe, explore, explain, measure or predict observable or measurable conditions with as much objectivity as possible. **Qualitative research** allows investigators to identify, examine and explain the experiences of an individual or group from a number of subjective viewpoints. Quantitative and qualitative research approaches are presented in more detail in later chapters and, as will become clear, each can use both inductive and deductive methods.

STUDENT CHALLENGE

Identifying Sources of Knowledge

Read the following scenario containing examples of each of the sources of knowledge described above and identify them as they occur.

Ginny Saunders, a community nurse, had been visiting Ms Chan on and off for a year to dress an ulcer. Even though Ginny was quite busy, each visit they would sit together chatting until Ms Chan said: 'Let's get started'. It was, after all, her house.

On the surface, nothing appeared to be different this day, but Ginny could not shake a feeling that something might be amiss. Ms Chan talked about her great grandchildren. She mentioned the youngest wouldn't settle and she had told her granddaughter (the child's mother) to try leaving the light on in the hall, and if that didn't work, maybe alter the child's bedtime.

Ginny changed the dressing and reapplied the pressure bandages and explained the latest evidence about the healing of venous ulcers. She gently asked questions that enabled her to assess Ms Chan's activities of living (as she always did with older clients). She explained to Ms Chan why it was important to keep the foot elevated when she was sitting.

When she finished, Ginny packed up the dressing equipment and shut her bag. For some reason Ginny could not shake her feelings of unease and wondered if Ms Chan really was 'fine', as she had claimed.

'You know what, Ms Chan?' she said, 'if you don't mind I think I will just check your vital signs before I leave'.

Tradition and custom are the predominant sources of knowledge for Ginny's decision to wait for an invitation to start. This has probably become an unconscious part of her everyday practice in the community. The advice to try leaving the children's light on was trial and error on the part of the grandmother. The latest evidence on wound healing was drawn from research. Managing to assess Ms Chan while chatting was something Ginny learnt in her personal practice. By explaining why she should keep her foot elevated, Ginny was reasoning with Ms Chan. Finally, before she left, Ginny had a feeling that all was not quite right and stopped to check Ms Chan's vital signs. In this case, Ginny was acting on intuition.

You could try this exercise out again using a scenario from clinical practice.

What is nursing and midwifery research?

Nursing and midwifery research addresses problems or questions that are encountered in practice, the answers to which inform and guide future actions, whether the users of research findings are in management, education, scholarship or clinical situations. Nursing and midwifery research uses the research process as a tool to search for, develop, refine and expand a body of knowledge that shapes and enhances professional practice. It also challenges and provides evidence to reject practice based solely on tradition. Research can be classified as nursing and midwifery research when the research endeavour produces knowledge relevant to either discipline.

The research process is used as a tool to search for, develop, refine and expand a body of knowledge that shapes and enhances practice. In today's world, nursing and midwifery research per se is difficult to define; the scope of nursing or midwifery practice tends to overlap sometimes with medicine and allied health because of increasing numbers of shared interventions and therapies. The rise of teamwork in the health field means many questions that arise in practice are of an interdisciplinary nature and involve a team of researchers from a range of disciplines, including nursing and midwifery.

Interdisciplinary teamwork is viewed as a positive development, as patients require a service that is streamlined and does not appear to be fragmented into a whole host of different bits of care and treatment. It is therefore reasonable that health professions create new knowledge about health services together. Nurses and midwives collaborate and make important contributions to interdisciplinary teamwork. For example, an exploratory study of women's choices around breastfeeding was undertaken by a team made up of midwives, a sociologist, a social worker, a diabetologist and an obstetrician (Stenhouse & Letherby 2010). The researchers described how the different opinions, informed by the team members' varied backgrounds caused the group to reflect more deeply on the wider perspective surrounding infant-feeding, including the issue of infant-feeding for women with diabetes.

Research is a process of systematic discovery undertaken in order to establish things such as: the incidence of problems, effectiveness of interventions, the appropriateness of interventions and the feasibility of implementing interventions. Box 1.2 connects the examples above with the aim of finding out how often things occur (incidence), whether things work (effectiveness), whether they are acceptable (appropriateness) and whether it is possible to implement them (feasibility).

Box 1.2
Connecting the examples

Research Examples	Findings	Questions
Breastfeeding	Health issues, medications	What are some of the circumstances in which breastfeeding may be difficult?
Wound healing	Effectiveness of dressing	Is there an association between moist wound dressings and improved healing of wounds?
New practices	Feasibility	How will a team accept, implement and evaluate change?

Why is research important?

Ultimately, the importance of research is found in its definition – 'diligent and systematic inquiry or investigation into a subject in order to discover facts or principles' (from the *Macquarie Dictionary*). The development of knowledge that is evidence-based allows professionals to make better-informed decisions and choices in relation to their practice as nurses or midwives. Research findings may validate existing practices created from tradition, intuition and personal experience. Importantly, research may examine tried and true practices and make them more efficient, less expensive or less complicated. It may explore ways of tackling newly evolving problems in an increasingly complex world. Ultimately, nursing and midwifery research ought to contribute to better healthcare outcomes for consumers.

Overall, healthcare research is big business and billions of Australian and New Zealand dollars are invested in the future through the funding of research studies each year. Imperatives that drive healthcare research include the pursuit of knowledge to improve health, minimise risk and alleviate suffering, and profit resulting from research undertaken to develop new drugs and innovative technologies. Nursing and midwifery research studies are important because they contribute another dimension to the information generated in relation to health and welfare.

Nursing and midwifery research serves several purposes for both professions and for nurses and midwives as individuals. Research findings provide standard and reliable evidence bases upon which to develop professional practice. This in turn ensures the care given to clients is practice-based on the best available evidence. So, nursing and midwifery research plays an important role in guiding and improving the delivery of client care.

Professions are commonly judged by the body of knowledge they generate, and a clearly defined evidence base built on a strong research foundation lends credibility to nursing and midwifery as distinct professions. If this evidence base is clearly defined, the role of the nurse or midwife in the delivery of healthcare will also be clear. If clinicians can define their roles, then they can articulate distinctions and similarities between their roles and those of other healthcare professionals, which, in turn, allows consumers of healthcare to see and value the contributions of nurses and midwives and the professional group of which they are a part.

The practice of nursing or midwifery in today's litigious society demands increasing accountability for one's actions. Consumers demand reasons for nursing or midwifery interventions and clinicians need sound rationales for their decisions and actions. An evidence base grounded in the findings of sound research provides such rationales. Individual nurses or midwives need a current knowledge base drawn from research findings in order to be responsible and accountable to the consumer. This connection is the nub of evidence-based practice (Fig 1.1) and is written into the Australian Nursing and Midwifery Council and the Nursing Council of New Zealand competencies for beginning practitioners.

As well, nurses and midwives are increasingly called on to document the cost-effectiveness of the care they provide. Many healthcare facilities have tried to reduce costs by substituting nurses, in particular, with untrained personnel. In part this is because nursing and midwifery services consume such a large part of an institution's budget. Interestingly, research demonstrates effective nursing care leads to fewer patient complications, shorter hospital stays and fewer readmissions, and that nursing cutbacks actually increase overall institutional costs (Aiken et al 2010).

In the next section the development of nursing and midwifery research is plotted internationally, with a particular focus on Australia and New Zealand. Mapping these historical moments helps to build an understanding of how relatively new nursing and midwifery research is in Australia and New Zealand and how important it is to build capacity strategically and network nationally and internationally with colleagues to sustain the existing momentum.

Historical influences

The first research efforts in nursing can be traced back to Florence Nightingale. After this first flurry of success, relatively little formal research was carried out by nurses until the late 1940s. Even though the development of **nursing research** has been relatively brief, its evolution has been exciting.

Nursing schools in New Zealand and Australia evolved from military and religious roots that stressed order and obedience, which is similar to the historical roots of nursing schools in Europe and North America. Nurses with inquiring minds who asked challenging questions had little place in this system of education. Instead, dedication to hard work and submission to authority were valued and promoted. Training was viewed as an apprenticeship, with long hours, rote learning and repetition the order of the day. Nurses had little free time or say in their own training or work. The traditional subservient role of women in society reinforced the values promoted by hospitals and hospital schools of nursing.

Progress of nursing research has been closely tied to the development of nursing and nursing education. Only when nursing began to move towards advanced education and affiliation with university settings did a research culture begin to emerge. This move began in the USA. Ironically, it was research by investigators in other disciplines that exposed deficiencies in the preparation of nurses and urged better educational opportunities and a move to university settings. Sociologists found the study of nurses and nursing as a work culture particularly fascinating and, as a female-dominated occupation, nursing held special appeal for sociological investigation. Nursing work, habits, roles and attitudes were dissected and reported for decades in sociological literature.

World War II increased the demand for nurses and sparked interest in nursing as a profession. Nurses and nursing were in the spotlight. In the USA, funds for the development of nursing to professional status were suddenly available from government and private sources and US nurses began to push for basic and advanced education in university settings. Nursing research got a major boost in that country with the establishment of a nursing research centre and a nursing foundation to promote nursing research. A journal was created to publish the results of that research. More nurses were receiving advanced degrees and had expertise in research, although most of these degrees were in fields other than nursing. Thus, early research efforts by nurses tended to ask questions about the education, psychology or sociology of nurses.

During the 1960s and 1970s in the USA, the number of nurses with advanced degrees and research skills continued to increase and the push for doctoral preparation in nursing began. Formal support mechanisms for research and research funding in nursing increased and stabilised. Nursing practice became more standardised, complex and specialised. Nursing education at master's level became more common and emphasised specialisation in rapidly emerging specialty areas. Research was carried out to establish standards for specialty practice. Nursing researchers began to turn to nursing care and clinical practice to provide questions for research and the focus shifted from the study of nurses to the practice of nursing. Nursing theories evolved that attempted to describe and explain the practice of nursing. These theories began to be tested by nurse researchers. Practice-related research flourished and, by the end of the 1970s, two new research journals were launched in the USA to handle the nursing research explosion. In 1988 the US National Center for Nursing Research was federally mandated and funded under the National Institutes of Health and in 1993 it was named an institute in its own right.

In Australia and New Zealand, such developments took longer. The move to tertiary education only began in earnest in the mid-1980s. In the USA there was already a critical mass of nurses with doctoral degrees and research skills by the 1980s, and many Australian and New Zealand nurses went to the USA to study for higher degrees. The Dawkins reforms in the late 1980s saw the merger of colleges of advanced education and universities and resulted in the basic entry for nursing in Australia becoming an undergraduate degree, with nursing research identified as a crucial component of this process of professionalisation. The inception of postgraduate degrees led to further growth in nursing research, although in the early stages much of this research was about nursing education and nurses themselves (Roberts & Taylor 2002).

As increasing numbers of nurses (mostly academics at this stage) conducted research, the Royal Australian Nursing Federation (now known as the Australian Nursing Federation [ANF]) launched the *Australian Journal of Advanced Nursing* in 1983, to create an outlet for research publication. Since that time, other key nursing bodies have also committed to encouraging research activity. The Australian College of Nursing (ACN) and the ANF have developed a position statement on nursing research that can be accessed online (www.acn.edu.au). The ACN and the ANF have funding available nationally for research and scholarships. The incorporation of a competency statement about nursing research into the Australian Nursing and Midwifery Council competencies for beginning practitioners confirms the profession's commitment to research (Roberts & Taylor 2002; Australian Nursing and Midwifery Council 2006a). The New Zealand Nurses Organisation (NZNO) has a well-developed nursing research section.

In much the same way as in the USA, nursing research in Australia and New Zealand has been through a process of evolution. Much work has been done in refining and expanding nursing research efforts. Through such international and national efforts, nursing today has established a firm foundation for its practice through research. The National Review of Nursing Education (Commonwealth of Australia 2001) and the Senate Inquiry into Nursing (Commonwealth of Australia 2002) came out strongly in support of nursing research and urged the development of strategies to enhance research capacity and attract research funding for nursing. The previous Research Quality Framework and the current Excellence in Research for Australia strategies have had a significant impact on research in Australia and New Zealand. The introduction of these strategies caused nursing and midwifery research to come under much closer scrutiny, and to be judged alongside other disciplines.

University disciplines, including nursing and midwifery, are required to subject the research of their staff to internal self-assessment and international and/or national peer review, as well as provide evidence of impact on policy and/or practice. In most Australian and New Zealand universities and colleges, undergraduate students study research as part of their degrees, and honours programs are available for talented students to develop research skills early in their careers. In Australia and New Zealand, there are numerous doctoral programs in nursing and midwifery. Centres for nursing and midwifery research are beginning to proliferate in many hospital and university settings, and clinical professors of nursing and midwifery have been established through university and health service partnerships. The quality and quantity of nursing and midwifery research continues to grow and an increasing number of research journals have been launched to help disseminate their respective research findings. Clinical practice specialty groups progressively fund, promote and publish research in their respective specialty areas.

Around the beginning of the 21st century, the focus of nursing research, particularly in the West, shifted to the exploration of nursing practice. Much health-related research is now driven by national health priority areas; the funding is strategically aligned. While research remains predominantly initiated and conducted by people affiliated with the university sector (academics and students), research questions (the substance of research) are being generated by clinicians to a much larger extent. More clinicians are joining with academics to form research teams. Moreover, research teams are expected to be multidisciplinary and cross-institutional. Traditionally, Australian and New Zealand researchers have relied on the Australian Research Council, the National Health and Medical Research Council (NHMRC) and Health Research Council of New Zealand, Te Kaunihera Rangahau Hauora o Aotearoa, to support research. Now research teams must look increasingly to international or non-traditional sources. It is a challenging, exciting and optimistic time for research in the two fields. A review of research published in nursing journals between 1985 and 2010 indicates a decrease in descriptive studies, theory-testing research, and theory-based studies, and an increase in qualitative studies, correlational and experimental designs (Yarcheski, Mahon & Yarcheski 2012).

Table 1.1 presents some highlights in the development of nursing and midwifery research in Australia. NZNO, the New Zealand College of Midwives,

Table 1.1
Nursing and midwifery highlights in Australia and New Zealand

Date	Event
1868	Lucy Osborne arrives at the Sydney Infirmary to establish the first hospital-based school of nursing based on the Nightingale system
1899	Formation of the New South Wales Trained Nurses Association, which later became the Australasian Trained Nurses Association
1901	New Zealand Nurses Registration Act September 12
1904	New Zealand Midwives' Registration Act
1903	*The Australasian Nurses' Journal* first published
1908	*Kai Tiaki* journal published in New Zealand
1915	Midwives' Registration Bill passed in Federal Parliament, resulting in the establishment of a Midwives' Board in Australia
1923	The Australian Nursing Federation becomes the first national nursing organisation
1924	Nurses Registration Act passed through Parliament in Australia
1926	Establishment of the New Zealand Nurses and Midwives' Board
1928	New Nurses' Act results in the abolishment of the Midwives' Board, bringing midwifery under the regulation of the nursing body
1931	NSW Nurses' Association founded
1943	The Kelly Report published by the Committee for the Reorganisation of the Nursing Profession in New South Wales
1949	The NSW College of Nursing established
1950	The College of Nursing Australia, established in Victoria, begins offering postgraduate courses
1950s	*Journal of Nursing Research* established
1967–74	Nine reports published on the issue of the education preparation of nurses and nursing in New South Wales
1967	First combined degree and nursing course offered at University of New England, Australia
1967	New Zealand nursing undergo changes from being hospital-based apprenticeships to tertiary education courses
1969	Truskett Interim and Matron's Reports released, Australia
1970s	New Zealand nursing education moved to polytechnics and universities
1970s	*Advances in Nursing Sciences, Research in Nursing and Health, Western Journal of Nursing Research* established
1971	The Carpenter report released in New Zealand, centred around the nursing education system, advocating training nurses in an educational environment; the government, however, decided that polytechs rather than universities were more appropriate for this, but as a consequence nurses obtained a diploma rather than a degree
1972	Nurses Education Board established in New South Wales
1973	Nurses Education Board Act passed through Parliament in New South Wales
1978	Six colleges of advanced education offer undergraduate courses in nursing in Australia
1978	Sax Report on Nurse Education and Training: Report of the Committee of Inquiry into Nurse Education and Training to the Tertiary Education Commission released in Australia

Table 1.1
Nursing and midwifery highlights in Australia and New Zealand—cont'd

Date	Event
1979	Inaugural conference of the National Association of Midwives (Australia)
1983	*Australian Journal of Advanced Nursing* established
1983	Sydney hosted the International Confederation of Midwives conference, leading to the national body becoming registered as a college
1984	Australian College of Midwives established by the amalgamation of state midwifery professional bodies
1984	The Australian Medicare tribunal recommended health program grants be made available for the purpose of evaluating independent midwifery practice
1985	Nurse education and training moved to the tertiary sector in New South Wales; Diploma of Applied Science (Nursing) offered at colleges of advanced education
1987	The National Health and Medical Research Council (NHMRC) (Australia) set up working parties, which, through investigation and examination of midwifery practice, established professional guidelines for midwives in relation to birth centres and home births
1987	First working party of the NHMRC recommends setting up an accreditation process by the Australian College of Midwives Incorporated
1990s	*Contemporary Nurse, Nursing Inquiry, International Journal of Nursing Practice* established; last student graduated from New Zealand hospital program
1990	Amalgamation of colleges of advanced education with universities; Bachelor degree in nursing becomes requisite for registration as a nurse in Australia
1990	Midwifery regains its status as an autonomous profession in New Zealand
1992	The Australian and New Zealand national governments sign a Mutual Recognition Agreement
1993	Full transfer of nursing education across Australia to the tertiary sector
1994	Transition of midwifery training from hospital-based to tertiary education in Australia
1996	Joanna Briggs Institute for Evidence Based Nursing (now known as the Joanna Briggs Institute) set up in South Australia at Royal Adelaide Hospital and University of Adelaide
2000	KPMG Strategic Review of Undergraduate Nursing Education, New Zealand
2001–2	Senate Inquiry into Nursing and National Review of Nursing Education, Australia
2001	First direct-entry 3-year Bachelor of Midwifery course started in Australia
2004	The Health Practitioners Competence Assurance (2003) Act comes into full power on 18 September in New Zealand, requiring nurses to have current competences relating to their scope of practice
2005	Research Quality Framework proposed by the Australian Commonwealth Government
2006	Council of Deans of Nursing and Midwifery Australia and New Zealand establish the Research Advisory Group
2009	Excellence in Research for Australia established
2009	Midwives and Nurse Practitioner Bill introduced into Australian Federal Parliament
2010	National Maternity Reforms set up; a national registration for all nurses and midwives came into force in Australia in July 2010

and the Nursing Education and Research Foundation offer advice about research activities and some offer grants and scholarships. NZNO has an excellent index of New Zealand nursing research that can be accessed free of charge.

Questions nurse and midwife researchers ask

Earlier in the chapter, it was stated that research is a systematic way of generating knowledge in response to questions posed about nurses and midwives and their practices. It would appear reasonable to suggest nursing and midwifery research questions arise from curiosity or a practical need. Developing a good question and refining it for the purpose of research requires a person to have a good grasp of practice and research. Undergraduates are required to be able to recognise a research question; they are not necessarily asked to pose research questions as yet.

Nursing and midwifery research questions can arise from a number of different sources (Box 1.3). Often the researcher's personal experience as a clinician leads her or him to identify a question that can be investigated. Other times, research questions are identified in the literature where recommendations have been made for further studies to be undertaken. In addition, the context of nursing and midwifery practice, and existing theories about various aspects of practice, can prompt questions for research.

For example, to form a research question, a nurse may have been exposed to any of the sources listed in Box 1.3. Perhaps she was a nurse experienced in the field of caring for women with gynaecological cancer and she might have suspected, through her work, that Aboriginal and Torres Strait Islander communities were not deriving as much benefit from a partner support program as non-Indigenous women in remote Australian communities. Or she may have recognised this problem when reading research literature in the area. Or it may be the nurse is aware that in Australia, there is a social shift towards involving partners in healthcare services and decision-making. She might also

Box 1.3
Sources of research questions

- Clinicians' experiences
- Literature
- Patients' experiences
- Theories
- Context of practice

be aware of the recognition Aboriginal and Torres Strait Islander communities have culturally distinctive needs in this area. Or this experienced nurse is led to ask a research question by referring to a study of Orem's (1991) self-care theory of nursing, which may lead her to think of partners as self-care agents. Or lastly, it may be that the government has identified support of family health in rural communities and the health of Aboriginal and Torres Strait Islander people and communities as a national research priority.

When writing about a study the researcher presents a problem statement and associated research question either at the beginning of the research paper or at the end of the literature review section. It is up to the researcher to present a problem statement in such a way as to convince the reader of the magnitude or significance of the problem. A researcher will generally refer to the source of the research question in the problem statement, for example, that it is a problem the researcher has experienced in practice, it is stressed in the literature as a known social problem or it is considered to be an area of national priority.

Once the problem statement has been written, the researcher can write a research question. For example, here is a research question that could have emanated from the problem above: How can a partner support program, designed for rural women with gynaecological cancer, be customised by Aboriginal and Torres Strait Islander communities to respect the distinctive nature of their ways of life? On the other hand, the nurse might have chosen a different perspective on this research and asked the following question: How do women and their partners in one rural Aboriginal and Torres Strait Islander community experience support while the woman undergoes treatment for gynaecological cancer?

To demonstrate how the research question leads the researcher to the next step in the research process, it is necessary to introduce the major classifications of research. They are qualitative research, quantitative research and **mixed methods research**. Those readers who have already studied research will know these categories are an oversimplification but, because they are commonly used and relatively easy to understand, they are adopted in this book.

Quantitative and qualitative research approaches are explained in more detail in Chapters 5 and 6 respectively so, for now, the following brief descriptions should suffice. Researchers undertaking quantitative studies aim to test ideas and generate information that is exact and useful for a broad number of people; they collect numbers and do statistical tests under controlled circumstances in order to predict and control what occurs. Qualitative researchers aim to understand things as they naturally occur in context; they collect words rather than numbers and create rich descriptions of experience. Researchers who use mixed methods use elements of quantitative and qualitative research to find answers to complex questions (see Chapter 7). This multi-perspective view of health service research is becoming more common as multidisciplinary and cooperative research teams become more common. Here are some examples of how different research approaches may be used:

- How do women and their partners in one rural Aboriginal and Torres Strait Islander community experience support while the woman undergoes treatment for gynaecological cancer? The best way to find this out is to ask the community members so the research study would probably involve interviews and use a qualitative design.
- Does a partnership support program reduce stress and improve feelings of control for women receiving treatment for gynaecological cancer and their families? The way to address a 'how effective is this' question is to make a comparison and therefore this would be set up as an experiment with a control group and a group participating in the partnership support program. This would be a quantitative study.
- How can a partner support program, designed for rural women with gynaecological cancer, be customised by Aboriginal and Torres Strait Islander communities to respect the distinctive nature of their ways of life? The best way to answer this question is to take it to the community and generate data from their discussions and understandings of the problem and its solutions. The data collected might be a mixture of qualitative and quantitative. This would be a mixed methods study.

Evidence-based practice

Evidence-based practice can be defined as a 'life-long problem-solving approach to the delivery of health care that integrates the best evidence from well-designed studies (i.e. external evidence) and integrates it with a patient's preferences and values and a clinician's expertise' (Melnyk, Gallagher-Ford, Long, Fineout-Overholt 2014, p.5). Current competency standards for Australia and New Zealand nurses and midwives include a requirement to implement evidence-based practice based on an understanding of research findings. As well, nurses and midwives are expected to be actively involved in research studies wherever possible. For example, the Australian document states that the nurse 'practises within an evidence-based framework' (Australian Nursing and Midwifery Council 2006b) and a midwife 'uses research to inform midwifery practice' (Australian Nursing and Midwifery Council 2006c). This means a nurse will be able to access research findings, often called 'evidence', demonstrate an ability to evaluate the research study that produced the findings, and then make a decision about using these findings at the point of care. The thought processes involved in reading, appraising and making a decision about using research findings in practice are called knowledge translation. Deciding to go ahead and use research findings in practice is called research utilisation, which is explored more fully in Chapters 9, 10 and 11.

Figure 1.1. demonstrates clearly how each of these three components – accessing research, knowledge translation and research utilisation – link together to influence patient or client care. Researchers produce findings that are usually published in journal articles, textbooks and research reports. Nurses and midwives read these findings or attend continuing professional development (CPD) sessions in order to develop their level of knowledge and skills based on this evidence. The current annual requirement for nurses and midwives is 20 hours of CPD (Nursing and Midwifery Board of Australia 2010). An example of how this could be partially achieved in a nursing workplace might be the establishment of a journal club, aimed at the presentation of research findings of interest to peers and colleagues, information on new research, and clinical trials. Members of the club could attend, present and/or manage the journal club's program and these activities would be counted in their 20 hours of CPD.

To bring evidence to the point of care, nurses and midwives need to translate research findings into practice by appraising their value. The nurse or midwife will utilise research findings in practice if he or she decides the evidence is strong, will lead to positive outcomes for patients or clients, and if their work environment is receptive to change. In order to decide the worth of a research study, nurses need to know how it was undertaken and what the findings comprise. Clinicians must not change practice based on poor quality research. Practising nurses are expected to incorporate research findings into practice and this is called practising from an evidence base, or evidence-based practice.

It is important to realise, however, that nurses and midwives take into account a number of things when making a decision to change their practice. As well as current research findings, nurses and midwives consider patient, client and carers' preferences and concerns, clinical experience and local context (Rycroft-Malone et al 2003) when deciding on a pathway of care. Even though research findings are the strongest form of evidence, they are not normally sourced from only one research paper. There may be a number of studies that have addressed the same question and, to make life even more confusing, they may even present conflicting findings. Luckily, there are a number of institutions and organisations around the world dedicated to finding and disseminating the best available evidence, such as the Joanna Briggs Institute – an international collaboration involving nursing, medical and allied health researchers, clinicians, academics and quality managers across 40 countries in every continent (HealthDirectAustralia 2012). These groups are made clearer in Chapter 10.

A physician called Archie Cochrane coined the term 'evidence-based practice' in the 1970s (Sackett 1996). Cochrane appreciated that with advances in medical science, it was becoming increasingly difficult for doctors to keep up-to-date with the latest evidence for practice (we would argue nurses and midwives have similar difficulties) and they needed a support system to assist them. Some of the barriers to evidence-based practice are time pressures, limited access to electronic databases during work hours and insufficient skills to access and appraise all of the evidence required to answer a focused clinical question. Cochrane set up a systematic process for research teams to find, appraise and summarise research evidence ready for use by clinicians. This process became known as the systematic review and is explained more fully in Chapters 9 and 10. Reports of systematic reviews can be found in a range of evidence-based practice sites listed at the end of this chapter. For everyday use, the systematic review report may be too long to digest, so summaries of evidence are also prepared and come in a range of guises such as best practice information sheets and practice guidelines. These materials are a valuable resource for nursing and midwifery students, as well as busy clinicians who are not yet skilled enough to access and critique research for themselves.

'Levels of evidence' is a phrase that refers to the trustworthiness of research findings. Level 1 evidence indicates the findings are robust and should be applied in practice. There are a number of ranking systems; for example, the Cochrane Collaboration ranks evidence of effectiveness from level 1 (best) to level 4 (expert opinion). The Cochrane Collaboration has a variety of examples of different ways of conducting reviews of qualitative studies and quantitative studies at the following website: www.cochrane.org.

STUDENT CHALLENGE

Understanding the Research Process

1. Go to the following website: www.joannabriggslibrary.org/jbilibrary.
2. Register and log in to the JBI Database of Best Practice Information Sheets and Technical Reports.
3. Scroll through the titles of the sheets and choose one of interest.
4. Look at the back of the sheet to find the information source for the information sheet and identify whether the sheet is based on a systematic review of the literature. (Chapter 10 discusses evidence-based practice and research utilisation in greater detail but we suggest you work your way through the book first because by then you should have a much better understanding of how researchers actually conduct research through what we call the 'research process'.)

Professional nurses and midwives need to keep an eye on the research outputs in their particular specialties by subscribing to journals either personally or through the hospital or university library. When reading papers, one must critique the quality of the research before making a decision on whether to consider adopting the findings into practice. Please be aware that not everything published is necessarily good research. If a nurse judges the research to be of a high quality, the nurse might then consider relevance and workplace policies, practices and processes before deciding whether and how to adopt the findings into practice. A framework for critique of quantitative and qualitative research papers is included in Chapter 9. Even without research training nurses will be able to make some judgment about the quality of research reports such as journal articles. Try the next challenge: it gives you guidelines on how to identify and critique a research report.

STUDENT CHALLENGE

Identifying Parts of a Research Report

1. Find a research report in the form of a journal article. Check the journal to see whether the papers included in it are peer-reviewed before publication, as this is an indicator of quality.
2. What year was the paper published? As a rule of thumb the research should be as up to date as possible.
3. As you skim-read the paper, ask yourself: are the sections of the paper clearly marked (introduction/background, literature review, research design/methodology, results, discussion, conclusions)?
4. Early in the paper can you find the research question and are you persuaded by the author's claims about the significance of the work?
5. Turn to the results and findings and check to see whether the author has written a critique of the work telling the reader where it is limited and what it adds to current knowledge.

The point of this exercise is to make you aware that, even at this early stage of your studies, you are able to identify parts of a research paper and to make preliminary judgments about the quality of the findings. With more research training you will become more confident in critiquing the design of the study. It is useful to read the abstract of a research paper, as this should include a sentence on all of the major features of the research study such as the research aims or question, the methodology, the data collection and analysis, the findings and the recommendations.

Ethics

Nursing and healthcare research often involves the use of humans as research participants. It is important that all research involving human participants is conducted in such a way as to do no harm to the participants. All nursing and midwifery research must be conducted in accordance with the relevant ethical codes and guidelines (www.nhmrc.gov.au/guidelines-publications/r39) and subjected to rigorous review by an institutional review committee (see NHMRC guidelines). For further reading on ethics, see Chapter 4.

Conclusion

Research is an important source of knowledge to be used not only by qualified nurses or midwives but also by students learning in an undergraduate degree program. Research is a complicated process in which one cannot expect to be an expert straight away. However, there are many commonsense elements to research that can be grasped immediately. Completing the challenges in this chapter will enable a student to learn how to appraise a research report. Evidence-based practice centres, such as the Joanna Briggs Institute, have repositories that are a great resource for students; this site and others are listed as a resource at the end of the chapter. Students must develop an appreciation of the importance of research to nursing and midwifery in the delivery of quality care.

RESOURCES KIT

Useful evidence-based practice sites

Cochrane Collaboration. www.cochrane.org.

Excellence in Research Australia. www.arc.gov.au/era/default.htm.

Joanna Briggs Institute. www.joannabriggs.org.

Recommended tool for critical review of academic papers

Critical Appraisal Skills Program (CASP) www.casp-uk.net/#!casp-tools-checklists/c18f8.

Recommended reading

Creswell JW: *A concise introduction to mixed methods research*, Thousand Oaks, California, 2015, SAGE Publications.

Nagy S, Mills J, Waters D, et al: *Using research in healthcare practice*, Sydney, 2010, Lippincott, Williams and Wilkins.

Mills J, Birks M: *Qualitative methodology: a practical guide*, Thousand Oaks, California, 2014, SAGE Publications.

References

Aiken LH, Sloane DM, Cimiotti JP, et al: Implications of the California Nurse Staffing Mandate for Other States, *Health Services for Research* 45:904–921, 2010.

Australian Nursing and Midwifery Council: *The competency standards for registered nurses (RN) can be accessed by choosing the RN option at the following address*. 2006a. www.nursingmidwiferyboard.gov.au/Codes-Guidelines-Statements/Codes-Guidelines.aspx#competencystandards.

Australian Nursing and Midwifery Council: *National competency standards for the registered nurse*. 2006b. Online. Available: www.nursingmidwiferyboard.gov.au/documents/default.aspx?record=WD10%2f1342&dbid=AP&chksum=N5ws04xdBlZijTTSdKnSTQ%3d%3d 27 March 2011.

Australian Nursing and Midwifery Council: *National competency standards for the registered nurse*. 2006c. Online. Available: www.nursingmidwiferyboard.gov.au/documents/default.aspx?record=WD10%2f1342&dbid=AP&chksum=N5ws04xdBlZijTTSdKnSTQ%3d%3d 27 March 2011.

Benner PE: *From novice to expert: excellence and power in clinical nursing practice*, Menlo Park, California, 1984, Addison-Wesley.

Benner PE, Tanner CA, Chesla CA: *Expertise in nursing practice: caring, clinical judgment, and ethics*, Springer Publishing Company, 2009.

Commonwealth of Australia: *National Review of Nursing Education*. 2001. Discussion paper. Canberra: Commonwealth of Australia. Online. Available: http://www.aph.gov.au/Parliamentary_Business/Committees/Senate/Community_Affairs/Completed_inquiries/2002-04/nursing/report/index 14 August 2014.

Commonwealth of Australia: *Report on the Inquiry into Nursing – The Patient Profession: Time for Action*. 2002. Online. Available: http://www.aph.gov.au/Parliamentary_Business/Committees/Senate/Community_Affairs/Completed_inquiries/2002-04/nursing/report/index 27 March 2015.

Estabrooks CA, O'Leary KA, Ricker KL, et al: The internet and access to evidence: how are nurses positioned?, *Journal of Advanced Nursing* 42(1):73–81, 2003.

HealthDirectAustralia: *Joanna Briggs Institute*. 2012. Online. Available: www.healthdirect.gov.au/partners/joanna-briggs-institute 14 August 2014.

Melnyk BM, Gallagher-Ford L, Long LE, et al: The establishment of evidence-based practice competencies for practicing registered nurses and advanced practice nurses in real-world clinical settings: proficiencies to improve healthcare quality, reliability, patient outcomes, and costs, *Worldviews on Evidence-based Nursing* 11(1):5–15, 2014.

Ministry of Health: *The Health Practitioners Competence Assurance Act*. 2003. Online. Available: http://www.health.govt.nz/our-work/regulation-health-and-disability-system/health-practitioners-competence-assurance-act 27 March 2015.

Nursing and Midwifery Board of Australia: *Continuing professional development registration standard*. 2010. Online. Available: www.nursingmidwiferyboard.gov.au/documents/default.aspx?record=WD10%2f135&dbid=AP&chksum=8UL9PD4%2byPR9h99u%2b6alcA%3d%3d 27 March 2011.

Orem D: *Nursing–concepts of practice*, ed 4, New York, 1991, McGraw Hill.

Roberts K, Taylor B: *Nursing research processes: an Australian perspective*, Melbourne, 2002, Nelson.

Rycroft-Malone J, Seers K, Titchen A, et al: What counts as evidence in evidence-based practice?, *Journal of Advanced Nursing* 47:81–90, 2003.

Sackett D: Evidence-based medicine: what it is and what it isn't, *British Medical Journal* 312:71–72, 1996.

Stenhouse E, Letherby G: Multidisciplinary research in midwifery: reflecting on a collaborative relationship, *Evidence Based Midwifery* 8:17–20, 2010.

Yarcheski A, Mahon NE, Yarcheski TJ: A descriptive study of research published in scientific nursing journals from 1985 to 2010, *International Journal of Nursing Studies* 49(9):1112–1121, 2012.

CHAPTER 2

USING LIBRARY RESOURCES: WHAT, WHEN AND HOW!

Kath Peters, Judy Mannix and Lucie Ramjan

CHAPTER OUTLINE

KEY TERMS

- call number
- catalogue
- citation database
- electronic database
- grey literature
- index
- information literacy
- interlibrary loan (document delivery)
- journal (periodical or magazine)
- microform
- reference collection
- reserve collection
- search engine
- search strategy

LEARNING OBJECTIVES

After reading this chapter and following critical reflection the student will be able to:

1. Use the different services and resources offered by the library
2. Understand how the library filing/classification systems can assist to locate resources
3. Access, compare and contrast electronic databases to obtain nursing, midwifery and healthcare-related information
4. Conduct a basic information search using library resources
5. Identify which electronic databases and other electronic resources, such as e-books and the like, will best help with regard to their studies.

STUDENT QUOTE

I couldn't believe the amount of information I have access to via the library! This will definitely benefit my studies and improve my grades.

ABSTRACT

Libraries collect, store and organise information and make it readily accessible for use. Libraries can also direct users to other profession-specific repositories of information. Hard-copy materials within the library are organised using a classification system and located by searching the catalogues. Electronic data is accessed using electronic databases or, in some cases, can be accessed via a library catalogue. Successful searches for information about a particular topic demand certain skills. These include the ability to define the topic of interest, select appropriate electronic search tools, and conduct a basic search of databases and the catalogue system to identify and access the information required.

How can this chapter help you?

Take the following quiz to find out if this chapter will help you.

1. Do you know what libraries are available in your area and if there are resources available to you electronically?
2. Do you know what kinds of materials they have and what kinds of services they offer?
3. Do you have library privileges and if so, what do they entitle you to?

4. Do you find it easy to locate what you are looking for when you use a library?
5. Can you use computerised search systems?
6. Do you know what an electronic database is? Can you provide a list of the most appropriate databases for nursing, midwifery and allied health?
7. Do you use the same small set of resources for all your work and not look further afield?
8. Do you know the advantages of using CINAHL, MEDLINE, SUMSearch or the TRIP database, relative to internet search engines such as Google?

If you answered 'yes' to most of these questions you may want to skim this chapter, but if you have answered 'no' or if you have ever said to a lecturer or colleague, 'there wasn't any information available on the topic', then it would be useful for you to read this chapter and complete the student challenges.

Types of libraries

In the 21st century almost limitless access to information via the internet is taken for granted and an expectation for many students enrolled in education courses. With access to these vast amounts of information students need appropriate skills to determine in a timely manner which information is useful and appropriate for use in their studies. Central to these skills is **information literacy**, which has been defined as 'the ability to search for, select, critically evaluate and use information for solving problems in various contexts' (Limberg et al 2012). Possessing these skills can also enhance lifelong learning beyond completion of courses.

Present-day libraries can be described as either virtual libraries or physical libraries. The physical library is the actual library building with the collections of different resources for borrowing and library staff to assist you in person, whereas the virtual library is the electronic library that consists of online resources where library users can access resources at any time via a computer (PC) with an internet connection. Online resources, for example, e-books, online journals (full text), newspaper articles and various other documents, can be available via library homepages. These types of resources do have an advantage over print as they cannot be misplaced on the shelves and more patrons can use the resources from distant locations. To access some of these electronic resources you may be prompted for your username and password as some titles may only be available to particular users. Always check with your library if you have any problems accessing and using e-books. Many libraries offer specialist librarians in nursing and midwifery, an online chat service or even online question services to assist you with your information needs. Blogs and Twitter can also be available for use. These services can assist you outside the library. Overall, the traditional view of a library as a place where information is physically housed has been relegated to history and libraries are now places that facilitate information access.

Academic libraries are connected to academic institutions and collect information of interest to staff and students. The types of material collected are strongly associated with the degrees offered at that academic institution; in other words, the resources held support the curriculum taught. In some cases, at a multi-campus university the library has a physical presence on campuses where students are attending classes. Specialty libraries are formed by organisations with specialised information needs. They collect information on specific topics dictated by the needs of the organisation that funds them. These may include business and corporate libraries, or professional libraries, such as hospital libraries. The information collected is based on the needs of the special population being served. If you are located in a hospital or other care facility you may have access to an onsite library, which is usually a cross between an academic and a specialty library.

What's in the library?

Libraries use very precise systems to organise all the information they collect. These organising systems are called classification schemes. Libraries use two major classification schemes: the Dewey decimal classification (DDC) and the Library of Congress classification. Both systems use number–letter combinations to label their collections. These labels are known as **call numbers**. Some libraries put call numbers on all their materials, while others label only books. Each hard-copy book has a unique call number and ranges of call numbers are clearly marked on library shelves to make a particular book or a range of books about a specific subject easy to locate. As a rule of thumb, in Australia and New Zealand most public and academic libraries use the DDC. Specialty libraries may use a scheme adapted to handle large volumes of material in relatively few subject areas. Medical libraries may use the National Library of Medicine classification system, adapted from the Library of Congress system. The key point is that all the physical material in the library is carefully organised to make it easy to find and use.

Library users need to know what physical and human resources exist within the library as well as what external resources may be accessed from the library. Every library is arranged differently but there are usually some common features. The main section of the library typically contains a loans (circulation) desk, an information/reference/research inquiries desk and an area set aside for computer workstations where you can search in catalogues, **indexes**, abstracts and full text databases. Other key areas include a **reference collection**, a current and bound periodicals section and the main collection shelves. Most libraries also have a media or audiovisual centre, **reserve collection** section and special collections. Most modern libraries have a variety of learning spaces to accommodate individual student's study needs. Students can access computers, with internet, printing and photocopying facilities, and space is available for interactive learning with others as well as space for private reading time.

The loans (circulation) desk is where you borrow books and other circulating materials to use outside the library. The information/reference inquiries desk is the place to go when you don't know where to look for needed materials or when you have questions about various library services and resources. Many libraries combine the functions of the information/reference research inquiries desks. The names used to describe these services may vary between libraries. Most libraries have help guides in print or available online from the library homepage, including virtual tours of the library. Library staff will demonstrate how to access various databases and may offer consultations for further assistance or there may be generic classes where you can attend and learn about the services the library offers. iPhone/iPad apps are another option to give library users access to information.

The reference collection contains materials such as encyclopedias, dictionaries, statistical reports, directories, handbooks and other materials that are handy for quick reference. These materials are referred to as 'library use only' because they are for use within the library and may not be borrowed and taken outside the library. The current periodicals section displays the newer issues of journals and magazines and may be organised alphabetically by title or call number. These issues frequently start with the first issue of the current year and contain all the issues for the year to date. The bound periodicals contain single issues of a particular **journal** or magazine published in previous years, bound together in book form, called a volume. The number of years contained in a volume depends on the size of the journal and number of issues published annually. Typically, one year of a journal constitutes a volume and the specific volumes or issues of periodicals the library owns are referred to as its holdings. This section is usually arranged by call number (e.g. DDC) but in some libraries it is arranged alphabetically by periodical title. It is common practice for libraries to have current and bound periodicals housed together on the same shelf. Most periodicals are also available online via the online library **catalogue** record. It is useful to find out what resources are available in full text in the libraries accessible to you.

In addition to books and periodicals, many libraries have an audiovisual section containing DVDs and computer software. Some libraries may also have a **microform** section consisting of microfilm and microfiche that allow the reader to view different documents stored on film; for example, newspapers. The reserve section contains materials that have been put aside by the library or faculty staff for special use. The function of the reserve section is the sharing of limited resources needed by a number of users. Typically, these materials can only be checked out of the library for a few hours, overnight, or for one or two days. Some material can only be viewed in the library. These materials are often heavily used, so a reserve system allows a greater number of people to access them. Special collections, or archives, contain rare materials that are not easily replaced. These might include collections of items such as government and professional documents, old, rare or one-of-a-kind books, or materials of historical importance. Access to these materials may be restricted and they may not be borrowed.

You may have visited your university or health centre library; however, if you have only a sketchy idea about where things are located or how to use the library in general, please take time to do the following student challenge. It can save you a lot of time and energy when you need to use the library and want to locate the resources or services you need quickly.

STUDENT CHALLENGE

Exploring Library Layouts

Make a visit to your university or health centre library. Allow an hour for this experience.

- Wander around, explore and browse.
- Pick up any handouts that are available to users as helpful hints or guides.
- Skim the brochures you've collected.

Become comfortable with the space and with the library, before attempting to undertake the following tasks.

1. Make a mental note of the physical layout (the library may already have a map for users). Then:
   a. Locate and visit the loans desk, information/reference/research inquiries desk, reserve desk or other operational groupings.
   b. Find a library workstation. Find the search tool section (e.g., indexes, abstracts, databases and catalogues) available via the internet.
   c. Find several periodical titles and their holdings that are available via the library catalogue for your area of interest.
   d. Find the bound periodicals (they may be with the single-print issues on the shelf or in a separate area).
   e. Visit the reference collection.
   f. Visit the special collections and archives.
   g. Locate the section containing government documents.
   h. Locate the section containing theses and dissertations.
   i. Visit the media centre.
   j. Locate the audiovisual resources collection (microfilm, microfiche, CDs, DVDs).
   k. Find the photocopy machines, change machines, vending machines and recharge card machine.
   l. Locate the study areas, lounges and toilets.
2. Find out about library operations.
   a. What are the library's opening hours?
   b. When are generalist library and specialist nursing and midwifery library staff available to help?

c. What sort of help do they provide?
d. Are library tours or classes available in the library and, if so, when?
e. How do you obtain borrowing rights? Identify what interlibrary loan or document delivery privileges you can access.
f. What are the policies for borrowing and returning materials? Is there a self-checkout system, text reserve system or loan extension system?
g. Is this library connected with other libraries you can use?
h. Can you access library search tools from computers in other locations on campus or from your home computer?

3. How is the library collection classified?
4. Where are the nursing or midwifery resources located? Locate the following: nursing/midwifery books, nursing/midwifery journals, professional documents (such as those from the Australian Nursing and Midwifery Council, Nursing Council of New Zealand, Australian College of Nursing or New Zealand Nurses Organisation) and government publications (such as those from the Australian Institute of Health and Welfare – nursing and midwifery labour force).

Searching for information in catalogues

Libraries have specific filing systems called catalogues to assist you in locating specific materials so you may retrieve the information you seek. It is worthwhile spending time exploring your library's catalogue, as it will list all items held in the library including books, videos, CDs, and DVDs. The titles of newspapers, scholarly journals, popular periodicals and other library materials, such as government or professional documents, may also be listed. However, information about the specific content contained in those periodicals or documents is not usually in the catalogue.

Books are listed with bibliographical information, location, collection, call numbers and borrowed status. Books may be located by searching for a specific title, author, keyword/s, call number, International Standard Book Number (ISBN), government document classification number or subject matter.

Using electronic catalogues

Most catalogues are now available electronically. They may be accessed directly from library workstations or from any internet connection either on or off-campus. Using the latter you may be asked to provide a username and password to authenticate yourself as someone authorised to use the system. This connection to the catalogue enables you to search for books and other library materials. You simply need to follow the onscreen directions, which tell you how to search for a book by title, author, keyword and so on. Many libraries external to your own university also offer free access to their catalogues where you can search and discover what resources are held.

Such online systems offer the added advantage of providing the latest information on all new materials coming into the library, and usually carry additional useful information such as whether a book is available on the shelves or if it has been borrowed. In cases where books have been borrowed, the due date for return will be indicated in the catalogue. Catalogues may have a holds/reservations system that you are able to use when an item you require is out on loan. This will allow you to place a reservation on the resource when it is returned. Some catalogues may also allow virtual shelf-browsing that allows you to see what resources are shelved nearby; for example, naming the five books held on either side of a selected text.

Using your library's electronic catalogue, complete the following challenge.

STUDENT CHALLENGE

Scanning Electronic Catalogues

1. Sit down at one of the computer workstations in the library or use your own personal computer.
2. Examine and try the different options available for searching the library catalogue including searching different library locations.
3. Use the online catalogue to locate one of your nursing, midwifery or healthcare textbooks by using a keyword in the title.
4. Try locating it by author.
5. Try locating it by subject matter.
6. Which way was easiest? Did you have any problems using one of the search options? How did you solve them?
7. Locate the book in the library. What information did you use from the library catalogue to find the book?

Indexes, abstracts and electronic databases

Historically, the term 'index' was used for a list of citations to periodicals and other publications such as newspapers and government or professional documents. It is important to note that terminology has changed over the years. While the electronic versions of the subject-specific indexes listed below still perform the same function as their paper-based predecessors, they are now more commonly referred to as **electronic databases**. Several different databases exist for a wide variety of specialty areas.

An abstract is a short summary of a publication and is useful in helping you decide whether the publication contains the information you are seeking. These summaries are virtually always available as part of the citation information provided to users as part of their search results after they search a database. The library will probably not hold full text versions of all the materials identified in search results but it should have access to them through **interlibrary loan/document delivery**. Some databases may provide links to other databases, which may enable you to access the full text of an article.

Some common and useful databases are listed in Boxes 2.1 and 2.2. Please note that, although the word 'index' remains in titles, these electronic resources are also known as databases.

Electronic healthcare databases

A major advantage of electronic databases is that they are available online and offer access to a wider range of information. Cumulative Index to Nursing and Allied Health Literature (CINAHL) and MEDLINE are the two main databases that provide online access to materials related to research and practice in the disciplines of nursing, midwifery, medicine and allied health care.

CINAHL includes indexing for over 5000 journals, and provides full text articles for more than 1300 journals in the areas of nursing, midwifery, consumer health, medicine, complementary medicine and 17 other allied health disciplines (CINAHL 2014). Journal articles, eBooks, book chapters, practice guidelines, dissertations/theses, conference proceedings, educational software and audiovisuals can all be accessed via CINAHL. While various types of literature are available, some have not been subject to peer review (e.g., theses and government reports), and therefore may not be as suitable to inform practice or for use in academic studies. This information that is not formally published is called **grey literature**. While CINAHL focuses on nursing, midwifery, allied health and psychosocial issues, MEDLINE focuses on biomedicine and health. MEDLINE, a **citation database**, contains more than 21 million citations from journals in life sciences including, but not limited to, medicine, nursing, dentistry, veterinary medicine and behavioural sciences (Fact sheet MEDLINE 2014).

Another useful electronic database is ProQuest Health and Medical Complete, which provides access to more than 2800 reputable clinical, health and biomedical publications (ProQuest Health and Medical Complete 2014). Various other electronic databases are available covering a variety of disciplines; for example, Intermid is a database that allows browsing of two reputable midwifery journals, and each operates in a slightly different way.

Most electronic databases have introductory lessons to guide you in your search and a help function to troubleshoot any difficulties you may encounter. However, if you require additional support, you may wish to contact the library staff at your university.

Box 2.1
Nursing, midwifery and health specific databases

Aboriginal and Torres Strait Islander Health Bibliography (ATSIHEALTH)
Australasian Medical Index (AMI)
Australian Education Index (AEI)
British Nursing Index (BNI)
CINAHL (Cumulative Index to Nursing and Allied Health Literature)
CINAHL Plus with Full text
Clinical Evidence (BMJ)
Cochrane Library
Education Resources Information Center (ERIC)
Embase
Health Source: Nursing/Academic Edition
Index New Zealand on Te Puna (INNZ)
Intermid.co.uk
International Pharmaceutical Abstracts
Maternity and Infant Care
MEDLINE
MIMS Online
Proquest Central
Proquest evidence-based resources from the Joanna Briggs Institute
PsycINFO
PubMed
Science Citation Index (SCI)
Social Services Abstracts
Social Sciences Citation Index (SSCI)
Sociological Abstracts
SUMSearch
TRIP database – clinical search engine

Online systems allow you instant access to a wide range of electronic databases. One particularly useful feature of some electronic databases is the ability to run a search for a topic of interest on one database and if further reference material is sought then the user can select additional databases to search and re-run the current terms without retyping the search terms of interest.

Box 2.2
Other helpful databases

Australian Bureau of Statistics (ABS) 2014: www.abs.gov.au

Australian College of Midwives (2011): www.midwives.org.au/scripts/cgiip.exe/WService=MIDW/ccms.r?pageid=10062

Australian Institute of Health and Welfare (AIHW) (2013). Authoritative information and statistics to promote better health and wellbeing: www.aihw.gov.au

Google Scholar: http://scholar.google.com.au

INFOKOORI: an index of Australian Indigenous Affairs – an index to the *Koori Mail*, a national fortnightly newspaper published in Lismore, NSW, for Aboriginal and Torres Strait Islander people: www.sl.nsw.gov.au/infokoori

LactMed: A TOXNET database: toxnet.nlm.nih.gov/newtoxnet/lactmed.htm

National Guideline Clearinghouse (NGC) 2014: www.guideline.gov

National Health Service (NHS) 2014: www.nhs.uk/Pages/HomePage.aspx

National Institutes of Health (NIH) (2014): www.nih.gov

New Zealand College of Midwives (Inc) (2014): www.midwife.org.nz

Public Library of Science (PLOS) 2014: www.plos.org

Statistics New Zealand: www.stats.govt.nz

The Joanna Briggs Institute library: a database of Best Practice Information Sheets and Technical Reports: joannabriggs.org

Dissertations (Theses)

Australasian Digital Theses Program – will provide a range or resources: adt.caul.edu.au

NZ theses – The University of Auckland provides access to dissertations at various levels: www.library.auckland.ac.nz/services/research-teaching-and-learning/finding-theses-and-dissertations

Using apps to search

There are now dedicated academic literature search applications (apps) available for most mobile internet access devices. Increasingly, these apps are being used by healthcare professionals to access literature to enhance both their research and clinical practice (Mossa et al 2013). While there are many apps available, one notable app is Article Search, which is designed for both iPhone and iPad. The Article Search app is user friendly and allows you to search multiple search engines, libraries and databases simultaneously which can save you time (iTunes Preview 2014). Another app available for searching literature for

Android users is Academic, which searches around 20 prominent **search engines** including Google Scholar, JSTOR, Medline Plus and Microsoft Academic Search (Google Play 2014). The search apps allow you to view and download PDF versions of articles returned by your searches. There are also apps that allow access to specific journals; for example, *The Journal of Obstetric, Gynecologic & Neonatal Nursing*, and *MCN: The American Journal of Maternal/ Child Nursing*.

STUDENT CHALLENGE

Examining Electronic Databases

Sit down at one of the computer workstations in the library or use your own personal computer.

1. Does the same computer allow you to do catalogue and electronic database searches? If so, how do you go from one type of search to the other?
2. Look at all the electronic databases available online. Which ones look like they would be relevant to nursing, midwifery or healthcare?
3. Explore at least two databases you consider relevant to your discipline. Can you locate a description of each database? Can you find a list of the journals that are indexed?

Tips for successful searching

As previously discussed, a search can be conducted using electronic databases, internet search engines and catalogues to find information about specific subjects. Searching for a particular book or article by title or by author is fairly straightforward. Searching for unknown materials on a subject or topic you have interest in is slightly more complicated. If you have ever tried to do a search and received a message that says, 'there are 21,346 matches', or 'there are no matches meeting your search parameters', this can be very frustrating. This section is designed to provide tips for effective searching so that you are more successful and productive and can develop a **search strategy**. During your search you need to be mindful of publication bias (where knowledge published may be misleading for a variety of reasons including flawed methodologies, see Rothstein et al 2005; Schmitt 1998), and salami slicing (where multiple publications from the one study dominate the area, see Jackson et al 2014) both of which either skew or provide an inaccurate representation of results.

Clearly define your search

Start the process by having a clear idea of your search topic or subject. What is your subject area or topic? Tip: It can be helpful to write down what you would like to explore in sentence form (written description) or summarise your topic in the form of a question. What are the key concepts and subconcepts for that subject or topic? Which concepts are most important? Concepts should usually be verbs and nouns. Tip: It can be useful to underline or highlight the main concepts in your written description and in the question you have developed. Next think of other keywords that mean the same as your key concepts or subconcepts (synonyms) – think of the alternative spelling of these words; for example, paediatrics or pediatrics, labor or labour. Truncate words or use wild cards to expand a search. Truncation involves formulating other words by using the base of a word (e.g. Nurs* = nurse, nurses, nursing, nursery). Wild cards are symbols that replace characters in a word (e.g. Wom?n = woman or women) (Harvard 2007). Tip: It is worthwhile to create a table with the key concepts and associated subconcepts, and to list truncated words and/or wild cards that you may decide to use in your search. What information do you currently have? Reading your own textbooks, reference books or articles you may already have for background information before you access databases and catalogues can help focus and direct your search. Look at the references listed in these books and articles. You may find pertinent sources on your topic that you can look up electronically or in the library. You should also refer to subject guides produced by your lecturers, as these guides are often a good starting point to find the information you need. If you are using an evidence-based frame of reference you may prefer to adopt the PICO(T) or SPIDER approach to searching for specific knowledge (see Chapters 10 and 11).

Choose appropriate resources

Books tend to provide good reference information on a particular subject or topic, particularly if the subject area is new to you. It is important that the books you use are current unless they are seminal works. Journals provide more current and specific information than books as they report changing trends and practices. Research journals are particularly valuable in providing the results and outcomes of the latest research studies (Harvard 2007). If you require definitions, statistics, trends, professional or government documents or policies, then these are usually found in electronic reference materials available on the internet (e.g. Australian Bureau of Statistics: www.abs.gov.au, or Department of Health: www.health.gov.au). Alternatively, they may be found in the special documents sections of the library. Dictionaries and encyclopedias can also provide definitions and overviews of your subject matter.

Choose appropriate databases

Choosing an appropriate database is imperative for success in searching. Each database has a primary area of focus, plus advantages and limits. A description of the purpose of a particular database may be listed in the catalogue or there may be further information next to or underneath the name of the database on the library homepage. A list of the journals may be listed with the database. Think about three issues when selecting a database: Firstly, what subjects are covered in the database? Tip: As indicated the database description will help you decide which database to use and provides information on subjects. Secondly, what years does the database cover? Tip: Some databases only index recent articles while others index older publication years. For earlier seminal publications you may need to source the print index. Thirdly, what sources does the database include? Tip: The database description should provide this information and indicate whether the database searches articles only or other sources such as book chapters, theses or newspapers (The University of Chicago Library 2013).

A useful database is the Evidence-Based Medicine Reviews (EBMR). This is a specialised database for locating full-text evidence-based publications by searching seven evidence-based medicine reviews databases, which includes Cochrane Database of Systematic Reviews and The Database of Abstracts of Reviews of Effectiveness (DARE) (Ovid Technologies, Inc. 2014). Other useful databases for Nursing and Midwifery subject areas include ProQuest Health & Medical Complete (ProQuest), CINAHL Plus with full-text, MEDLINE and PubMed.

Define your search parameters

Electronic databases operate with a special vocabulary. However, the computer helps you define the preferred terms to use in a search. If you enter a term, it will supply alternative terms for use. It will also let you view the entire directory if you want to see how it is organised. Different databases use different listings of terms. MEDLINE uses a medical subject–heading directory (MeSH Subject Heading). CINAHL uses its own built in specialised thesaurus and other databases have their own specialised subject directories, referred to as 'controlled vocabulary'. Tip: Use an advanced search option when available as it allows greater flexibility and scope for entering various parameters such as search terms, author, title and so forth (The University of Chicago Library 2013).

Place limits on your search

Use limits to narrow your search so it is as precise as possible. If you have several key terms, use them. Limits you can apply include language, type of resource, publication date, and full text only (The University of Chicago Library 2013). You can always remove some of the limits if the results are not what you want. For example, say we want to find out the latest information on the effects of menopause on individuals with diabetes mellitus. If we enter the word 'diabetes' to search in MEDLINE (EBSCOhost, EBSCO), we will get more than 441,000 different citations. If we use the words 'diabetes mellitus' we come up with about 303,000 citations. If we combine the words 'diabetes mellitus and menopause' it narrows the search down to 691 citations. If we limit the search to include only adult females, we get 252 citations. If we further limit the search to articles written in English and published from 2005 to current, we get a manageable 95 citations (see Figure 2.1).

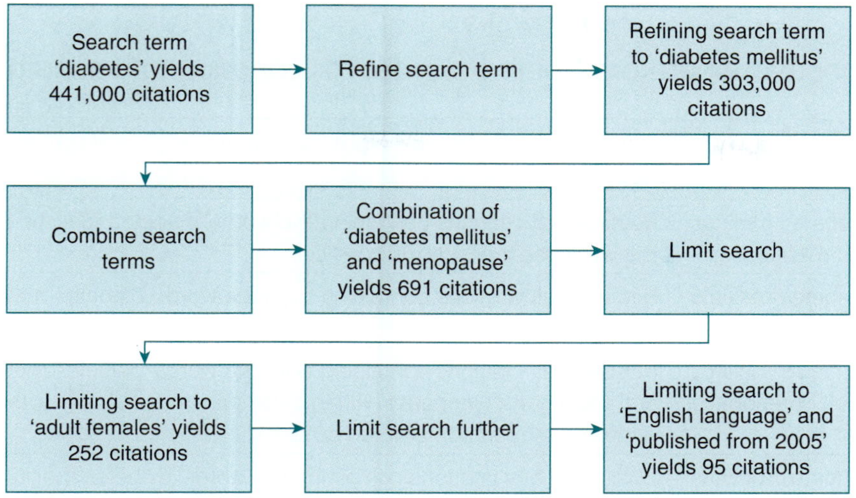

FIGURE 2.1
Limiting your search

All computerised search databases have rules for use that can save time and effort when searching. The more you know about these rules and how to use them, the more successful you will be with refining your searches. For instance, most databases use Boolean operators (named after George Boole. 1815–1864) (Redshaw 1996). These operators or joining words allow you to combine terms with the words 'AND', 'OR, 'NOT' 'NEAR' to retrieve a specific result. The term 'AND' narrows a search by ensuring that all search terms are present. The term 'OR' broadens a search by ensuring that any of the search terms are present. However, this term needs to be used with caution as it retrieves multiple categories, some of which may not be relevant to your search. The term 'NOT' limits a search by removing a particular search term that you do not want (The University of Chicago Library 2013). Finally the term 'NEAR' ensures the search terms are found within close proximity (usually within 10 words) of each other. Review the diabetes and menopause example shown in Table 2.1. You can see, 'OR' is the least restrictive link and 'NOT' is the most restrictive link. (To remember this, think 'OR' is 'MORE'.) Other operators or joining words may be used to place limits on things such as age, gender, type of journal, years of publication, and so on. Note that it is not always necessary to use uppercase.

When searching within a database you may find a limit option, which will only return references in your search results that are peer-reviewed. Peer-reviewed articles are articles that have been subjected to a process of critical evaluation by one or more experts on the subject material.

A few databases use a technique that gives you a list of articles ranked in order of relevancy; that is, from most to least likely to be relevant, based on a set of supplied search terms (e.g. diabetes mellitus, menopause, female, adult).

Table 2.1
Examples of boolean operators (joining words) for conducting a search

Boolean operator (joining word)	Example	What happens
OR	Diabetes mellitus OR menopause	Retrieves all citations containing the words 'diabetes mellitus' or the word 'menopause' in an article
AND	Diabetes mellitus AND menopause	Retrieves all citations containing both the words 'diabetes mellitus' and the word 'menopause' in an article
NEAR	Diabetes mellitus NEAR menopause	Retrieves all citations containing both the words 'diabetes mellitus' and the word 'menopause' within close proximity (usually within 10 words) of each other in an article
NOT	Diabetes mellitus NOT menopause	Eliminates any citations containing the words 'diabetes mellitus' that also contain the word 'menopause'

Articles containing all the terms would be high on the results list and those containing one term would be at the bottom of the results list. You can even weight the terms to indicate which are more important in the search (e.g. the terms 'diabetes mellitus' and 'menopause' could be more heavily weighted than 'female' or 'adult').

The best way to increase proficiency with using search operators is through regular practice. Many students do not make full use of the electronic database's system capabilities so make sure you use these resources and review the available materials on conducting a search to guide your practice. Library assistance is always available if you are experiencing difficulties.

An equally important skill is locating electronic repositories of professional data and knowing what types of data may be found in these repositories. The next chapter deals specifically with issues relevant to surfing the internet; however, it is important to realise at this point how public-access internet search tools can assist you in literature searching. One highly recommended search tool is SUMSearch, a free medical meta-search engine (Crom 2007), which simultaneously submits your search terms to some highly reputable medical information within, for example, Cochrane Library's Database of Abstracts of Reviews of Effectiveness (DARE), National Guideline Clearinghouse and PubMed. These sites are government-sponsored and therefore likely to have limited bias due to conflicts of interest.

View your search results

Once you have defined and run your search, you will want to view the results. The first page of results will list each citation with the option to view an abstract or full text if available. Simply looking at article titles or journal names helps you eliminate more articles from your search. If a citation seems promising, you may want to look at the abstract. You should save, email, export or print the PDF version if available, to retain the original pagination, tables and figures. As you build your personal library on this search it can be stored electronically using software programs such as EndNote and RefWorks. These software-referencing programs can help you manage the literature and citations.

In the example about menopause and its effects on diabetes, a preview of results led to the identification of approximately 20 articles worth further examination. The next step is to access the full text; however, if it is not available, check your online library catalogue for the journal in which the article is published. Sometimes the library will have a print copy or full text access via another means. If the article is only offered in print it will require a visit to the library. The library may also have special library services such as document delivery to assist you in accessing a full text copy from another library.

Looking at the citations may also give you clues about making a search narrower. For example, when we did the search using just the word 'diabetes', the vast number of returned citations lead us to add 'mellitus' to the term 'diabetes' to be more specific.

Another tip is: If you do find important and relevant articles on your topic, check the reference lists at the end of each article. A reference list will guide you to other good topic-specific resources. Additionally, some search engines identify related articles to the one you are reading. If any of the references, be they in the reference or related article lists, look useful, check and see if you can access the full text. Check the source (the journal in which the article is published) in your catalogue to see if your library has full text access either electronically or in print. These references could be very useful when writing up your paper. Check with your library if you are having difficulties finding the references.

Now that you have had step-by-step practice, try the following student challenge and do another search using the computer and whichever electronic resources you deem most appropriate. Use the information from the successful search section and the knowledge gained from the previous student challenges to assist you.

STUDENT CHALLENGE

Use your Knowledge to Practise Doing a Basic Search

Search for updated information on a basic nursing or midwifery skill (such as hand-washing, blood pressure readings or taking a fetal heart rate).

1. Define what you are looking for.
2. What resources will you use? Why did you choose them?

3. Describe how you conducted your search. What parameters did you use? How did you limit the search? Did you limit your results to peer-reviewed articles?
4. How many different searches did you do? What guided your decision-making processes during the search process? What aspects of your search approach worked and what aspects did not work?
5. Print the results of your search. Locate the articles you think are most pertinent to your selected topic. Do they contain the information you need?

RESOURCES KIT

Help button: Electronic databases have an online help button. It is designed to help you make the best use of that database. Click on it whenever you require assistance and need guidance while conducting an electronic search.

Librarians: There are specialist librarians for nursing and midwifery – seek their expert help. They field all kinds of questions and are very willing to assist. Librarians also run classes on conducting searches and specialist librarians offer consultations by appointment. There are also online librarians available on most electronic library websites where a chat facility is available to seek advice. Alternatively, you can phone or email for support.

Library help guides: Many libraries offer a range of guides (print and online) to make library use easier. Both print and electronic guides will assist you with your research.

Acknowledgements

This chapter has been revised from previous editions and the authors would like to acknowledge the previous contributions of Dr Les Fitzgerald, Jill Stokes and Dr Bill Koch.

References

CINAHL – Cumulative Index to Nursing and Allied Health Literature (2014). Online. Available: www.ebscohost.com/biomedical-libraries/the-cinahl-database 26 July 2014.

Crom V: SUMsearch, *Journal of the Medical Library Association* 95(4):471–473, 2007.

Fact sheet MEDLINE. (2014). Online. Available: www.nlm.nih.gov/pubs/factsheets/medline.html 26 July 2014.

Google Play (2014). *Academic*. Google. Online. Available: https://play.google.com/store/apps/details?id=com.sebkabuto.academic&hl=en.

Harvard L: How to conduct an effective and valid literature search, *Nursing Times* 103(44):32–33, 2007.

iTunes Preview (2014). *ArticleSearch by Foreminds by Bottosso Ltd*. Apple Inc. Online. Available: https://itunes.apple.com/au/app/articlesearch/id401914624?mt=8 27 July 2014.

Jackson D, Walter G, Daly J, et al: Editorial: Multiple outputs from single studies: acceptable division of findings vs.'salami'slicing, *Journal of Clinical Nursing* 23(1–2):1–2, 2014.

Limberg L, Sundin O, Talja S: Three theoretical perspectives on information literacy, *Human IT: Journal for Information Technology Studies as a Human Science* 11(2):93–130, 2012.
Mossa ASM, Yoo I, Sheets L: A systematic review of healthcare applications for smartphones, *BMC Medical Informatics and Decision Making* 12:67, 2013.
Ovid Technologies, Inc. (2014). *Evidence-Based Medicine Reviews*. Online. Available: www.ovid.com/site/catalog/databases/904.jsp 18 July 2014.
ProQuest Health and Medical Complete (2014). Online. Available: www.proquest.com/libraries/academic/databases/pq_health_med_comp.html 26 July 2014.
Redshaw K (1996). *George Boole (1815–1864)*. Online. Available: www.kerryr.net/pioneers/boole.htm 19 July 2014.
Rothstein HR, Sutton AJ, Borenstein M: Publication Bias in Meta-Analysis. In Rothstein HR, Sutton AJ, Borenstein M, editors: *Publication Bias in Meta-Analysis: Prevention, Assessment and Adjustments* (1–7), West Sussex, 2005, John Wiley & Sons Ltd.
Schmitt M: Publication bias in nursing research, *Research in Nursing & Health* 21:383–384, 1998.
The University of Chicago Library. (2013). *How do I find articles?* Available: guides.lib.uchicago.edu/articles 18 July 2014.

CHAPTER 3

UNDERSTANDING AND NAVIGATING THE NET: A SOURCE OF NURSING AND MIDWIFERY KNOWLEDGE

Bob Ribbons

CHAPTER OUTLINE

KEY TERMS

blogs
browser
critical reader
evidence-based practice
information-literate
information quality
internet
search engines
social media
wikis
world wide web

LEARNING OBJECTIVES

After reading this chapter and following critical reflection the student will be able to:

1. Understand the internet's components and functions
2. Explore the services and resources available on the internet
3. Understand the basics of web searching and navigation
4. Locate and interrogate professional databases and electronic journals for evidence-based information
5. Understand the need to check web-based material for quality
6. Begin to explore the notion of critical reading and how it can be done
7. Learn to summarise to avoid plagiarism in a web-based culture.

STUDENT QUOTE

I feel like an explorer setting out in uncharted territory ... It's exciting and scary at the same time.

ABSTRACT

Technology and the internet have changed the way we find, use, store and share information. The **internet** is a worldwide, interconnected network of computers where you can tap into vast amounts of stored information and databases. Searching for resources and navigating the internet is made easier by using web browsers and **search engines**. Library catalogues, indexes and a myriad of other resources are available, including quality health-related databases such as MEDLINE and Cumulated Index to Nursing and Allied Health Literature (CINAHL). As the majority of journals are available online in electronic form, many libraries are no longer renewing paper journal subscriptions. The internet has become an incredible communications tool. It enables you to communicate with individuals or groups across the globe in real time or at a time that suits. You can take a course, observe surgical procedures, explore the human body in three-dimensional images, search for evidence for your practice and hold interactive meetings. The internet has revolutionised the way in which information is managed.

The knowledge economy

Easy access to affordable, powerful and user-friendly computer technology has changed the way we interact with the world around us forever. Computers are used in nearly every aspect of our lives and have pushed all boundaries of communications and data management. We have moved from an industrial economy based on capital in the form of machines and factories to a digital economy based on computerised networks, information and knowledge. One of the early, most enduring and dynamic outcomes of this has been the internet, which instantly links us to people and resources around the world. The explosion of social networking technology in the past few years has fundamentally changed the way our society functions, just as the industrial revolution changed society in the 19th century. Recent decisions relating to the rollout of Australia's National Broadband Network (NBN) should provide fast, reliable high-speed communications and internet services. This will transform almost every aspect of our lives – the way we conduct business, obtain healthcare and education and access government services.

Already, we can buy almost anything or complete a tertiary course without leaving the house. In fact, at some stage in the not-too-distant future, it is conceivable the vast majority of all commerce will be conducted electronically. We can find information about almost any subject and access the latest available evidence for our clinical practice. At the tap of a screen or the push of a button, we can meet and chat with new friends from around the world and access and exchange any material we wish. This has major implications to how we work, learn, communicate and manage our ever-growing access to information.

What's this chapter all about?

You have explored the library as a resource that can help you become and remain **information-literate**. This chapter introduces you to the modern, value-added library – the internet. It enables you to explore the **world wide web** (WWW) and to investigate what it is, what it can offer and how to use it.

It will introduce you to the internet as a tool for locating and accessing valid information and evidence-based resources on which to ground your practice. The ability to use the internet effectively can extend and enhance your research skills and make finding appropriate information easier, less time-consuming and more convenient.

Picture this: you are a typical student and have a tendency to procrastinate when it comes to assignments. It is late on Friday night and, in a panic, you realise you have an assignment due on Monday and you haven't started it yet. Not that long ago because the library was closed you would have spent a restless night knowing you were unable even to begin your literature search. Nowadays, you can sleep easy knowing that in the morning you can retrieve the aggregated web feed you set up when you first received the essay topic. Your literature search has been automatically completed and it is waiting for you!

If you are already an accomplished internet user, you may want to skim the first part of this chapter and concentrate on the section that addresses use of the internet for professional purposes.

The need for information literacy

There is now little doubt that all healthcare professionals require computing and information technology (IT) skills. As the use of IT in clinical practice increases, so too does the need for nurses and midwives to possess the skills and knowledge to use and manage digital information effectively. As a student you have a responsibility to incorporate evidence-based information into your study and practice (Aveyard & Sharp 2013). However, simply providing computer literacy in the form of word processing, database or clinical systems skills will not be sufficient in itself to facilitate the development of healthcare professionals working in an information age. It does not necessarily follow that teaching these skills results in sufficient knowledge management skills for healthcare practitioners to critically evaluate and apply this knowledge in clinical practice. Given the imperative for **evidence-based practice** (EBP), it is clear that nurses and midwives working in increasingly complex technical environments require well-honed skills in the formulation of questions, hypothesis testing, data analysis and other appropriate cognitive processing related to problem-solving and decision-making within an information systems framework.

As a student, you need to use the appropriate tools to find information quickly and easily and, having found it, you need to be able to discern the quality of the information retrieved. The emphasis for all health professionals must be on those skills required for the effective use of IT, information management, utilisation and knowledge synthesis. Effective use of such skills results in the ability to reorganise new data, critically analyse the data, synthesise the resulting new knowledge with the existing body of knowledge and, if appropriate, apply it to practice.

What exactly is the internet?

The internet (the net) is, in the broadest sense, a microcosm of our world. It reflects a vast variety of cultural and societal views and allows people across the planet to share ideas on a personal level never before possible. In a more literal sense, the net is a mass of networks that interconnect computers and mobile devices located all over the world. It does not contain information itself but is the vehicle for transporting the information stored in files or documents on other computers. Some of the computers in the network are known as hosts or servers, because they 'serve' information in various ways to computer owners, known as clients or users. The use of the net has expanded rapidly, with the Internet Domain Survey (Internet Systems Consortium 2014) reporting there were 1,010,251,829 host servers on the net in January 2014, an increase of 46,733,231 servers compared with the same time in 2013. A recent survey by Netcraft revealed responses from 958,919,789 unique uniform resource locators (URLs) (Netcraft 2014).

The internet is a mass of networks that interconnect computers and mobile devices located all over the world.

Although the most common net interactions are made by people with a computer, modem and an internet service provider (ISP) account, internet protocol television, mobile devices and smart phones are alternative ways of viewing content on the net. You can also access a vast array of information and resources stored on other people's computers. No one knows how many computers are connected on the net but the server numbers above can give us an idea.

The most common net interactions are made by people with a computer, modem and an ISP account.

The net began as a highly specialised network of computers designed by the US military in the 1960s. The initial aim of this network was to provide connectivity for US military computers in the event of nuclear strike. Academic institutions were granted access to this military network in the late 1960s and by 1974 the term 'internet' was coined – a contraction of international networks. Use of the internet widened to governmental agencies, universities and research institutions in the 1970s and, by the 1980s, libraries and other professional associations began using it to exchange scholarly information. The explosion of personal computers (PCs) and their increasing affordability marked a rapid evolution of the net in the 1990s. The internet now functions as a personal communication exchange, commercial marketplace and an information resource. It has revolutionised communications, created businesses and transformed society.

Given the genesis of the net, it remains relatively lacking in structure and control. There is no single governing body that controls what happens on the internet. For the most part it is self-moderating. One disadvantage is there is no single authoritative internet information source outlining who is connected and what is available. One advantage is that, with a few notable exceptions, no person, group, government or country is able to impose censorship or restrict access to network resources. The internet is not free, even for those with access through a hospital or university; it's just that these institutions do not pass on the cost to the users. Some individuals have described the internet as anarchic, and to some degree this is true.

As a result, there are few rules and the only organising concept that exists is domain naming. Each computer on the internet has an address – an internet protocol or IP address. This is a unique identifying number given to every machine on the internet. It consists of four parts separated by dots, for example, 131.234.245.7. This addressing convention is fine for computers but creates difficulty for humans (it's easier to remember a name than a 10-digit number). The domain-naming system is a method of managing the names of networks and computers on the internet. As with the IP number, the domain name is separated by full stops, for example, www.acu.edu.au. The suffix (extension) after the organisational name, acu (Australian Catholic University), is known as the top-level domain (Table 3.1).

As the internet became more internationalised, a country code top-level domain (ccTLD) was required as an additional identifier and this is used or reserved for a country, a dependent territory or a sovereign state (Table 3.2).

One area of rapid development is the platform on which internet content can be delivered. Smartphones (iPhone, android), touch screen devices such as the Apple iPod Touch and larger-sized tablet computers (Apple iPad, HP Dream Screen, Amazon Kindle), gaming devices (X-Box, Play Station, Nintendo DS, Play Station Portable), global positioning systems and internet protocol television all provide some form of internet connectivity. There are now homes

Table 3.1
Original top-level domains

Suffix	Usage	Example	Name
.com	For commercial organisations	http://www.proquest.com	ProQuest
.edu	Educational organisations	www.acu.edu.au	Australian Catholic University
.gov	Government	www.health.qld.gov.au	Queensland Health
.mil	Military	http://www.navy.mil	US Navy
.org	Non-profit organisation	http://www.redcross.org.au	Australian Red Cross
.net	Network resources	http://www.abc.net.au	Australian Broadcasting Corporation

The Whole Internet User's Guide & Catalog, 2nd Edition. By: Ed Krol. Copyright © 1994 O'Reilly Media, Inc. All Rights Reserved. Used with Permission.

Table 3.2
Country top-level domains

Suffix	Country	Example	Name
.au	Australia	www.sydney.edu.au	The University of Sydney, Australia
.ch	Switzerland	www.icn.ch	ICN Switzerland
.cx	Christmas Island	www.shire.gov.cx	Shire of Christmas Island
.de	Germany	http://www.mercedes-benz.de	Mercedes Benz
.nz	New Zealand	www.immigration.govt.nz	New Zealand Department of Immigration
.uk	United Kingdom (UK)	www.nhs.uk	UK National Health Service

where the domestic appliances, heating, cooling, lighting and security functions can be controlled remotely via the internet.

Although the potential of the net seems limitless, that very potential presents challenges (Box 3.1). The biggest challenge when using the net, particularly for research, is learning to navigate it efficiently and effectively. Although the net can be difficult to navigate and the lack of regulation can be problematic, these are the elements that also make the net a dynamic space and fertile resource for research. Think of searching as an exploration, because the net, while providing you with a powerful tool for research, communication and learning, will also test your ability and resolve.

Most education providers have a code of conduct regarding people's use of their computer networks. This includes rules regarding what can be downloaded and uploaded from sites. Check your organisation's code of conduct before using their network. Moreover, the Australian Health Practitioners Regulation Agency (AHPRA) has recently released a new social media policy that applies to all health practitioners (AHPRA 2014).

What does the internet offer?

The internet represents potentially the most powerful research and educational tool to emerge since the invention of the printing press. The expansion and adoption of the internet and WWW have opened up vast communication, information and educational possibilities for the healthcare sector and for health professionals. Tele-health is just one example of the technological developments made possible by the internet and the WWW. Increasingly, both consumers and health professionals are utilising the internet for health-related information. As we already know, the internet and WWW are growing at a remarkable rate. Not surprisingly, with this volume of information there are serious issues around the quality, reliability, accuracy, authenticity and currency of health-related sites and the information they disseminate. For health professionals, this means the added responsibility of ensuring that the material

Box 3.1
Some issues encountered when using the internet

Confusion and Chaos

The internet operates in a freewheeling culture with few rules, limits or boundaries. No entity exercises control over net offerings and, although some have tried, there is little regulatory control over net transactions.

Needle in a Haystack

The number of internet websites is growing at an incredibly fast pace. No single search device has been devised that allows efficient access to everything on the net. Sometimes you have to wade through a mass of useless and irrelevant pages to find the one you need.

Time Drain

Although touted for its instant access and speed, it is easy to spend hours moving and scrolling through various web pages on the internet, with little to show for the effort.

Questionable Reliability of Information

Anyone is free to post information and this leads to a dilemma about the accuracy and reliability of such information. The exact source and that source's credibility are often hard to determine on the internet.

accessed for use in professional and client information is evidence-based; and also, that you as a health professional are able to help consumers assess material they have accessed themselves. To do this, you will require a good working knowledge of search strategies, search engines, reliable databases and sites, as well as evaluation tools and other quality safeguards, such as gateways.

There are many services on the internet. Each service is essentially a separate protocol of the internet. The WWW (hypertext transfer protocol or HTTP) and electronic mail (email; simple mail transport protocol or SMTP) are probably the best known. Other applications include listservs, **blogs**, **wikis**, **social media** sites, newsgroups, chat rooms, audio and interactive video. Each of these is described in the following sections.

World wide web

The WWW or 'the web' is an information service that supports multimedia content on the internet. It is a rich source of healthcare information for the healthcare consumer and the health professional. This information can be accessed via electronic databases, web directories, search engines, and online publications and journals.

Although the web is a single protocol within the internet (i.e. the web is a subset of the internet), in reality, it consists of two separate webs. The first, the surface web, is a visible web that can be accessed by regular search engines. The second, the deep web, remains mainly hidden because of the inability of many normal engines to access the type of material held there. The deep web was first described in 2001 (Bergman 2001) and is the most rapidly growing portion of the internet.

The surface web is a huge, loosely organised collection of documents on thousands of topics, written in hypertext mark-up language (html). The deep web contains a sizeable proportion of government resources, databases and similarly structured materials that are not written in html. It is estimated the deep web is 500 times larger than the surface web; it is highly specialised, 95% cost-free and is the largest growth category on the web (Conrick 2002). The collections from the two webs are located on various websites, each containing numerous web pages of material. These web pages use a variety of multimedia resources with a mixture of text, colour, sound, graphics and video. However, the more elaborate a site is, the more time it can take for the web page to load.

The surface web is the most commonly used by search engines to trawl for information. The remaining four-fifths or 80% of the web is referred to as the deep web, the hidden web or the invisible web. The web is therefore analogous to an iceberg; the bulk of which lies below the surface. It is made up of information locked away in password-protected databases, white papers and grey literature. The term 'grey literature' refers to material that is either unpublished or has been published in non-commercial form. Examples of grey literature include government reports, issues papers, market reports, conference proceedings and research theses. Grey literature tends to be of a high quality, although much of this literature has generally not passed through a peer review process. The importance of this information lies in the fact that much of it represents the most up-to-date research in any given area of interest.

Web pages on the surface web are linked by hypertext, which allows you to move from one page to another or from one website to another by clicking on a highlighted word.

Honing your internet skills

Using your education provider's computers is a good way to hone your skills in navigating the net to gain knowledge. Most campuses provide hands-on tutorial sessions or provide downloadable guides to using their computers and the net.

To use the internet from your home, you need a computer, smart phone or tablet, an internet connection and an ISP. Some universities provide ISP services, so you may not need to sign up with a commercial firm.

An ISP is a company that provides internet access, usually for a charge. Charges vary and can be based on downloads/uploads, volume or time. Most connections require a modem or Network Termination Device (NBNCo 2014) and can be made through satellite dishes, cable television and digital subscriber lines, which include the very popular asymmetric digital subscriber line (ADSL) or via the National Broadband Network. A modem is used to connect to your ISP. Some ISPs provide free connections but these often contain advertisements, which you will regularly receive. The resource kit at the end of the chapter lists several online services and ISPs but before committing you should read more about ISPs. The Australian Competition and Consumer Commission website (http://www.accc.gov.au/consumers/internet-phone/internet-phone-services) provides good guidelines to help with this.

Once you have a connection, you are ready to log on to the net. The easiest way to do this is with a web **browser**. Mozilla Firefox and Internet Explorer (Microsoft) are popular browsers and both will run on Windows or Macintosh systems. Opera is a standards-compliant web browser. Opera is the preferred browser for a number of small devices like mobile phones and hand-held computers. The search engine company Google has developed Google Chrome, a free, open-source web browser while Safari is the default browser for Mac systems.

These browsers can send and receive email, access blogs and newsgroups, edit web pages and facilitate the use of internet telephones. A browser is usually bundled with your computer or provided by your ISP but can also be downloaded for free from the web. Browsers often have a similar look and feel but Mozilla Firefox, because it is open-source, is not subjected to as many viruses.

Navigating the web

The browser serves as your guide to the WWW. It allows you to track the websites you visit, to revisit previous sites and to save your favourite sites so you can find and visit them easily.

When you first connect to the internet, you will automatically connect to the front page of your provider's homepage via your web browser program.

Uniform resource locator

There are three major ways to move around the web from your initial page. Because each page on the internet has an address or a URL, direct access to that page can be gained by entering its address into the location bar and pressing go. For example, http://www.cochrane.org/reviews is the URL for the Cochrane Collaboration review page.

You must enter the address exactly as it appears. If you add a space, omit a dot or misspell a word, the site cannot be located. However, you can skip the 'http://www.' because the web browser will insert it for you. The White Pages

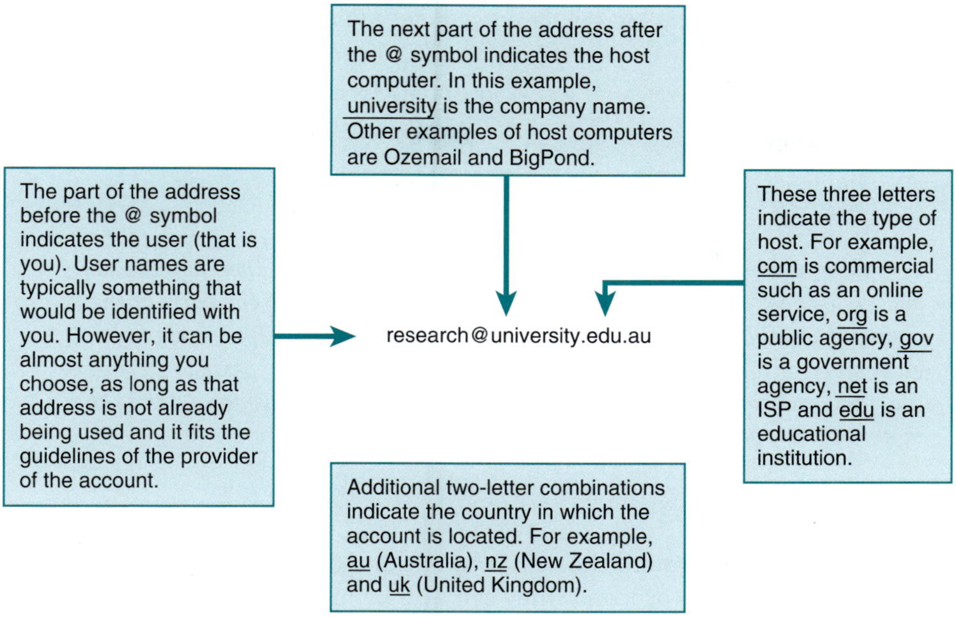

FIGURE 3.1
Elements of a uniform resource locator (URL)

list web addresses and there are also website Yellow Pages. Most businesses and organisations routinely post their URLs. Examining a URL can tell you something about the site. Figure 3.1 presents the elements of a URL.

1. *If you want to find an organisation and do not have a URL, type the name of the organisation into the location bar and you will be directed to its home page (try ACN).*
2. *If you type a question into the location bar and press the go button your browser will take you to the site that can answer your question. Begin your query with 'What is ...'*

To see how URLs work, try the following student challenge.

STUDENT CHALLENGE

Using URLs

On your PC, tablet or smart phone try the following:

1. Collect three or four URLs you have seen mentioned here or from another source.
2. Enter one of the URLs in the address or location text box on the browser (long, rectangular white area). You may have to highlight and type over or erase an existing URL before entering the new URL.

3. Click the 'Go' button to the right of the text box, or press 'Enter' ('Return' on a Macintosh) on your keyboard.
4. You should now be at the page of the site for which you entered the address.
5. Try entering an organisation's name and see if you can find its homepage.

Computer addresses do not change very often but pages can. Therefore the site address is most reliable. If a page does not open try removing the parts of the address from the end. For example, if http://www.ahrq.gov/clinic/epcix.htm gives an error message, then remove: /epicix.htm. If the error persists go back to the next / and so forth until the page opens. Look on that page for a link to the material you want.

Hypertext links

Another way to move around the web is by clicking on the web page's hypertext links. These may be text or icons. They can also be highlighted, underlined or may only display as an active link when you take your mouse pointer over the top of them (roll over).

Lost? Luckily your browser keeps a record of where you have been. This trail is available in the History button in Mozilla, the Favourites, Feeds and History icon in IE, the Customise and Control icon in Google Chrome or by using the 'Back' button. Try the following student challenge.

STUDENT CHALLENGE

Leafing Through Links

Using one of the sites you found by entering a URL, try the following:

1. Look at the web page. Note the hypertext links (when the pointer changes to a hand). Clicking or tapping on one of these links will take you to a different location.
2. Check the address window on your web browser. Note how the URL has changed. If the address has been added to, you have moved to another page or place on the page. If the information right after 'www' has changed, you have accessed a new site.
3. Explore the pages for this website by clicking or tapping on various links and viewing several web pages.
4. If you are using a mouse, try 'rolling over', hovering the mouse pointer over the text, icons and boxed text to see if the pointer changes to a hand shape. If it does, click on these, as they are links.
5. Play around; enjoy being on the move from link to link and page to page.

Search engines

A third way to navigate the web is by using a search engine. Search engines are tools that allow you to search the web for information by using keywords. You will find they resemble the search tools you used in Chapter 2 when doing index searches. Various search engines are available and some of the most used engines are described in Box 3.2.

There are hundreds of other search engines. Some of these search only certain segments of the web, which is helpful for narrowing a technical or specialised search. For example, some search engines search only health sources or reference resources. There are a few sites such as Beaucoup that list thousands of specialist search engines. There are engines that allow you to use a number of different search engines at once for a more global search. These are the 'metasearch' tools. Box 3.3 presents examples of specialty and metasearch engines.

You have access to all these engines through your ISP or by using their URL addresses. Each search engine uses slightly different search methods and indexing systems and some will list the pages retrieved based on payment for prominence.

Box 3.2
Sample search engines

The website for each of the following search engines is accessible through this book's Evolve website.

General search

- Google is the most popular search engine. It provides comprehensive coverage of the web. It also offers advanced searching and a specific academic search engine (Google Scholar).
- ASK was one of the first natural language search engines.
- ANZWERS and Web Wombat are Australian cluster search engines. These are great if you are looking for specific Australian content.
- Bing is Microsoft's replacement for its old MSN Search.
- IXQuick does not record your IP address or your search strings. It claims to be the world's most private search engine.
- Hotbot provides easy access to the web's three major crawler-based search engines, Yahoo!, LyGO and MSN. Very user-friendly and guides you through the process. Yahoo! allows you to use a subject index or keyword search approach. You can conduct a keyword search within a selected index category. Yahoo! has hypertext links to other engines and rates as the second most used search engine.

Box 3.3
Specialised search engines

The website for each of these search engines is accessible through the Evolve website.

Metasearch: search using multiple engines

- Dogpile sends a search to a list of search engines, directories and specialty search sites that you can customise and then displays results from each search engine individually.
- Vivisimo searches the major search engines and also automatically organises the pages into categories. Slick and easy to use.

Deep web

- Complete Planet, Infomine and Deeperweb are tools designed specifically for searching the deep web.

Specific

- bmjupdates provides access to current best evidence from research for medicine, nursing and midwifery. You can tailor the search to your own healthcare interests, to support making evidence-based clinical decisions.
- Google Scholar broadly searches for scholarly literature across many disciplines and sources: peer-reviewed papers, theses, books, abstracts and articles, from academic publishers, professional societies, preprint repositories, universities and other scholarly organisations.
- @nursing is a search engine for internet and MEDLINE for Nursing resources.
- TRIP Database – Clinical Search Engine is a search engine specifically designed for health professionals wishing to access high-quality EBP publications.
- Healthline is a consumer-oriented engine that searches the top health sites.

A perfect search system would find all the relevant information available in one sweep but, regrettably, such an engine does not exist. If you use different search engines, you will get differing results and sometimes different presentations of the search. Some use Boolean search logic and others use probabilistic methods. Some allow you to search only by keywords; others index the first 250 words. The presentation of results also varies between those using flat lists of sites and those that cluster the information. However, your results are very closely tied to the search algorithm and keywords you use. (You might like to refresh your memory on using Boolean searches by referring back to

Chapter 2.) If you wish to locate grey literature, it is interesting to note that much of this information is stored on the web in Adobe Acrobat (PDF). This means it is relatively easy to find recent examples of grey literature using the Google Advanced search (www.google.com.au/advanced_search). Once at Google Advanced, scroll down and click on File type and select Adobe Acrobat (PDF) from the dropdown list. This restricts your results to Adobe Acrobat (PDF) documents and consequently will increase the number of grey literature items that appear in your search results.

If you want further information on search engines and how they work, log on to this book's Evolve website at http://evolve.elsevier.com/AU/Borbasi/maze and then link to the Spider's Apprentice website. This site explains how search engines work, gives you tips on conducting and refining a search, provides ratings for several popular search engines and even lets you try out several search engines.

Ultimately, the best way to view how search engines work and to see the difference in results is to use and explore a few of them. Try the following student challenges.

STUDENT CHALLENGE

Sampling Search Engines

Decide on the specific subject area on which you would like information. Then, log on to your ISP and web browser. Then do the same search using at least one search engine from each group.

1. Note the rules for searching for each search engine you try.
2. Try a specialty health topic and use a general search engine (note the number of sites returned).
3. Try the same again but use a specialty health search engine.
4. Do the same with a metasearch engine.
5. Note the different special features available.
6. Compare the results from the various searches.
7. Which search engine was the easiest to use? Which gave you the best results?

Communicating on the net

There are a number of ways to communicate with others over the internet.

Email

All email programs have common features. They allow you to compose and send messages to anyone with an email account (provided you know the email

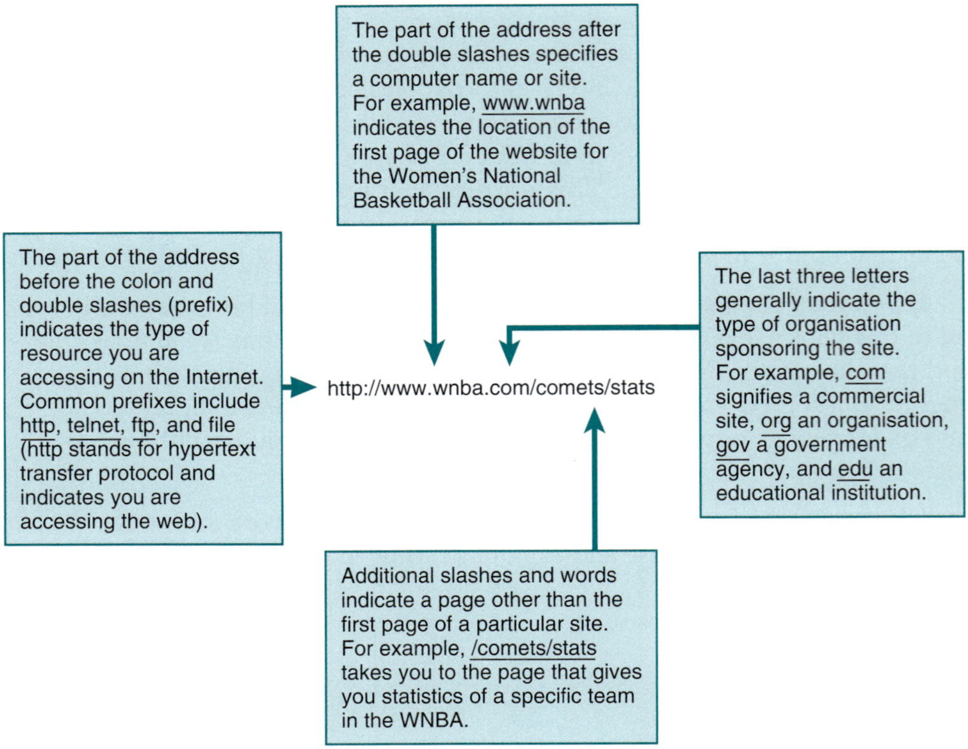

FIGURE 3.2
Elements of a sample email address

address), to read and save or print messages sent to you by others. They also let you keep an electronic address book. All these features are easily accessible through various menu options or toolbar buttons. An email address consists of two basic parts: the user name and the host name. These two parts are connected by an '@' symbol. You determine the first part of the address. The second part of the address is dictated by the service that supplies your internet account. Examining an email address reveals information about the location of the account (Fig 3.2).

Newsgroups and chat rooms

Newsgroups and chat rooms also allow you to communicate over the net. Newsgroups allow you to post and receive messages from participants in that group. Messages and replies are clustered together to establish a conversational flow. Newsgroups revolve around particular interest areas. Chat rooms are similar to newsgroups, except that you can carry on typed conversations with people who are logged on to their computers at the same time as you. Feedback in a chat room is immediate (synchronous) whereas feedback in newsgroups, wikis and blogs is delayed (asynchronous). Yahoo! offers a number of chat rooms and allows you to search for others. You might want to explore these further but remain vigilant and cautious. If you do not know the other person, think before you release any personal information.

Blogs and wikis

The internet also opens up the world of blogs and wikis. A blog, short for weblog, is like an electronic diary. Blogs take up space in the blogosphere (collective term encompassing all weblogs). If you have a blog, you can write, reflect, publish your thoughts and understandings, then receive comments and feedback from others. This can provide information for you to construct further knowledge (Conrick & Foster 2006).

You can either begin your own blog or interact with someone else's. You can find blogs through a search engine such as blogsearch.google.com and leave your comment on a blog by simply clicking on the comment area at the end of a posting and following the prompts. Begin your own blog at Blogger, or start a nursing or midwifery-specific blog at Mediblogopathy. These sites are easy to use and guide you through the steps.

A wiki is a website that allows users to create and edit any number of hyperlinked web pages via a web browser using a simplified text editor without having to use a programming language. Wiki comes from a Hawaiian word meaning 'quick'. Anyone can revise wiki pages and, because of this, wikis are becoming known as the tool of choice for large, multiple-participant projects and research.

Wikis are typically powered by wiki software that facilitates the development of collaborative wiki websites used in corporate intranets, education and to drive knowledge management systems. The concept is based on a technology that provides a quick and easy method of information capture, editing and dissemination. Perhaps the best known wiki is Wikipedia. Since its creation in 2001, Wikipedia has grown rapidly into one of the largest reference websites, currently boasting in excess of 4,562,196 articles with over 21,835,582 registered users (Wikipedia: Statistics 2014).

Google Blog search and Feedster are effective blog and wiki search engines.

Social media

The past few years have seen the explosive growth of social network services on the web. Social media outlets, platforms and applications, including blogs, social networking sites, video and photo sharing sites, and online chat rooms and forums are now very much a part of social interaction. Services such as Facebook, Twitter, LinkedIn, Tumblr, Bebo, MySpace and Google + have changed the way people interact online forever. Most social network services are accessed using a web interface or via a Short Message Service (SMS) or mobile device application (app). Social network services allow individuals to create a representation of themselves on the web, usually in the form of a profile. Social media sites allow users to share ideas, activities, events and interests within their individual networks. Technologies such as Twitter have even been adopted by political parties as a way of connecting with their constituents.

The judicious use of social media can be of benefit in health care in a variety of ways. A number of authors have indicated social media is increasingly used to encourage professional connections and promote time effective communication with patients/clients and family members (Farrelly 2014; Costello 2014). These networks may also be effective in educating and informing consumers and healthcare professionals (West & Verran, 2013).

Nurses and Midwives are increasingly using blogs, forums and social media sites to share workplace experiences, particularly events that have been challenging or emotionally charged. As students many of you would be familiar with journaling and reflective practice as critical to the development of professional practice. Sites such as Mahara provide a journaling and portfolio service that is transportable, much like LinkedIn. While the concept of netiquette is not new there are a number of other traps as an internet user you should be aware of. In the author's experience several students have breached standard practice by posting unprofessional material and comments on to social networking sites (such as Facebook and Snapchat). Comments denigrating teaching and clinical staff or fellow students have been placed in the public domain. Once material has been posted on to such sites, it tends to remain there in some form, even if the original posting is deleted.

The same applies to internet or cyber bullying. Cyber bullying is not just confined to high-school children as it also affects many adolescents and teens on a daily basis. Cyber bullying involves the use of some form of technology such as mobile phone SMS, as well as the internet through sites such as Facebook, Twitter, mySpace and blogs, to bully or harass another person. Internet users need to be aware that anonymity is often not the case when such material is posted. There will always be an audit trail back to the original posting. Students really need to think about what they intend to post to social networking sites and be sensitive to the effect this may have on others. They also need to be aware that anything posted into the public domain may return to haunt them one day! Under no circumstances should patient or client cases be discussed on any internet site as this is clearly a breach of patient/client confidentiality.

The ease with which data, images, videos and grey literature can be found and copied is also a trap, particularly for student researchers. It is becoming increasingly easy to plagiarise material unwittingly from the net. At the same time, with the advent of plagiarism detectors such as Turnitin, academic staff are in an even better position to detect plagiarism. More about plagiarism later.

Fraud or theft committed using online technology is yet another threat that students need to bear in mind. Internet banking fraud is one example and represents a form of identity theft. The theft of such data is made possible through a number of relatively well-known techniques, including:

- phishing – emails claiming to be from banks
- Trojans – usually downloaded as 'shareware', purporting to be a useful application
- key logging programs (worms)
- man in the middle attacks (when the connection between a client and a host/server is compromised).

Internet users need to remain vigilant to subtle, or not so subtle, changes in the way their computer is operating. If the computer is freezing consistently, or files and folders seem to disappear or will not open, or shows other signs of malfunctioning, the user should suspect some form of viral infection. The most effective way of dealing with these threats is to limit the amount of personal data disclosed over the internet and to install and keep updated antiviral software.

How do you use the net for professional purposes?

The greatest challenge with accessing professional information on the net is deciding its validity and filtering out the rubbish. Because you now have access to such a huge variety of databases and other resources, being able to search for information effectively from either your library or the web is essential. Universities have facilities for online off-campus searches or remote access to their databases via student portals.

If you do not have remote capabilities through your local academic or health sciences library, do not give up just yet. You can conduct comprehensive searches on the net. Over the last few years many evidence-based electronic journals and websites have become available.

To access these sites just type the name into your search engine and hit the go button. Or take the easy way – explore the Evolve site.

Evolve will link you to a special website set up just for this learning package. It contains hypertext links to the resources mentioned below as well as other sites that will help with your research.

Journal indexes give you a listing of journals and journal articles; because most have specific focuses you will not find all journals in the one index. You are able to access MEDLINE and PubMed at no cost through the National Library of Medicine Gateway. PubMed includes over 16 million citations from MEDLINE and other life science journals for biomedical articles back to the 1950s and has recently released apps for iPhone and Androids. It also includes links to full text articles and other related resources, including from the PreMEDLINE database. PreMEDLINE allows you to search basic citation information and abstracts before the full citation record is generated and added to MEDLINE. This means you can find the most current material available because new records are added to PreMEDLINE daily.

CINAHL is also accessible from a website but, because it is a commercially maintained index, an access fee is charged, although student discounts are available (CINAHL Information Systems 2006). Medbioworld is a site to explore for research articles and many on this site are free.

Evidence-based practice

There are a number of online evidence-based journals. Some are free and others not. You may like to explore some of these. There are so many journals on the web, both free and commercial, that it is difficult to sift through them. However, Google Scholar can really help with this. It provides a simple way to search for scholarly literature. You can search across disciplines and sources for peer-reviewed papers, theses, books, abstracts and articles, from academic publishers, professional societies, preprint repositories, universities and other scholarly organisations. You can also download citations to your bibliography software, like EndNote. Many universities now offer free access to bibliography software.

Evidence-based sites abound on the internet. The most used for research are the Cochrane Collaboration and the Joanna Briggs Institute (JBI). The Cochrane Collaboration and library are available for free, courtesy of the Australian government. This is one of the leading evidence-based sites for quantitative, mostly randomised control trials, while the JBI engages in a collaborative approach to the evaluation of mostly qualitative evidence. The JBI has access restricted to subscribers, although there are some free resources available.

In addition to these well-known EBP sites, students who have access to CINAHL via the EBSCOhost research database system will also have access to the CINAHL information system's evidence-based care sheets. There are more than 150 evidence-based care sheets on this site for students to access.

The web also hosts other free resource sites and organisations such as the Australian Institute of Health and Welfare, the Australian Bureau of Statistics and the Centers for Disease Control in the USA. These are all very rich sources of information and statistics. The Australian Digital Thesis Project provides access to hundreds of Australian postgraduate theses, while some online bookstores enable you to read books online or download them for later use. Evolve has links to some of these areas.

The National Institute of Clinical Studies (NICS) produces evidence-based resources for nurses, midwives and other health professionals, as does the Western Australian Centre for Evidence Based Nursing and Midwifery.

HealthInsite (an Australian government site) provides access to quality information about human health for both consumers and professionals. Universities are beginning to upload staff papers to the net; for example, the Queensland University of Technology has a site called QUT ePrints and this page has links to others you might like to explore.

Finding peer-reviewed journals in library databases is easier than locating them on the web. For example, ProQuest has a box you can tick to search just for peer-reviewed articles. On the internet, most journals will tell you whether or not they are peer-reviewed. Look for text saying 'peer review' or 'double-blind peer review'. If it's not obvious on the page, all browsers have a 'search in page' (or similar term), which may help. Failing this, such information may be located in a section of the journal called 'about this journal' or 'information for contributors'.

It is just as important to test the validity and reliability of electronic journals and web resources as it is for paper resources because one cannot assume that something is either valid or reliable because it is in print or on a website. This is particularly so of sites that use testimonials, which may not be valid or reliable.

When trying to determine the validity of information on the WWW it is critical first to test the source of the information. If you are accessing information from textbooks or peer-reviewed journals you should be able to be confident that the information obtained from such sources will fulfil the criteria for validity. More often than not this information has been published by reputable authors, often leaders in their chosen discipline. Reference texts and reviewed journal articles have better credibility as their content has gone through a vetting process in which other experts on the topic critically review the material before it is published.

On the other hand much of the material on the WWW has not been through this process. In fact, the bulk of material on the WWW has been placed there often by well-meaning, but far from expert, individuals. The amazing thing about the WWW is that it essentially allows anyone with an internet connection to publish on the web. Clearly no review process is ever undertaken with this material. Content of blogs, chat rooms, listserves, wikis and the like should be used with the utmost caution in academic writing given the lack of critical analysis evident in much of this type of content. Even seemingly reputable websites can often be the work of one or two individuals with some sort of agenda to propagate.

With an increasing number of individuals sourcing their health information from the web, it is more important than ever that health professionals have the skills to perform some level of critique on the material our clients often obtain. General practitioners are now routinely presented with reams of paper containing 'health information' their patients have downloaded from the WWW. We need to ensure this information is evidence-based, and also, that as a health professional, you are able to help health consumers access material from reputable sources. You will require a good working knowledge of search strategies, search engines, reliable databases and sites, as well as appropriate evaluation tools. As a student you are probably accessing numerous journal articles from the internet; these too need to be evaluated and critiqued. This chapter has addressed the issue of finding information on the net. Now we are going to discuss how to decide whether the information we locate is adequate and how we can begin to evaluate it for quality and read with a critical eye.

Factors affecting information quality

The nature of the internet and the ease with which material can be created means it has become increasingly difficult to judge its quality. One of the critical issues facing us is how to assess the quality of the information to which we are exposed.

Several factors – accuracy, adequacy, balance, currency, presentation and reliability – affect the quality of information. Accuracy is associated with the content of the material. Accurate information is the result of an active effort to confirm or verify and shows conformity to existing facts (which can be verified through other sources).

Adequacy refers to the scope and depth of information presented. Adequate information provides the reader with materials that are sufficient in scope and depth for the specific purposes of that reader.

Balance deals with acknowledgement and presentation of competing points of view. Lack of balance leads to bias.

Currency addresses the immediacy of the material and whether it accurately reflects ongoing changes in a particular field of study.

Presentation has to do with whether the content is presented in a well-organised manner. Reliability is often connected with the source of the material.

Reliable information is consistently dependable and comes from a generally proven and trustworthy source.

Several considerations can help you make judgments about the quality of the information you have accessed. The first consideration is the source of the material. If you have tapped into e-materials from published textbooks, reference books or recognised journals, there is a reasonable expectation the material has been reviewed and edited by authorities in the area. You may wish to check this out. Many text and reference books list contributing authors or reviewers and their credentials in the front of the book. Journals may be refereed or peer-reviewed (meaning that the article is sent for critique by one or more experts in the field before being accepted for publication). This is an additional sign of quality. This means that most traditional sources (textbooks and journals) have been adequately reviewed and evaluated by a reputable publisher and are more trustworthy. There is more on this in Chapter 9.

However, if you have pulled the information from a general site on the internet, evaluating the source requires more effort. Look first at the three letters in the URL, which tell you what type of organisation is sponsoring the site. (Note: some sites don't use this identifier.) If it is a commercial organisation (.com), ask yourself what it is selling and whether this might bias the presentation of data. In other words, treat the information like you treat advertisements. If the address is for an organisation (.org), ask yourself what its purpose and agenda are and what audience the materials are geared towards. Government (.gov) and educational (.edu) sites are generally good sources of reliable information.

Whenever possible, check the author's credentials and affiliations. Although this is often difficult on the internet, the more reliable sources usually provide this information on the site. Because there are no editors or quality checkpoints for much of the material on the internet, you need to exercise greater caution and scepticism about the information you find. The second thing you can do is evaluate the types of materials you are using. Is the information from a primary or a secondary source? A primary source is the original source of the data. A secondary source secures the data from the primary source. The secondary source should cite the primary source when securing such data. This allows you, the reader, to access the primary source, if you wish, for more information about a specific point. (Note: footnotes or cited references tell us when data are from another source.) Is the material intended for a professional or lay audience, or the general public? This often changes the presentation manner, breadth and depth of coverage. You need to decide whether the material contains enough information for your purposes.

Third, evaluate the timely nature of the information. Check the publication date and see how current the information is. If you are seeking information in a rapidly changing field or subject, this step is crucial. Remember that information in a book may already be 3–5 years old when it is first published, so sometimes data in textbooks are dated. It can be a worthwhile exercise to check the reference list of e-books to see just how current the information is that the authors drew on when the book was put online. On the other hand, information in journals tends to be from 6 months to 2 years old when published. However, this is not always the case. Close reading of research papers can sometimes reveal a long lapse in time between collection of data and publication. The internet, with posted conference proceedings and electronic journals, has the potential to provide the most current resources available. Of course, again, this is not always the case, as some web pages are not updated regularly. When you are looking at internet sites, check to see when the information was last updated. This is usually posted on the site's homepage.

Try the following student challenge and see what you discover.

STUDENT CHALLENGE

Checking Sources

1. Look at two or three nursing or midwifery journals and locate their policies for manuscript acceptance. Did you find any that were peer-reviewed? If not, check the *Maternal and Child Health Journal* or *Journal of Advanced Nursing*. How could you tell they are peer-reviewed? How do peer-reviewed journals look compared to a journal like the *Australian Nursing Journal* or *Midwifery News*? What are the most noticeable differences between them?
2. Check out some of the health-related websites on the internet. What information is available about the source of the information? Could you distinguish professional and academic sites from general sites? Could you tell how current the data were?
3. Check out one of the internet sites that post professional conference proceedings. Find a newsgroup or other forum on the web that is for healthcare or midwifery professionals. Explore it and see what it has to offer. Did you find any ground-breaking information?

The final step in assessing the quality of the material you find lies in looking at the content of the material itself. Is it presented in a well-organised and straightforward manner? Are major points adequately illustrated and explained? Are arguments backed up with supporting material such as referenced citations? Is the presentation balanced and does it include alternative points of view? Does the material make sense? Is the material logical? Is the material adequate, or does it leave the reader with partially answered or unanswered questions? Compare the content with other sources. Look for similarities and differences. How do various sources agree or disagree? What common ground can you find?

Conrick (2002) provides a useful framework for testing the validity of electronic resources (Table 3.3).

Becoming a critical reader of net material

Determining the quality of a piece of writing you find on the net ought to go hand in hand with reading the material critically. This is especially important if you are to avoid the trap of non-critical readers who think that material/texts simply provide facts. These types of reader tend to focus on memorising and repeating the statements they have read. Since you are embarking on the journey of becoming a researcher or user of research yourself, your challenge is not simply to accept the beliefs and texts of the material you source, but also to find the weaknesses in the arguments therein and to find your own position on an issue.

Table 3.3
Framework for testing validity and reliability of resources

Challenge the source	Who says so? Why do they say so? Why should I believe it? Why should I trust this research or source? How do I know that it is authentic and accurate? Does it give the whole picture? Is the argument reasonable? Who supports this research?
Criteria for evidence-based resources online	Describe explicit criteria for how the evidence is retrieved and appraised for the resource and adheres to these criteria. List the authors/developers of the resource. Provide a date for the most recent update of the site.
Credible resources	Includes the source, currency, relevance/utility and editorial review process for the information.
Author's credentials	Should show evidence of being knowledgeable, reliable and truthful.
Disclosure	Includes informing the user of the purpose of the site, as well as any profiling or collection of information associated with using the site. Lists any conflict of interest.
Caveats	Clarification of whether the site's function is to market products and services or is a primary information content provider.

From Conrick, M Looking for a needle in a haystack: Searching the internet for quality resources, 2002. Reprinted with permission from *Contemporary Nurse*, http://www.contemporarynurse.com/archives/vol/12/issue/1/article/1806/looking-for-a-needle-in-a-haystack

Non-critical readers might think they have nothing to say on a topic because other writers have already said it all, whereas critical readers understand that readers are quite capable of making their own interpretation of the texts they read. Different people will interpret what they read in different ways and put 'their own spin' on it. Your 'spin' may be just as valid as theirs – it is OK to challenge different 'takes' on a subject. Furthermore, there's always something more that can be said about something. That's why conversations and debates are so interesting!

A **critical reader** is someone who thinks that a text might have something to say, but who also believes that texts vary in their believability and in their relevance. A critical reader might be aware that texts are constructed by a writer and that texts can sometimes say more about the writer of the text than they do about the facts. Texts may be shaped by a particular bias or world view and the writer may have a subliminal intention in the message.

For example, a non-critical reader might read a book on Aboriginal history to learn the facts pertaining to populations, languages, customs and the effects of white settlement to discover an accepted interpretation of those events. A critical reader might read the same work to appreciate how a particular perspective (e.g. a white European view) on the events and a particular selection of facts (such as considering Aboriginal history only after white settlement) can lead to particular and incomplete understandings (Chapter 8 explores this subject more fully).

In order to move on to becoming a critical reader, ask yourself questions like: 'What is the author trying to prove?' and 'What is the author assuming I will agree with?'

Then consider your responses:

- Do you agree with the author?
- Does the author adequately defend the argument?
- What kind of proof was used?
- What kind of language is used?
- Is there something the author has left out that you would put in? Would including this invalidate the writer's argument?

As you get used to reading critically, you will start to see the sometimes hidden agendas of other writers and you can use this skill to improve your own ability to argue.

For example, imagine an author categorically states:

It is a well-known fact that private hospitals provide better care than public hospitals.

A critique of this statement would include the following:

- Where is this well-known? In Australia? In New Zealand? In the UK?
- By whom is it well-known? Who is the person making this statement? Is the author, for example, the chief executive officer of a private hospital?
- Why should private hospitals offer better care than public hospitals?
- What evidence/proof does this writer offer to back up such a statement?

Once you know the limits, weaknesses, omissions or particular frame of reference influencing the author's arguments, you will have produced precision and clarity, two useful skills to use in your own writing.

So, a good argument:

- is a claim backed up by evidence
- is not just a collection of facts or details
- may include other authors' arguments and research findings

- is inclusive of evidence valued in your field
- is inclusive of stories, anecdotes and verbal quotes from your experience.

In becoming a critical reader, the skill rests in recognising the author's purpose, the elements of persuasion that have been used and any bias. So next time you read a text, try to be a critical reader and attend to these three tasks:

1. What the text says: restatement. Restatement may be in the form of a summary or paraphrase. See http://www.criticalreading.com/restatement.htm.
2. What the text does: description.
3. What the text means: interpretation.

Being a non-critical reader and simply repeating phrases from a text contributes to the perpetuation of untruths and misinformation. Repeating ideas and presenting them as one's own is an even more serious problem, called plagiarism. As previously stated, the advent of abundant sources of information on the internet that can easily be 'cut and pasted' has made plagiarism a particular problem and one that you will need to avoid. Table 3.4 explains plagiarism.

Useful professional websites and databases

A wide range of other healthcare-related databases and professional sites are available to you via your computer and internet account. A brief sample of some of these is provided in Box 3.4.

If you have not already done so, take a minute to use Evolve and log on to explore the website. Then try the following student challenge.

STUDENT CHALLENGE

Advance with Evolve

1. Log on to the Evolve website at http://evolve.elsevier.com/AU/Borbasi/maze.
2. Add the website to your Favourites or Bookmarks list.
3. Explore the site and see what is offered.
4. Find out a little about us (your textbook authors).
5. Read up on some frequently asked questions.
6. Check out available links and activities.

STUDENT CHALLENGE

Communication Contingencies

1. Explore professional listservs and blogs on the net.
2. See what discussion groups your education provider has on the web.

Table 3.4
Identifying and avoiding plagiarism

A definition of plagiarism	Using other people's work without due acknowledgment or permission.
An example of plagiarism	Jane cuts and pastes a paragraph from a website into her own essay and tries to pass it off as her own work.
Another example	Con borrows his friend's essay and realises he couldn't have said it better himself. So he copies it into his own work and changes one or two of the words.
Another example	Maya researched in books, journals and the internet to provide a lot of backup to her argument. But she forgot to keep a record of who said what and when. So she inserts the phrase 'research has found …'. She believes that at least she isn't attempting to pass off others' work as her own. But she didn't include the research references.
Another example	There have been many lawsuits for copyright infringement in the music industry.
Avoiding plagiarism	Authors don't mind students quoting their work. It shows they have influence. But be sure to acknowledge them in the reference list and in the text you are writing. Whenever you use words straight from a text, put quotation marks around them and give a reference to show where the text came from. Even if you summarise or paraphrase someone else's ideas, acknowledge them through an in-text citation. Remember that words found anywhere that are not your own need to be referenced. That includes: websites, journal papers, newspapers, videos, textbooks, magazine articles and even personal communications. Always keep a record of the author, title, publication, location and date details. As much as possible, reference the original author of the idea, or the primary source. That way you can be sure that the author's words haven't been misquoted by someone else. It is now very easy for instructors to detect plagiarism. The most widely used software to detect plagiarism is Turnitin. This cloud-based application is now used not just to detect plagiarism but can also be used to manage all aspects of students' assignments. Google also has excellent tools. So if you use words that are obviously not your own, or that look similar to those the instructor has already seen, it is likely it will be discovered.

Box 3.4
Selected professional websites and databases

The website for each of these is accessible through this book's Evolve website.

- Australian Nursing Federation (ANF): Australia's nursing union. The ANF website provides access to policies and reports and tables of content and information about the *Australian Nursing Journal* (ANJ) and the *Australian Journal of Advanced Nursing* (AJAN).
- Look at the Australian Health Practitioners Regulation Agency (AHPRA) website with links to the Australian Nursing and Midwifery Board of Australia.
- The Nursing Council of New Zealand and the Midwifery Council of New Zealand sites.
- Australian Institute of Health and Welfare provides access to a wealth of health- and welfare-related statistics.
- HealthInsite: wide range of up-to-date and quality-assessed information on important health topics such as diabetes, cancer, mental health and asthma.
- Australian College of Nursing (ACN): Australia's professional organisation. This website offers conference information, online forums, educational opportunities, a substantial resource list of publication information and information about scholarships.
- The Australian College of Midwives similarly has professional news and updates.

International

- Hardin Meta Directory of Internet Health Sources: a meta listing with links to indexes that index healthcare sites. A huge listing of nursing indexes is found here.
- Nursing Society: the website for Sigma Theta Tau. It contains information about the Society, grants and research activities, online publications and eligibility requirements, among other topics.
- Nursing Net: one of the indexes from the Hardin site. This provides an electronic guide to nursing journals and other publications and references, including journals, continuing education sites and employment postings. It also links to an online discount bookstore.
- Nursing World: the website for the American Nurses Association (ANA). You can link to state nursing association sites, check nursing and healthcare policy, read up on credentialling issues and do much more.

Continued

Box 3.4
Selected professional websites and databases—cont'd

- The International Alliance of Midwives provides a forum for midwives to share what they have learned in their practice, bringing together knowledge and techniques from around the world.
- StudentMidwife.net provides support and access to educational information and facilitates participation in discussion and debate.
- US Library of Congress: an online government catalogue with links to other library catalogues, search mechanisms and resources.
- US National Institutes of Health: the home of the National Institute of Nursing Research (NINR) and the National Library of Medicine (NLM).

Conclusion

The information explosion that has occurred in recent years with the advent of the internet, with universal access to education and rising literacy levels, has made greater amounts of information far more accessible and allowed us to become much more connected to it. In summarising this chapter, there are a few key ideas. Can you figure out what they might be?

The internet is here to stay – the limits of technology appear boundless. The information and knowledge it enables you to access will continue to grow exponentially. The key is to be constantly on top of the databases and to continue to upskill yourself on how to access the best sites – prepare yourself for a life of learning! (See more in Chapter 10.)

Be discerning. Just because information is published or appears on the internet in electronic form does not necessarily mean it is correct or current. So use the tips and strategies discussed in this and other chapters to help you gauge the merit of the texts you are reading. Ask questions, crosscheck resources against one another and bring a healthy degree of scepticism to your reading. Ultimately you must make a judgment about whether a particular resource can be trusted to provide the quality information you need.

Be critical. Find out the limits of the author's ideas and try to suggest ways the conversation could move on.

RESOURCES KIT

Finding internet service providers

If you have a computer with Microsoft Windows, you can find out about major ISPs by using the Internet Connection Wizard located in your Internet Explorer program (look under Tools, Internet options). The wizard will also help you to download the software and to make the connection to your chosen ISP.

You can also find local ISPs in the Yellow Pages telephone directory under the heading 'Internet Services'. With your now well-honed skills you might like to browse the web for providers; start with a web search or type in Broadband Guide.

Easy-to-use guides to help you log on to and use the internet

The Australian Communications and Media Authority (2014) has produced a number of fact sheets which may help you to choose the best-value products and services to meet your home office needs, including your internet connection. Go to www.acma.gov.au.

Levine, JR, & Young, ML: *Internet for Dummies*. Indianapolis: Wiley Publishing, 2011. Comprehensive reference, easy to follow, economical.

Check out the puzzles, activities and links on the Evolve website.

References

Australian Health Practitioners Regulation Agency: Social Media Policy, 2014. Online. Available: http://www.nursingmidwiferyboard.gov.au/Codes-Guidelines-Statements/Codes-Guidelines/Social-media-policy.aspx. 30 June 2104.

Aveyard H, Sharp P: *A Beginner's guide to evidence-based practice in health and social care*, ed 2, Berkshire, England, 2013, Open University Press.

Bergman MK: The deep web: surfacing hidden value, *Journal of Electronic Publishing* 7(1):2001.

CINAHL Information Systems: The CINAHL Database, 2006. Online. Available: http://www.cinahl.com. 18 September 2006.

Conrick M: Looking for a needle in a haystack: Searching the internet for quality resources, *Contemporary Nurse* 12(1):2002.

Conrick M, Foster J: Healthcare Education. In Conrick M, editor: *Health informatics: transforming healthcare with technology*, Melbourne, 2006, Thompson/Social Science Press.

Costello K: Social media: used with care, it's a friend, used carelessly, it's a foe to your business, *Journal of Aesthetic Nursing* 3(4):200–201, 2014.

Farrelly R: Nurses and social media, *British Journal of Nursing* 23(6):343, 2014.

Internet Systems Consortium: Internet Domain Survey (2014), 2014. Online. Available: http://www.isc.org. 22 July 2014.

NBNCo: Installation Guide, 2014. Online. Available: http://www.nbnco.com.au/connect-home-or-business/information-for-home/fixed-line/installation.html#.U84PuKOKAv0 22 July 2014.

Netcraft: April 2014 Web Server Survey, 2014. Online. Available: http://news.netcraft.com/archives/2014/04/02/april-2014-web-server-survey.html. 22 July 2014.

West C, Verran D: Something to tweet about: incorporating social media into your nursing practice, *Transplant Journal of Australasia* 22(1):10–12, 2013.

Wikipedia:Statistics: Statistics – Wikipedia, the free encyclopaedia, 2014. Online. Available: http://en.wikipedia.org/wiki/Special:Statistics. 28 June 2014.

CHAPTER 4

NAVIGATING NURSING AND MIDWIFERY RESEARCH ETHICS

Wendy M Cross

CHAPTER OUTLINE

KEY TERMS

autonomy
beneficence
ethical codes of conduct
fraud
human rights
privacy
risks
values
vulnerable groups

LEARNING OBJECTIVES

After reading this chapter and following critical reflection you will be able to:

1. Identify the rights of human participants in research
2. Describe the ethical issues pertaining to nursing research
3. Discuss what constitutes a vulnerable group of participants
4. Understand the relationship between the risks and benefits of research
5. Describe the process of obtaining ethical clearance.

STUDENT QUOTES

I didn't realise the importance of human rights in research before. Those early studies were shocking.

Working out how to complete the ethics form is very helpful in clarifying the other parts of the research plan because you need to have all the methods right and work out what you will be expecting from participants.

ABSTRACT

Before undertaking a research project, at the planning stage, consideration must be given to the methods of data collection. Researchers must also consider the applicability and efficacy of the research because all research must have significance for the community otherwise it is unethical. Most nursing and midwifery research will be undertaken using humans as participants. Those participants might be adversely affected by the procedures involved such as distress (direct or indirect) during an interview, sharing sensitive information, being deprived of an intervention or suffering the side effects of an intervention. This means that the researcher must be mindful of the ethical standards for research. As a researcher or research consumer you must be concerned for the welfare and rights of participants.

This chapter is designed to help you understand the issues related to human participants in research and to navigate the processes involved in producing an ethical research project. Any research you are involved in conducting or any research you draw upon to inform your practice must conform to ethical codes of practice.

Values and ethics

Values are the beliefs that members of a group agree about in terms of what is imperative, has merit, is decent or is immoral. They set standards and the criteria for judging behaviour. Nursing and midwifery research comprises both **values** and ethics. For example, as nurses and midwives we value evidence. We therefore pursue such evidence through research. Ethically, we must obtain the evidence in a way that ensures human participants are informed and consent to the activities involved in collecting the evidence in question. Otherwise a tension between scientific inquiry and human rights may result.

Basic human rights in research

> ***Human rights*** *are rights inherent to everyone regardless of our nationality, where we live, sex, race, religion, language, or any other status. Everyone is equally entitled to his or her human rights without discrimination. These rights are all interrelated, interdependent and indivisible (United Nations 2015).*
>
> *Human rights are often embedded in law, such as treaties. International human rights law lays down responsibilities of Governments to act in certain ways or to refrain from certain acts, in order to promote and protect human rights and the fundamental freedoms of people (United Nations 2015).*

There are four rights that must be observed when conducting a research project. They relate to the right not to be harmed (physically, mentally, dignity), the right to treatment, the right to self-determination and **autonomy**, and the right to **privacy**.

1. The right not to be harmed relates to ensuring that participants involved in research will have their physical and mental health protected and that their dignity is also preserved. Possible harm can occur where research interventions pose greater than normal exposure such as in the case of drug trials, or that the nature of the research causes distress to participants such as interviewing people following a disaster or other traumatic experience. Any procedure conducted in a study must maintain the person's self-respect and self-esteem. This right is related to the principle of **beneficence** and 'doing good'.
2. The right to treatment is a fundamental right in health care. In some instances when a person presents for treatment, a researcher might offer an alternative as part of an experimental trial. Any alternative treatment must be clearly matched by the traditional treatment so that participants are not denied a service to address their health problem. This right is linked to the principle of justice where all participants must be treated fairly.

3. The right to self-determination and autonomy is related to the principle of respect and includes informed and voluntary consent to participate, the right to refuse to participate, or to withdraw at any time without disadvantage. The researcher must make this known to the participant and dispel any worries they might have about refusing to participate. The researcher must not induce participation with promises of money or free care.

If a participant decides to withdraw from the project, the researcher must accept that decision and if data have been collected from that participant they are destroyed if they can be identified or have not already been aggregated into the findings of the project as a whole.

Informed consent relates to participants having full knowledge of the project including:

- the identity and credentials of the researcher
- its purpose and significance
- how they were selected to participate
- everything they will be asked to do
- the amount of time it will take
- any potential risks, discomforts, distress
- how the data collected will be used and who will have access to it
- how their privacy, confidentiality and anonymity will be maintained
- consent is voluntary and they may withdraw at any time
- any reimbursements for expenses or time
- the contact details of the researcher.

Informed consent means that the disclosures made to the participants are kept on file and they will not be deceived in any way. The participants' dignity and self-respect will be upheld at all times. An informed consent must be given without coercion or influence of any kind. Where a researcher has a relationship with a participant such as in the case of a university lecturer and students, that researcher must provide the opportunity for the participant to give the consent to another member of the research team.

Box 4.1 provides an example of a Participant Information Form (sometimes called the Plain Language Statement) and Box 4.2 provides an example of a Participant Consent Form.

4. The right to privacy is taken very seriously and there is privacy legislation to ensure that it is maintained (Privacy Act 1988). Privacy is also associated with respect. Any procedure to collect data that could be construed as invading privacy such as the use of digital recorders and taking photographs must be disclosed to the participant. All data that are collected must be stored safely so that only the research team has access to it. At the completion of the research and after the required

Box 4.1
Participant Information Form

Participant Information (*name of organisation*)

Full Project Title:

Principal Researcher:

Student Researcher:

1. **Introduction**

   You are invited to take part in this research project. This is because you (*reason for selecting the participant*).

   This Participant Information and Consent Form tells you about the research project. It explains what is involved to help you decide if you want to take part.

   Please read this information carefully. Ask questions about anything that you don't understand or want to know more about. Before deciding whether or not to take part, you might want to talk about it with a relative, friend or your local health worker.

   Participation in this research is voluntary. If you don't wish to take part, you don't have to.

   if you decide you want to take part in the research project, you will be asked to sign the consent section. By signing it you are telling us that you:

   - understand what you have read
   - consent to take part in the research project
   - consent to be involved in the procedures described
   - consent to the use of your personal and/or health information as described.

   You will be given a copy of this Participant Information and Consent Form to keep.

2. **What is the purpose of this research project?**

   The aims of the project are to:

   (*include the information about the study and its significance*)

3. **What does participation in this research project involve?**

   (*include everything the participant is required to do*)

   All information collected will be de-identified.

   You will not be paid for your participation in this research.

4. **What are the possible benefits?**

   It is anticipated that the outcomes of this research will assist to (*add the anticipated benefits*).

   There is likely to be no direct benefit to individuals involved in the research.

Continued

Box 4.1
Participant Information Form—cont'd

5. **What are the possible risks?**

   It is unlikely that this research will present any risks to you as an individual. All data collected during the research will be de-identified and recorded in terms of themes. Notes about a particular individual will not be taken.

   If you become upset or distressed as a result of your participation in the research, the researcher will arrange for counselling or other appropriate support. Any counselling or support will be provided by professionals that are not members of the research team.

6. **Do I have to take part in this research project?**

   Participation in this research project is voluntary. If you do not wish to take part, you do not have to. You are also fee to 'opt out' at any time during the project. You may choose to 'opt out' completely for the duration of the research project, or just 'opt out' for a particular time period.

   If you decide to 'opt out', please notify a member of the research team, so that you can be excluded from further data collection.

   If you decide to leave the project part way through, the researchers would be unable to destroy any data. Data already collected is de-identified.

   Your decision whether to take part or not, or to take part and then withdraw, will not affect your relationship with (*add organisation here*).

7. **How will I be informed of the final results of this research project?**

   At the completion of this phase of the study, a summary report will be made available via ... Also, a copy of any publications that are produced from this research will also be made available via ...

8. **What will happen to information about me?**

   All hard copy and electronic data will be stored in a locked filing cabinet in the locked office of the researcher, and will be accessible only to the researchers named on this project. The data associated with this research will be stored for seven years in accordance with the National Statement on Ethical Conduct in Research Involving Humans, 12.11. Seven years after the completion of this study, all electronic files will be deleted and all paper records will be shredded.

   Data collected in this study will not be included in any other research projects.

   This research does not involve the establishment of a data bank.

   In any publication and/or presentation, information will be provided in such a way that you cannot be identified.

Box 4.1
Participant Information Form—cont'd

9. **Can I access research information kept about me?**

   In accordance with relevant privacy and other laws, you have the right to access the information collected and stored by the researchers about you, however all information collected as part of this study will be de-identified, so it is not possible to identify which information relates specifically to you. Please contact one of the researchers named at the end of this document if you would like further information.

10. **Is this research project approved?**

    The ethical aspects of this research project have been approved by the Human Research Ethics Committee of (*insert name of organisation*).

    This project will be carried out according to the National Statement on Ethical Conduct in Human Research (2007) produced by the National Health and Medical Research Council of Australia. This statement has been developed to protect the interests of people who agree to participate in human research studies.

11. **Who can I contact?**

    For further information:

    If you want any further information concerning this project or if you have any problems that may be related to your involvement in the project (e.g. feelings of distress), you can contact the researcher: (*supply name and contact details*).

    For complaints:

    If you have any complaints about any aspect of the project, the way it is being conducted or any questions about being a research participant in general, then you may contact:

    (*supply name and contact details of ethics complaints officer for your organisation*)

period of storage (in most cases seven years), all data are destroyed using the appropriate means: recordings are erased, computer files deleted and paper records shredded.

Any participant identifiers (names or codes) must be kept separate to the research data and where data are shared between research teams they must have unique codes so they cannot be linked to the participant by anyone other than the research team. You should not be able to identify any participant in a research report (anonymity). Therefore all data are pooled and reported as an aggregate (group information). In the case of interview transcripts,

Box 4.2
Participant consent form

Project Title:

This research project is undertaken by: *[insert name of researcher]*

1. I have read the Information Sheet for this study and have had details of the study explained to me.
2. My questions about the study have been answered to my satisfaction, and I understand that I may ask further questions at any time.
3. I also understand that I am free to decline to answer any particular questions in the study.
4. I agree to provide information to the researchers under the conditions of confidentiality set out on the Information Sheet.
5. I wish to participate in this study under the conditions set out in the Information Sheet.
6. I understand that my participation is voluntary and I may withdraw at any time.

Contact details: [*insert researchers' contact details*]

Participant Name: ______________________________

Participant Signature: ______________________________

Date: / /

Researcher Name: ______________________________

Researcher Signature: ______________________________

Date: / /

pseudonyms are used. Any information the participant discloses must not be reported elsewhere except in the case of mandatory reporting requirements such as suspected child abuse. In this situation, the requirement for mandatory reporting must be disclosed to the participant before consent is obtained.

We must protect the rights of human participants and there are abundant examples from the past when these rights were violated. In particular, the atrocities of the Second World War committed by the Nazis, the Milgram behavioural experiment on student obedience (1963), the Tuskegee syphilis study with African-American men (Brandt 1978), the Willowbrook State School hepatitis study (1963–1966), and in the 1980s, the New Zealand experiment on women with cervical cancer (Johnstone 2009). Box 4.3 provides a summary of these studies.

Box 4.3
Examples of unethical research

Example	Description	Ethical Issues
Nazi experiments	Medical experiments performed on concentration camp inmates such as exposing them to freezing temperatures, malaria, poisons and incendiary bombs, among other things, without their consent and with blatant indifference to the suffering of the human participants by the researchers. Many inmates died, were disabled or disfigured.	Do no harm Right to self-determination Informed consent
Milgram study	An experiment of compliance with authority where student participants thought they were inflicting progressively stronger electric shocks to other participants. The authority figure (experimenter) urged and reassured participants there would be no damage to the person receiving the shocks. However, participants were clearly psychologically distressed at being urged to inflict pain on another person. The associated deception and the requirements of the study caused the participants embarrassment and distress.	Do no harm Right to self-determination Deception Withdrawal of consent
Tuskegee syphilis study	A 40-year study by the US Public Health Service (1932–1972) where poor rural black men with a diagnosis of syphilis were denied treatment (Penicillin) so researchers could study the progression of the disease. In addition, they were not told of their diagnosis and were recruited into the study with promises of free health care and other inducements.	Right to treatment Right to self-determination Do no harm
Willowbrook State School	Admission of severely disabled children to Willowbrook State School in the USA was granted on the proviso the children enter the hepatitis study. These children were placed in the isolation area and deliberately exposed to hepatitis. The parents of these children were previously told that there were no vacancies at the school.	Right to self-determination Do no harm Vulnerable groups Coercion and inducement
New Zealand cervical cancer study	Commenced in 1966, 948 women with cervical cancer in situ (CIS) were denied active treatment. By 1988 it was determined that these women were four times as likely to develop invasive cancer. It is unclear how many women died as a result of the study. Many were compensated following an inquiry in 1988.	Right to treatment Informed consent

Nurses were involved in these studies and whilst they were not the chief investigators, they were complicit in the unethical treatment of human beings. Nurses and midwives have a responsibility to raise awareness of the ethical conduct of research and to report incidents where research is unethical.

Unethical research might occur in other ways. Researchers themselves might not be ethical in their own conduct during research studies. Researchers must act with integrity and honesty during the study and in the reporting of the findings of their research. For example, there are a number of fraudulent studies where the research was never actually undertaken; there were faked trials and methods (Martin 1989); and the results were falsified or fabricated (Debaets 2006). The researchers found to be unethical in these examples of **fraud** were subject to what is known as research law. This law is drawn from the laws of consent, contract, negligence, and intellectual property. In addition, there are laws that govern human rights, the National Health and Medical Research Council (NHMRC), privacy and discrimination (Dawson & Peart 2003), which all directly influence research activity.

Considerable research is supported with funds from various organisations such as government agencies and departments, pharmaceutical and other companies, professional bodies and philanthropic trusts. These funds enable the development and evaluation of programs, the testing of products, the examination of the impact of a policy, or analysis of interest. As a consequence these funding bodies may exert various controls on the researcher including determining certain research designs be utilised or by placing restrictions on the publication of the research results. An acknowledgement of the funding source should be included in the research report. Any imposition placed on the research process impedes the collection and dissemination of accurate data and its interpretation is unethical. The NHMRC (2007 p. 79) states:

> *A conflict of interest may compromise the research process itself and/or the institutional processes governing research, and may lead researchers or institutions to base decisions about the research on factors outside the research requirements.*

Ethical codes of conduct

As the knowledge of those early experiments and breaches of integrity became public, inquiries were undertaken and codes of ethics were developed. The most notable is the Nuremberg Code of 1949 (US National Institutes of Health 2014). At Nuremberg, Germany, Nazis were tried for crimes against humanity including the unethical treatment of people in research studies (see Box 4.4).

Following the Nuremberg Code of 1949, the World Medical Association (WMA) was formed and by 1964 the Declaration of Helsinki was ratified (WMA 2014), which built on the Nuremberg code. The Declaration of Helsinki has been revised numerous times and now includes reference to:

Box 4.4
Criteria in the Nuremberg Code

Researchers must inform participants about their studies and obtain voluntary consent.

Research must be for the good of the society.

Where possible, animals should be used for experiments rather than humans.

Researchers must avoid harming participants.

No study must be undertaken where serious injury or death might occur.

The degree of risk must not outweigh the benefit of the study.

Proper facilities and preparation must be made to protect participants from harm.

Researchers must be qualified to undertake research.

Participants can stop the research if problems arise.

Researcher must cease the study if they believe that an unacceptable risk to participants has arisen.

From: Katz 1972, pp. 289–290.

- the duty of researchers to protect human rights
- research that is scientifically defensible
- research being reviewed by an independent human ethics committee
- research that is lawful
- special protections for children and other **vulnerable groups**
- research reports that are accurate and include both positive and negative results.

In Australia the NHMRC provides clear guidelines and codes regarding what constitutes ethical research (NHMRC 2007). The Health Research Council of New Zealand (2006) has published Guidelines on Ethics in Health Research. It is imperative that any research plan has accounted for the ethical considerations (Aita & Richter 2005). When you are reading research reports you will note that authors clearly outline how they managed any ethical dilemmas they anticipated or encountered.

Vulnerable groups

A number of groups that are of interest to nurse and midwife researchers are considered to be vulnerable because they have diminished capacity to give informed consent or are considered to be captive populations; that is, not completely free to give consent.

Children, fetuses, people with mental illness or intellectual disabilities, and those with impaired consciousness or cognition are assumed not to have the capacity to deliberate upon the **risks** and benefits of a research project and are therefore unable to give informed consent to participate. Consent to undertake research with these groups must be obtained from the parent or legal guardian. In the case of minors between 10 and 18 years of age, it is wise to provide them with the information about the study as they have the right to assent to participate so that a parent or guardian knows and understands the wishes of the minor before consenting for their child to participate.

People with life-limiting illnesses might also be considered vulnerable as their consent to participate may be predicated on the hope that they will be cured of their illness and, in their desire for such a cure, such individuals might agree to research procedures/treatments that could be harmful.

Prisoners are also considered vulnerable because they are not really 'free' to give consent. They might believe that agreeing to participate could lessen their sentence. In addition, ordinary financial compensation could be seen as a very large sum by people with limited earning capacity, which may place them in a precarious position in relation to other prisoners.

Members of the armed services are considered vulnerable as they might not question the researcher's intent or the procedures and agree to participate because it is customary for them to obey without question. They might not see that they can refuse to participate or can withdraw without penalty because they are trained to obey orders.

Other groups that might feel compelled to participate include students and employees. Both these groups could have a dependent or unequal relationship with the researcher especially if the researcher is the student's teacher or an employee's manager. Even if the research is being undertaken by another student or employee, the recruitment of these participants must be undertaken from classes or workplaces where the researcher has little or no involvement. In that way, participants will be free to consent or not, without feeling they have been coerced or influenced.

Lastly, we must also be sensitive to the cultural background of potential research participants. In some cultures it is seen as polite to agree to a request to participate especially if that request is made by someone who is deemed to be in authority. Therefore consent may be given even if the person is unclear or hesitant about the research. All information provided to people from culturally and linguistically diverse (CALD) backgrounds must be in a language they can understand and they must be given the opportunity to ask questions in the appropriate language. Unfortunately many researchers make the requirement to speak English an inclusion criterion for their research project and this eliminates a potential source of rich data from people whose primary language is not English.

In Australia and New Zealand, it is also important to recognise the special needs of indigenous people. There is great diversity across the many Aboriginal and Torres Strait Islander cultures and societies and research involving these groups requires special consideration and is governed by discrete guidelines (NHMRC 2014; Health Research Council of New Zealand 1998, 2004). The NHMRC Values and Ethics guidelines are based on six core values identified as being important to Aboriginal and Torres Strait Islander Peoples. The use of these core values, and of other cultural and local-language conventions, should be decided by the Aboriginal and Torres Strait Islander communities or groups involved in the research (NHMRC 2014). The six core values are:

1. reciprocity
2. respect
3. equality
4. responsibility
5. survival and protection
6. spirit and integrity.

See also Chapter 8.

Understanding the risks and benefits of research

Risk is the potential to harm participants. All researchers must balance the potential for harm against the overall benefits of the research to both the participant and to the broader community. There are risks associated with data collection methods, with special groups, between the researcher and the participant, regarding confidentiality and privacy, incentives and inducements, about the reporting of the outcomes of the research and where the study is located. The researcher needs to assess each of these risks and mitigate each one so that the rights of participants are not violated. Sometimes, an adverse outcome cannot be predicted. However, should this occur, the researcher must manage the outcome appropriately and notify the proper authority. When you read a research report, you will see the rationale for the project. This usually outlines the benefits of the study and any risks that might be involved. Figure 4.1 describes how to assess risk.

Human Research Ethics Committees

All institutions involved in research must convene an institutional ethics committee, commonly called Human Research Ethics Committees (HRECs) (NHMRC 2007). It is the responsibility of HRECs to assess the risk posed by a research project. HRECs have two functions: to assess the scientific merit of a project and to assess the risk to participants that the project

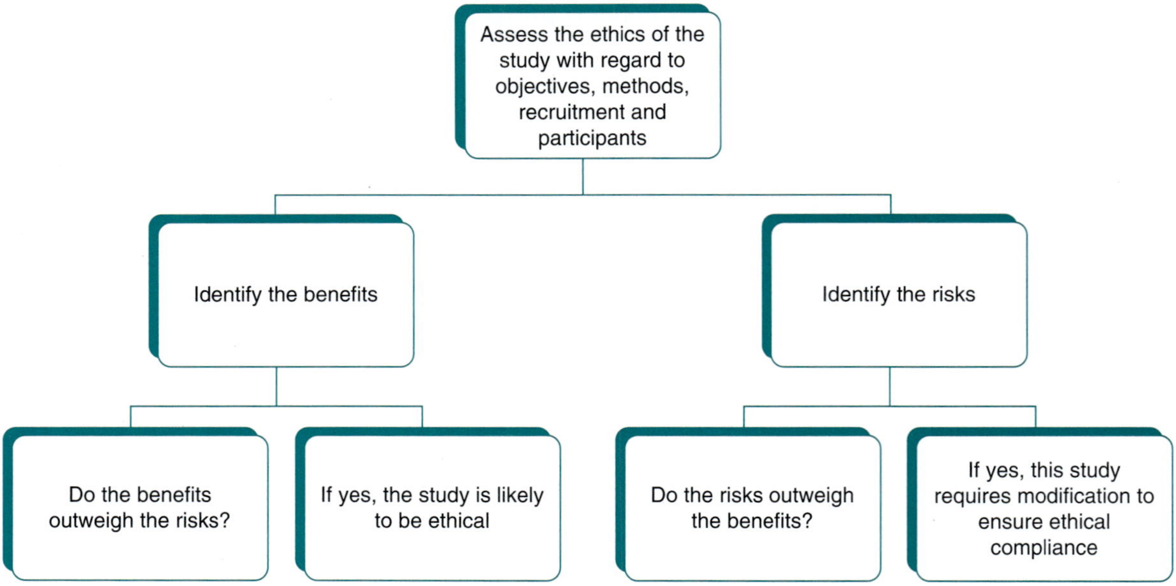

FIGURE 4.1
How to assess risk.

poses. Some have argued that as an ethics committee, their remit is to judge the ethical issues and not the scientific issues; that these should be left to another body. However, research that is not scientifically rigorous is also not ethical as it is inappropriate to expose participants to research that is poorly constructed and would have no clear knowledge generation (Horsfall et al 2007; Brand & Van Houwelingen 1994). The methods sections of research reports should clearly describe the design, methods, procedures and analysis undertaken within the project so that the scientific aspects of the project can be scrutinised. Authors also include any limitations of the project to explain aspects where the credibility of the research must be questioned. This is the ethical approach to reporting research findings.

In Australia, HRECs are composed of experts and lay people including scientists, statisticians, lawyers, clergy and consumers. Each member assesses the research project according to the rules that govern such committees and according to their own area of expertise and interest.

All research requiring human participants must secure ethical approval prior to the recruitment of any participant or the collection of any data. Institutional HRECs require the researcher to submit an application for ethics review of the study and may require the use of an application form that is produced by that institution or use of the NHMRC National Ethics Application Form (NEAF) (available at www.neaf.gov.au) or both. The NEAF is designed for projects that involve multiple committees and is intended to reduce the effort by researchers in completing multiple forms. However, it is generally the case that the researcher is required to submit the NEAF as well as the local form.

It is the responsibility of the researcher to identify all of the ethical issues and risks and state how each will be addressed. When the HREC is satisfied the research is sound methodologically and ethically, approval is given. The approval is for a defined period of time and the researcher must provide interim and final reports of the study to the HREC. Any unforeseen consequence of the research must be reported to the HREC immediately and any modification to the research plan must also be approved. You will note when you read research articles that the researchers often state ethical approval has been granted.

STUDENT CHALLENGE

Look at some quantitative and qualitative research studies and look for signs they were conducted ethically.

1. Were the rights of the participants protected? What evidence did you find that supports this?
2. Was the study approved by a HREC?
3. How was informed consent obtained?
4. How did the researcher manage sensitive issues?
5. Was there anything in the report that indicated the study might not have been conducted ethically?

Conclusion

This chapter has provided a basic overview of navigating the issues related to the ethics of research and the process of obtaining ethical authorisation for a research study. We have examined the relationship between ethics and values, the basic rights of humans, vulnerable and special groups, how studies have been conducted that have not been ethical and the process for achieving HREC approval for research. As you read research reports you should be able to identify the ethical issues that were addressed by the researchers. Scientific methods and ethics are fundamental to good research. They are inseparable and whilst navigating the ethics approval process might seem like a hindrance in undertaking your research, it is essential to protect the rights of the participant and of the researcher.

RESOURCES KIT

The following websites are helpful in understanding your ethical responsibilities in conducting research projects.

National Statement on Ethical Conduct in Human Research (2007). Updated March 2014

https://www.nhmrc.gov.au/guidelines-publications/e72.

Values and Ethics – Guidelines for Ethical Conduct in Aboriginal and Torres Strait Islander Health Research

https://www.nhmrc.gov.au/guidelines-publications/e52.

Australian Code for the Responsible Conduct of Research

https://www.nhmrc.gov.au/guidelines-publications/r39.

Guidelines approved under Section 95A of the Privacy Act 1988

https://www.nhmrc.gov.au/guidelines-publications/pr2.

The Privacy Act

http://www.oaic.gov.au/privacy/privacy-act/the-privacy-act.

National, State & Territory Legislative Framework for ethical review of multi-centre research

https://hrep.nhmrc.gov.au/toolbox/relevant-legislation.

References

Aita M, Richter C: Essentials of research ethics for healthcare professionals, *Nursing and Health Sciences* 7:119–125, 2005.

Brand R, Van Houwelingen H: Statistical and methodological aspects of clinical research protocols: a practical guide for review committees, *Monash Bioethics Review* 15:10–16, 1994.

Brandt AM: Racism and research: The case of the Tuskegee Syphilis study, *Hastings Centre Report* 8:21–29, 1978.

Dawson J, Peart N, editors: *The Law of Research: a Guide*, Dunedin, New Zealand, 2003, University of Otago Press.

Debaets AM: Korean cloning scandal and scientific fraud, *Ethics and Medicine* 22(1):61–62, 2006.

Health Research Council of New Zealand: Guidelines for researchers on health research involving Maori. 1998. Online. Available: www.hrc.govt.nz 31 July 2014.

Health Research Council of New Zealand: Guidelines for researcher on health research involving Pacific peoples resident in New Zealand. 2004. Online. Available: www.hrc.govt.nz 31 July 2014.

Health Research Council of New Zealand: Guidelines on Ethics in Health Research. 2006. Online. Available: http://neac.health.govt.nz/streamlined-ethical-guidelines-health-and-disability-research 31 July 2014.

Horsfall J, Cleary M, Walter G, et al: Conducting mental health research: Key steps, practicalities, and issues for the early career researcher, *International Journal of Mental Health Nursing* 16(Suppl 1):S1–S20, 2007.

Johnstone MJ: *Bioethics: a nursing perspective*, ed 5, Sydney, 2009, Elsevier.

Katz J: *Experimentation with human beings*, New York, 1972, Russell Sage Foundation.

Martin B: Fraud and Australian academics, *Thought and Action* 5(2):95–102, 1989.

Milgram S: Behavioral study of obedience, *Journal of Abnormal and Social Psychology* 67:371–378, 1963.

National Health and Medical Research Council (NHMRC): Guidelines for Ethical Conduct in Aboriginal and Torres Strait Islander Health Research. 2014. Online. Available: http://www.nhmrc.gov.au/guidelines-publications/e52.

National Health and Medical Research Council NHMRC (2007). National Statement on Ethical Conduct in Human Research. Updated May 2015. Online. Available: http://www.nhmrc.gov.au/guidelines-publications/e72.

U.S. National Institutes of Health: 'The Nuremberg Code'. 2014. Online. Available: http://history.nih.gov/research/downloads/nuremberg.pdf 31 July.

World Medical Association (WMA): Declaration of Helsinki 2008 (Sixth revision – Current). 2014. Online. Available: www.wma.net/en/30publications/10policies/b3/index.html 31 July 2014.

SECTION 2

Talking the talk

Health care and healthcare technology are becoming increasingly complex and expanding at a rapid rate. The practices of nursing and midwifery change on a daily basis. How do we cope? How can we keep our knowledge base and our practice current? Research is the key. It provides a solid foundation on which to base our practice. This means that as nurses and midwives we need to incorporate research findings into our practice settings. As you have learnt, this is commonly referred to as evidence-based practice. To do this we must be able to read, understand and apply the available research literature.

This section defines research, explores quantitative and qualitative research methodologies including mixed method and Indigenous approaches. Importantly, it provides you with the vocabulary and tools to read and understand research articles because in order to understand research it is important for you to learn about certain concepts (terminology) specific to the field and the relationships between them.

For example, knowing the difference between a paradigm, a methodology and the method is fundamental to research. See Chapter 6 in which we provide explanation of these terms in Table 6.5 in the Resources kit. Once you have read the chapters on each of the research paradigms you should have a much better understanding of some of the main concepts underpinning this thing we call research.

Afterwards, as you want to learn more, look at some of the excellent material available on the world wide web. Try a websearch for various terms and don't forget YouTube or iTunes or even a Massive Open Online Course (MOOC) as tool/s for learning more about research.

CHAPTER 5

QUANTITATIVE RESEARCH

Louise Hickman and Rebecca Disler

CHAPTER OUTLINE

KEY TERMS

data
descriptive statistics
inferential statistics
instrument
non-experimental research
problem statement
quantitative research
research
research design
research hypothesis
research process

LEARNING OBJECTIVES

After reading this chapter and following critical reflection the student will be able to:

1. Define quantitative research
2. Describe quantitative research classifications
3. Discuss the phases of the research process as they relate to quantitative research
4. Describe the steps involved in designing a quantitative study
5. Describe the steps involved in conducting a quantitative study
6. Describe the steps involved in analysing a quantitative study
7. Describe the steps involved in applying quantitative study results to practice
8. Discuss the relationships among phases of the research process using a quantitative method
9. Cite examples of steps and phases of the research process using a quantitative method.

STUDENT QUOTE

Once you understand what all those terms mean and learn that there is a set structure and defined process for doing a [quantitative] research study, it's not so hard to follow what's happening.

ABSTRACT

Quantitative research approaches follow systematic logical processes used to answer questions about measurable concepts. Quantitative projects can be classified in numerous ways, including classification by the stated goals of a specific research project or by the choice of research design. The research process comprises five phases that guide the researcher from the formulation of researchable problems to the confirmation of probable answers. The phases begin with conceptualisation and crystallisation of the problem grounded in literature from previous research and theory. A study plan is then developed that specifies a research design, the subjects to be studied, the instruments to be used for measurement and how the data will be analysed. The study plan is then implemented and data are collected adhering to a set of ethical guidelines. Data are analysed statistically and pre-defined research questions are answered and placed within a theoretical context. The findings are examined for their relevance to nursing or midwifery practice and future research. Results are compared to other findings, what is already known, implications for practice and recommendations for further research suggested, and communicated to research consumers.

Introduction

This chapter defines quantitative research, explores various ways in which quantitative research can be classified and identifies and discusses the specific steps of the quantitative **research process**. You may find some of the new language challenging to read and understand. That is to be expected because you are learning a new vocabulary and a new way of thinking about things. Don't panic. Take the time to read and summarise the material carefully. Chapters 9 and 10 provide the foundation you need to enable you to read and apply research results. Take a deep breath and attack this chapter one paragraph at a time. The more you read about and reflect upon a concept the easier it becomes to understand. Talking to your fellow students and comparing and contrasting understandings are also beneficial.

What is quantitative research?

Quantitative research is a systematic, objective process used to gather and analyse information that has been measured by some kind of instrument. Quantitative research can be used to describe and test relationships or examine cause and effect relationships. To do this it uses **instruments** (e.g. questionnaire) to collect information that is then converted into numbers (numerical data). Quantitative research uses descriptive and **inferential statistics**, which means briefly, to manage those numbers both in describing the results and analysing the outcomes of the research. Statistics allows the researcher to draw a numerical picture of the information collected, to look at how the things being measured are alike or different, to make decisions about whether things are related or different, or to determine whether one thing causes another to react in a certain way.

Quantitative research uses a systematic and logical approach that emphasises deductive reasoning. It has several identifiable characteristics. Which means briefly that it can either begin with:

- an educated statement (hypothesis) about how the concepts to be researched might be related, or
- with a question (research question) about what is to be explored or described.

Quantitative research investigates only quantifiable concepts (concepts that can be measured and turned into numbers). The process is very structured. There are a multitude of factors that could impact the way a study or person responds to an intervention. Quantitative research seeks to be objective by limiting or controlling the effects of things not being studied, so that you can understand the specific element in which you are interested. This approach yields results or findings that are specific to the question, clearly defined and easily interpreted.

The quantitative approach has limitations. Although objectivity is prized and strict controls imposed to limit bias, outside influences can never be entirely removed. In the context of health research, limiting the type of participant included in the study allows for safer comparisons, but can over-simplify the common complexities of comorbidity and outside influences. The researcher additionally brings a perspective that will influence the questions asked, hypotheses of predicted results tested and how the data is analysed and interpreted. There have been numerous reports about the conscious and unconscious influences that researchers bring to the interpretation and dissemination of results. Limiting influence is possible, but no person can exist outside of their own context. Compare this to the beliefs that underpin qualitative research.

Quantitative research classifications

Several different terms are used to describe or classify quantitative research. We will explore some of the more common classifications and terms so they will be familiar to you when you see them in research articles and literature.

Quantitative research may be classified in the following ways:

- the reasons for conducting the research
- the span of time in which data collection occurs
- the point at which data are collected
- the number of subjects sampled
- the purpose or aim of the research
- the research design or statistical method used (Box 5.1).

Studies may fall under several of these classification schemes. Thus, you might see a particular study described as a cross-sectional (time span), descriptive (aim), non-experimental (design) study.

Reasons quantitative research is conducted

Quantitative research is undertaken using a systematic process that involves gathering and analysing data for various purposes, including testing relationships, investigating cause and effect, and providing information to describe, explore, explain and predict (DEEP). Both qualitative and quantitative research approaches have the potential to create knowledge that can change practice. Quantitative research that is conducted systematically and uses robust research methods has the potential to be generalised to a large population. For this reason, quantitative research can more readily influence clinical practice. Qualitative and quantitative research can inform one another, to create new knowledge (see Chapter 7 Mixed Methods Research).

Quantitative research can be pure (basic) or applied. Pure or basic research is performed to establish or extend fundamental concepts and theories. It is a search for 'knowledge for knowledge's sake'. The findings may have no immediate practical application or benefit but act to extend our understanding.

Box 5.1
Classification systems for quantitative research

Reasons conducted
- Basic (pure) – theory-generating
- Applied – theory-testing

Time span
- Cross-sectional
- Longitudinal

Point of data collection
- Retrospective (ex post facto or after the fact)
- Prospective

Purpose or aim
- Descriptive
- Exploratory
- Explanatory
- Predictive

Research design
- Experimental/quasiexperimental
- Non-experimental

Applied research is conducted to solve immediate problems for practical purposes. Applied research is often based on a foundation of basic research. It may seek to test the boundary of explanation, and its results often suggest further areas for basic research study. Nursing and midwifery are practice-based disciplines and consequently the majority of nursing and midwifery research and journals are based on applied research. Being a consumer of research who desires to improve clinical practice, you will likely be most interested in applied research.

Time span and point of data collection

Research is sometimes described by the span of time used to collect the data for the study or to indicate when data were collected. Cross-sectional studies use data collected at one single point in time and provide a snapshot of the situation. Longitudinal studies use data collected at several time points over several months or years to measure the change in an outcome or context. Data can also be collected prospectively, with the study designed to analyse data collected on factors or events as they occur, or retrospectively, with data collected on factors or events that occurred before the onset of the research study.

Purpose

The two categories most helpful in describing a quantitative study are classification by purpose and classification by design. You may recall that we previously noted the general purpose of quantitative research can be classified as to describe, explore, explain or predict (DEEP) observable, measurable conditions.

Descriptive studies describe. A descriptive study does as its name implies: it describes the concepts under study. It commonly looks at the prevalence, magnitude and/or characteristics of a particular concept or of various factors in the study.

An example of a descriptive nursing research study can be found in Tsai et al's study (2013) that examined the factors associated with clinical nurses' innovation including individual characteristics, perceived worksite support and perceived personal creativity. Another example can be found in a study by Hickman et al (2010): these authors described how positive policy environments, interdisciplinary care collaboration, an emphasis on self-management strategies and empowered communities can improve the effectiveness of chronic care model for older persons. Furthermore, Wan et al (2014) described the stigma experienced by urinary incontinence patients, and determined that disease stigma impaired quality of life of women with stress urinary incontinence and mediated the association between symptom severity and quality of life.

Surveys, sometimes called questionnaires, are often used to collect data that describes a concept or health situation and are commonly used to investigate the attitudes, beliefs, characteristics and other phenomena of a population.

Wu et al (2014) used a survey design with four questionnaires to investigate factors that account for the differences between diabetic patients and nurses' perceptions of self-care, health education barriers and educational needs. Shelton et al (2013) similarly used a self-administered survey of nurses and doctors in the post-operative surveillance team program that sought to describe the attitudes of ward staff about medical co-management of high-risk, post-operative patients. The survey results allowed the researchers to identify the demographic characteristics of the staff and common characteristics of ward rounds that might influence management of high-risk patients.

Surveys are additionally useful for gathering information from a large body of people. Iglesias and Vallejo (2013) conducted a survey in Spain to determine the prevalence of burnout syndrome, job satisfaction, and job stress associated with stress disorders, and demonstrate the relationship between these variables among critical care nurses. Using surveys allows for easy distribution across many health sites not necessarily accessible if data collection relied on face-to-face collection by a researcher.

Exploratory studies explore. Exploratory studies are used to investigate a particular concept about which little is known. They go beyond describing concepts and begin to examine the relationships or differences between the concepts and other factors. For example, Spoelstra et al (2013) explored whether strategies for managing symptoms and adherence to oral chemotherapy agents can promote adherence and reduce adverse effects in patients with cancer. In another study, Williams (2014) used questionnaires to compare levels of stress of students undertaking an associate nursing degree before and after the implementation of an intervention and explored the students' perception of quality of care provided to patients.

Explanatory studies explain. These studies try to discover why a certain concept or phenomenon occurs. They search for cause and effect or interactive relationships between concepts and often act to link theory and to organise or integrate the relationships among various concepts or factors.

For example, in an explanatory study examining possible cause and effect, Adhikari et al (2014) looked at the factors that might cause or be associated with noncompliance of medications and particular lifestyle behaviour after renal transplantation. In this study the authors concluded that noncompliance is associated with the duration of dialysis and waiting time for transplant. Explanatory theory relating to postpartum fatigue was used by Song et al (2010) in an examination of the relationship between postpartum depression, sleep quality, childcare stress, the cultural phenomenon of Sanhujori and postpartum fatigue.

Predictive studies predict. Once events can be explained, the next step is to try to predict what will occur or what factors are likely to increase the probability of an outcome or situation occurring. For example, Hayes et al (2014) via an online survey tested how factors in the nursing work environment, job satisfaction, job stress and emotional exhaustion predicted emotional exhaustion among haemodialysis nurses.

Research variables

Variables are identified concepts or traits that are measured, manipulated or controlled in a research study. A variable is a concept or trait that varies. These traits may be associated with organisms or with the environment. For example, gender is an organism variable because some organisms are male and some female. Weather is an example of an environmental variable. Almost any concept, characteristic or trait that can be observed and/or measured can be considered a variable. When a characteristic or trait does not vary within a given research study context, it is called a constant. For example, if researchers wanted gender to be a constant, they might select only females as subjects for their study. Researchers often use constants to exert control over variables they don't want to study but that might otherwise interfere with the study results.

Variables may take different forms. They may be classified by quality or quantity. Qualitative (categorical) variables change in terms of the presence or absence of a specified trait (e.g. male or not male, married or not married, blue-eyed or not blue-eyed). Quantitative (continuous) variables change in terms of amount or degree (e.g. income, height, weight). These variables can be described in numbers and fractions of numbers. Classifying variables as qualitative or quantitative becomes more important in a later phase of the research study because researchers choose certain analytical tools based on this variable classification.

Another way to classify variables is to determine whether a particular variable is acting as an independent variable, a dependent variable or an extraneous variable in a research study. These distinctions in variables are usually used when the purpose of the study is explanatory or predictive, but they may be seen in exploratory studies in which relationships or differences are being researched.

The independent variable is used to explain or predict the change or variation in the dependent variable. For example, in a study that is researching whether a 'low-fat diet' will decrease 'cholesterol levels', the 'type of diet' is the independent variable and the 'level of blood cholesterol' is the dependent variable. The independent variable can be considered the cause, while the dependent variable is the effect.

An extraneous variable can also affect the dependent variable and interfere with the relationship of the independent and dependent variables. In the previous example, the extraneous variables 'exercise' and 'menstrual cycle' might also affect 'cholesterol levels'. Can you think of other extraneous variables that might affect 'cholesterol levels'? Researchers try to identify all potential extraneous variables so they can control them and keep them from interfering with the variables under study. The literature review helps them identify these extraneous factors. We discussed one form of control the researcher uses by turning an extraneous variable into a constant. Sampling and statistical techniques are also used to help the researcher exert control over extraneous variables. There are many types of extraneous variables and they may be associated with the sample, the researcher or the environment. An extraneous variable that reduces the positive outcome of the study is called a confounding variable.

When research questions are used, the purpose of the study is descriptive or exploratory. Research questions use an interrogative format to identify the variables to be studied and possible relationships or differences between those variables. Example 1 in Box 5.2 is from a descriptive study and shows questions used to identify and describe the variables (number of Emergency Department [ED] visits, chief complaints, time of day, season of year, ED category, payment method, gender and age) and the population (elderly persons using the ED). In the second example from an exploratory study, a question asks about differences on two dependent variables (anxiety levels, disruptive behaviours) for two different groups of individuals (children with and without parental

Box 5.2
Sample forms of problem statements*

Interrogative form

1. What characteristics are common among older individuals who seek care in an emergency department?
2. Does parental presence affect anxiety and behaviour of young children undergoing suture repair of a laceration?
3. Can oxygenation be improved in premature infants by use of extra tactile stimulation?

Declarative form

1. The purpose of this non-experimental study is to describe the characteristics of older individuals who use the emergency department.
2. The purpose of the study is to explore the influence of parental presence on anxiety levels and behaviours of young children who receive sutures for a laceration.
3. The purpose of this experimental study is to determine whether a stimulation protocol will improve the oxygenation of premature infants.

*Examples are taken from student theses.

presence). Parental presence or absence is the independent variable and young children with lacerations are the population. Research questions serve as queries about variables and how they might interact with one another. Research questions are used when no concrete information is available to predict an answer.

In a specific research study, variables come from the concepts identified in the **problem statement** and are specified in the form of research questions or hypotheses. The population to be studied is also specified in the research questions or hypotheses. (We discuss populations in the next phase of the research process.) Box 5.3 provides examples of research questions and hypotheses as derived from the problem statement.

A hypothesis is an 'educated guess' about the relationships between variables and the expected outcomes of the study. It tries to predict the nature of the relationship between variables. The researcher makes these 'educated guesses' based on the review of literature and the most appropriate methodology required to answer the question (i.e. randomised controlled trial). The results of the research study will either support or refute the hypotheses established in the first phase of the study. Research studies that use hypotheses are usually either explanatory or predictive in nature.

Box 5.3
Sample problem statements, research questions and hypotheses*

Problem statements

1. Common characteristics possessed by older individuals who seek care in an emergency department.
2. The effect of parental presence on anxiety and behaviour of young children undergoing suture repair of a laceration.
3. There may be a relationship between implementation of a stimulation protocol on oxygenation of premature infants.
4. Effect of meat eating on serum cholesterol in healthy men aged 55–60 years.

Questions/Hypotheses

1. What percentage of total emergency department visits are by older individuals over the age of 65? What are the chief presenting complaints of older people? Is use affected by time of day, season of year, availability of general practitioner, public or private status, gender or age of the person? (research questions)
2. Will there be a difference between the anxiety levels and disruptive behaviours of young children whose parents are present during laceration repair versus those with no parental presence? (research question)
3. Premature infants who receive extra tactile stimulation will have higher $P\text{O}_2$ levels than those who do not. (directional hypothesis)
4. There will be no difference in serum cholesterol in healthy meat-eating and non-meat-eating men aged 55–60 years. (null hypothesis)

*Examples are taken from student theses.

Apart from specifying the population, all hypotheses contain at least one identifiable independent variable and at least one dependent variable. Some hypotheses are labelled as simple. They contain one independent and one dependent variable. Other hypotheses are labelled as complex hypotheses because they contain more than one independent and/or dependent variable. Example 3 in Box 5.3 is from an explanatory study and shows a hypothesis that predicts one group of infants will be better oxygenated than another group. The independent variable in this hypothesis is the presence or absence of extra tactile stimulation and the dependent variable is $P\text{O}_2$ level. The population is premature infants.

Hypotheses can also be further classified (Box 5.3). A null hypothesis is one that predicts there will be no relationship between the independent and dependent variables in a specified population. An alternative hypothesis is one that predicts a particular relationship between the independent and dependent variables. A directional hypothesis specifies the direction of the relationship between the independent and dependent variables.

There are two important errors the can occur in this type of research. These are the type 1 error and the type 2 error. In a type 1 error, the researcher believes there is an effect, when in fact there is not; in this the researcher incorrectly rejects the null hypothesis. In a type 2, the researcher believes there is no effect, when in fact there has been an effect, and incorrectly accepts the null hypothesis.

Research design

There are three major **research design** categories: experimental, quasiexperimental and non-experimental. These approaches tell us how the research study has been designed.

Experimental research design

Experimental designs are characterised by three factors: (1) manipulation; (2) use of a control group; and (3) random assignment. All these factors allow the researcher greater overall control of the experiment and are used to ensure that changes in the dependent variable are not caused by influences outside the study (extraneous variables).

In manipulation, researchers examine how a particular concept (variable) under study will change or affect another concept (variable) under study. To make sure the change in the dependent variable is because of the treatment (manipulation) and not some other factor (extraneous variable), the researcher puts some of the subjects into a control group and some subjects into a treatment group. Control means an allocation into a group that receives the 'usual' or 'normal' treatment (control group) who are used to compare the outcome of those who receive the treatment under investigation (experimental group).

The control group does not get the experimental treatment (manipulation). The treatment group does get the experimental treatment (manipulation). If the dependent variable changes for the treatment group and does not change for the control group, then the treatment is probably causing the change. Look at example 3 in Box 5.3. This is an experimental study. The researcher had two groups of premature infants. The treatment group received the extra tactile stimulation treatment (manipulation). The control group got the usual care given by the nurses in the neonatal intensive care unit (NICU). Po_2 levels (dependent variable) were measured for both groups. The researcher was observing for a difference in Po_2 for the treatment group and for the control group. For example, Brettle and Raynor (2013) used an experimental, randomised control clinical trial to compare the effectiveness of an information literacy tutorial in which undergraduate pre-registration diploma nursing students were randomly allocated into an online tutorial group (experimental) or a face-to-face tutorial group (usual delivery). The information literacy of the two approaches (manipulation) was compared using a series of measures such as keyword selection, Boolean operators, truncation and synonyms. As previously discussed, manipulation is the treatment or intervention the researcher carries out on the independent variable to try to get the dependent variable to change.

Randomisation means there is an equal chance of being allocated into either the experimental or the control group, and that the allocation is done in a random way so that the researcher cannot bias the choice of individuals that are allocated into each group. Random assignment is the third characteristic of experimental designs. To guard against bias, the researcher randomly assigns subjects to a treatment or control group and randomly decides which group will get the treatment and which group will not. Random assignment means every subject has an equal chance of being in either group and each group has an equal chance of being designated as the treatment group. In example 3 in Box 5.3, the infants were randomly assigned to group 1 and group 2 using a table of random numbers (Box 5.4). The treatment group was then selected by placing two pieces of paper with the words 'group 1' and 'group 2' in a hat. One piece of paper was drawn and that group was designated as the treatment group.

Box 5.4
Sample of a section of a table of random numbers

77	51	30	38	20	19	50	23	71	74
21	81	85	93	13	51	47	46	64	99
99	55	96	83	31	86	83	42	99	01
69	97	92	02	88	93	27	88	17	57
68	10	72	36	21	62	53	52	41	70

Quasiexperimental research design

Quasiexperimental studies are also concerned with causality but unlike experimental studies, it is not possible to achieve a true control or complete randomisation. This may be because it is not always possible to have a control group or to decide who should go into one group or the other. When one of these two factors (randomisation or control) is missing, the design is called a quasiexperimental design. A quasiexperimental design must then use other ways to ensure that the study results are supported. One way to do this is to take extra measurements of the dependent variable, or to measure the dependent variable before and after the treatment. Quasiexperimental studies are one of the most popular designs used in quantitative nursing and midwifery research, as it is often not possible to hide the allocation of an active intervention and ethical considerations also limit the withholding of aspects of care in the healthcare or maternity workplace. Van der Riet et al's (2014) study provides an example of a quasiexperimental design in which pre-test and post-test measurement is used to determine the effectiveness of traditional Thai therapies on: activities of daily living; Barthel Index scores; and pain, emotion and sleep scores in stroke patients. It is not possible to hide the intervention from those receiving the treatment or hide the lack of intervention from those in the control group. While quasiexperimental designs are often used, the data is not as strong as that gained from experimental design and is more vulnerable to threats to validity and reliability.

Non-experimental research design

In **non-experimental research** the concepts are just studied as they occur naturally. Non-experimental designs do not use treatments or attempt to manipulate the independent variable. For example, Gray et al (2013) sought to describe the functional characteristics, occurrence of geriatric syndromes and the profiles of patients older than 75 years in 13 emergency departments in seven nations. The study had no control and only explored characteristics of individuals in metropolitan or large regional hospitals.

These designs use what is already occurring in a particular setting with a particular group of subjects to describe or explore relationships between certain variables. Descriptive non-experimental designs do not even have an identified independent variable to manipulate. Example 1 in Box 5.3 is a descriptive, non-experimental design. The researcher is simply collecting data on several variables and describing the results. Example 2 in Box 5.3 is an exploratory, non-experimental design with an independent variable – parental presence or absence. The researcher is looking to see if parental presence affects anxiety and behaviour (dependent variables). However, the researcher did not decide when the parents would be present or absent. She simply noted whether the parents were present or absent during the suturing procedure and measured anxiety and behaviour in the child.

When a study contains independent and dependent variables and the researcher chooses not to manipulate the independent variable, it is usually for one of three major reasons: (1) all events have already occurred; (2) the variable cannot be manipulated; or (3) it would be morally or ethically wrong to manipulate the variable. In a retrospective non-experimental study the researcher simply collects data on the variables after they have already occurred. Take the example of the infant stimulation study. Suppose the researcher located two different hospitals – one offered extra tactile stimulation as a part of routine care for all premature infants and the other offered no extra tactile stimulation. Further, suppose the researcher collected charts of premature infants in both hospitals, looked up recorded Po_2 levels and compared the Po_2 levels of a group of stimulated infants with a group of non-stimulated infants. This is a non-experimental research design in which the researcher is looking at variables that have already occurred.

Many variables cannot be manipulated. If researchers are interested in whether gender affects longevity, for example, they cannot manipulate the gender variable. They cannot make males become females to see if that change will make them live longer. If researchers are interested in whether ageing affects calcium levels in the blood, they cannot manipulate the age variable (i.e. they cannot make someone get older). In these instances, the researcher must examine the variables as they naturally occur.

Other variables can be manipulated, but to do so would present an ethical dilemma. When researchers were studying the effects of smoking on health, they did not manipulate the variable of smoking. They did not decide who would smoke and who would not smoke because it would not be ethical to force someone to smoke. So, smoking is a variable that can be manipulated, but for ethical reasons it is not. We discuss how subjects are protected against possible unethical treatments in phase 3.

When a variable cannot be manipulated or when manipulation would cause an ethical dilemma, non-experimental research designs must be used. This does not mean that non-experimental designs cannot be used to explain or predict. We can use sophisticated statistical techniques to examine relationships among variables and to predict how they should function under various circumstances.

A popular non-experimental design used in health, and also more broadly, is the survey design. Survey design studies are characterised by the use of a questionnaire as the data collection tool. All of you would have participated in a survey through participation in the population census. Surveys provide information about attitudes, beliefs, characteristics and other phenomena of interest. For example, Cho et al (2013) conducted a cross-sectional survey of nurses in acute hospitals via a questionnaire including items on the incidence of needle-stick or sharp injuries, use of protective equipment, nurse characteristics, and organisational characteristics. The authors identified the prevalence of and factors associated with such injuries among hospital nurses.

Non-experimental studies are sometimes referred to as correlational studies or non-intervention studies. 'Correlational' describes the statistical analysis used to determine if there is a relationship between variables. In Papastavrou et al's (2014) study, the authors sought to examine the relationships between nurses' perceptions of their professional environment and how they prioritise care within the constraints of a resource limited environment. The study found that teamwork, leadership and autonomy, and communication about patients accounted in total for 18.4% of the variance in prioritising overall patient care.

STUDENT CHALLENGE

For you as a beginning health professional it is essential that you start to learn how to translate information and evidence into clinical practice. There are many websites and tools you can use to help you understand the validity and reliability of the studies you read (see PICOT and evidence-based practice information in Chapter 10).

When developing clinical practice guidelines, all clinicians are expected to access the National Health and Medical Research Council (NHMRC) website, NHMRC levels of evidence and grades for recommendations for developers of guidelines (2009) (PDF, 140KB), and use the table named: NHMRC Evidence Hierarchy: designations of 'levels of evidence' according to type of research question. Please access this document and use the table to describe the characteristics of a quantitative published study of your choice.

1. Can you tell why they are classified as they are? Choose several other nursing or midwifery research articles.
2. Can you pick out the studies that are quantitative? (Look for studies that have numbers and symbols and discuss various types of statistical analysis.)
3. Could you determine any further classification of the quantitative studies you looked at? This can be more difficult. Some will tell you in the title or the abstract. Others give some clues but fail to identify the study classification. For example, an experimental study might talk about an intervention or use of experimental and control groups (e.g. randomised control trial).

What is the research process?

The research process is an orderly series of phases and steps that guide the researcher from asking a question to finding an answer. The answer, in turn, suggests new questions for future research. Thus research can be envisioned as a circular process with attendant phases and steps, as illustrated in Figure 5.1. These phases and steps guide the research process. Although they occur in the general order indicated by Figure 5.1, the order may vary, steps may overlap and the researcher may shift back and forth between various steps or phases. In some studies, certain steps are unnecessary and are omitted. However, we can use these phases and steps as a guide to paint a picture of the research process. This will help you understand how a researcher develops and conducts a study.

Phase 1: conceive the study

The first task for any researcher is to make a decision about what to study. The activities in this phase involve reading previous research and theory, theorising and thinking about the area of interest. The steps of problem identification, literature review, and conceptual and methodological considerations, are often developed simultaneously and lead to the formulation of research hypotheses or research questions that you intend to investigate.

Identify the problem

The problem statement describes the focus or intent of the research study. It identifies what concepts will be researched and is commonly undertaken using a Problem/Patient group, Intervention, Comparison, Outcome and Timeframe (PICOT) framework, as discussed in detail in Chapter 10. The purpose of the study (i.e. intent or goal) is also described and limits are drawn to ensure

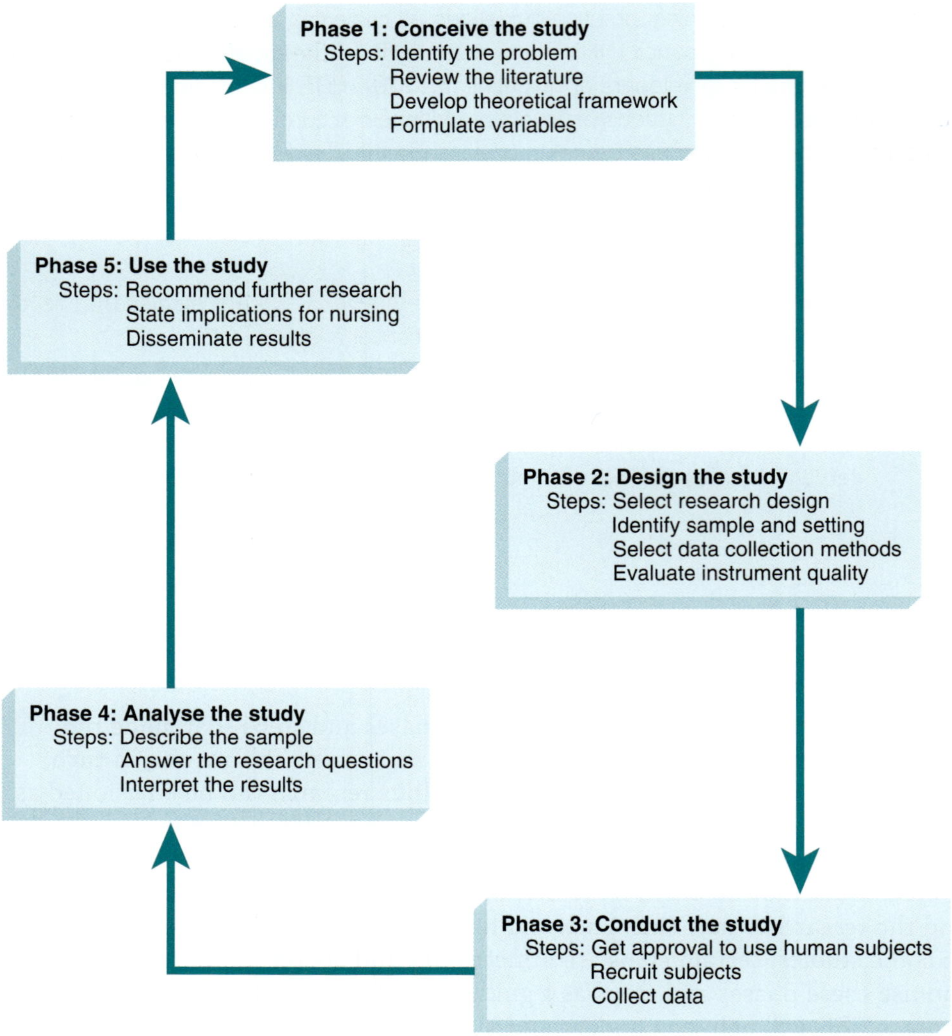

FIGURE 5.1
The phases and steps of the research process

the study is both relevant and achievable. Many research studies include more than one problem statement or statement of purpose. This may indicate increased complexity of the study. Whether the researcher uses a problem statement or a statement of purpose or both, the intent is the same. These statements guide and focus the research (see Box 5.2 for examples of problem statements).

Review the literature

The literature review involves a search for information that is relevant to the identified problem area. The literature tells us what is currently known about the area under study, where there is a gap in knowledge, and how this particular study fits into a larger picture. It is much like looking at the picture on the jigsaw box when trying to find how a single piece fits. The literature review may provide information about the best way to design the study or the best way to measure the concepts being examined. It may also serve to refine and define the problem being studied and help to develop the theoretical frame of reference for the study. Research studies that have examined some of the same or similar concepts are the most helpful and form the backbone of the literature review. The procedures used to conduct a literature review and sources used are outlined in Chapter 11.

Formulate variables

Variables are identified concepts or traits that are measured, manipulated or controlled in a research study and are discussed in detail above.

Once variables are identified in your study design, they must be defined. Variables are defined in two ways. The first is a conceptual definition. This is the type of definition you are familiar with, the kind you look up in the dictionary. It tells what the word means in the given context of a particular study. The second definition is an operational definition. This definition spells out how the variable will be measured. For example, the variable 'anxiety' might be conceptually defined as 'uneasiness or apprehension about an impending event'. The operational definition might state 'anxiety will be measured using the Clinical Anxiety Rating Scale'. Operational definitions are often decided in phase 2 of the study.

In a specific research study, variables come from the concepts identified in the problem statement and are specified in the form of research questions or hypotheses. The population to be studied is also specified in the research questions or hypotheses. (We discuss populations in the next phase of the research process.) Box 5.3 provides examples of research questions and hypotheses as derived from the problem statement.

A hypothesis is an 'educated guess' about the relationships between variables and the expected outcomes of the study. It tries to predict the nature of the relationship between variables. The researcher makes these 'educated guesses' based on the review of literature and the theoretical framework. The results of the research study will either support or refute the hypotheses established in the first phase of the study. Research studies that use hypotheses are usually either explanatory or predictive in nature.

Phase 1 can be thought of as the conceptualisation phase. It lays the foundation for the research study. When done well, the foundation is firm. When this phase is not well thought out, the study rests on a slippery slope, which makes the findings of the study suspect. Now you have read about phase 1, try the next student challenge.

STUDENT CHALLENGE

Perusing Phase 1

Select several quantitative research studies from the online databases available through your library.

Scan these studies and see if you can identify each of the elements we have discussed in phase 1. Remember, the studies may not contain all elements.

1. Find the problem statement. Can you find examples of the interrogative form and the declarative form? Did the studies label it as a problem statement? If not, look for a statement such as 'the purpose of the study was ...' or examine the title or the abstract.
2. Was a literature review present? Did it help you understand the context of the study better?
3. Can you identify the study design?
4. Can you identify the variables being studied?
5. Can you find the research hypotheses or research questions? Can you identify independent and dependent variables? What about extraneous variables? (Look for phrases such as '... was controlled using ...'.) Did the researcher state how the variables were defined?
6. What sort of hypotheses are used? Did they identify the null hypothesis or were the hypotheses alternative or directional in nature?
7. Were different elements easier to spot in some studies than in others? Were some elements obvious in all the studies? Were any elements missing in all the studies you looked at?

Phase 2: design the study

In phase 2 of a research study, the researcher makes decisions about how to conduct the study. The researcher designs the study and plans methods for conducting the study. The research question determines the research design. It is very important to achieve coherence between the aims of the project, the problem statement or research question, hypotheses and design of the study. The researcher selects the sample, determines the appropriate setting, operationally defines the variables, selects and evaluates the instruments and outlines procedures for data collection. These decisions have implications for the credibility of the results of the study. If the research design is flawed or inappropriate, then the findings are suspect.

Let's examine each step involved in making decisions about the study design. The order of the steps may vary slightly when making decisions, but all of the steps are crucial in the design process.

Select research design

The research design is the overall plan that guides how the study is conducted and analysed. As we stated earlier when discussing classifications of research studies, there are three major categories of quantitative research design: experimental, quasiexperimental and non-experimental. There is one important distinction between experimental/quasiexperimental and non-experimental designs. The researcher is an active agent in an experimental or quasiexperimental study, deliberately manipulating the independent variable in an attempt to change the dependent variable. This manipulation is often labelled a treatment or an intervention. In a non-experimental study, the researcher is an observer and recorder and there is no manipulation or treatment. Review the material previously presented in this chapter to understand the application of experimental, quasiexperimental and non-experimental designs.

Identify setting and sample

Once the research design has been established, the subjects and setting for the study must be considered. The setting is the physical location for and the conditions under which the study takes place and it is important to consider whether the site is appropriate for the intervention and whether the site will enable an appropriate sample to be included in the study. For example, the study in example 2 in Box 5.3 investigates children receiving suture repair (population) and measures their anxiety level and behaviour (dependent variable) depending on the presence or absence of their parents (intervention and independent variable). This study took place in the suture room of an emergency department in one children's hospital (site). Similarly, the study involving premature infants (population) and stimulation (intervention and independent variable) (example 3, Box 5.3) took place in a Neonatal Intensive Care Unit of a large teaching hospital (site). The location of this study is important in particular as the Neonatal Intensive Care Unit has computerised equipment capable of continuously monitoring $P\text{O}_2$ levels on all infants, is a tertiary referral hospital from the surrounding suburbs and will therefore be an appropriate location for both the intervention and the study population.

The subjects of interest for a research study are known as a population. These subjects possess certain common characteristics or traits that make them appropriate for inclusion in the study. For example, young children with lacerations that require sutures are the subjects of interest in example 2 in Box 5.3. Study subjects need not be human; they might be animals such as mice, bacteria colonies in Petri dishes, or data such as vital signs. Subjects are selected using a process known as sampling. Populations are usually large and it is not necessarily feasible to study every individual in that population. To overcome this, the researcher chooses a representative sample or subset of a population (Fig 5.2).

When selecting the sample, researchers try to make sure the included sample has characteristics that resemble the overall population characteristics

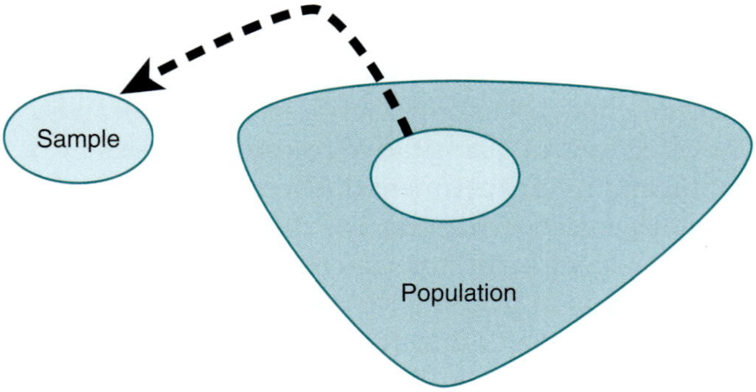

FIGURE 5.2
Sampling

as closely as possible. A sample that represents the larger population allows the study results to be applied to the whole population. For example, if the children in the laceration study were less anxious during the suturing process when a parent was present, it is helpful if this finding can be applied in many emergency departments and to all children receiving sutures for lacerations. The ability to apply study results from the sample to the larger population is known as generalisation. The ability for study results to be generalised from the sample to the broader population is determined by the sampling process chosen as part of the study design.

There are two major categories of samples: (1) probability; and (2) non-probability. Box 5.5 presents and defines sample categories and subcategories. Review these so you can recognise the vocabulary used to describe sampling in a research article and can distinguish between probability and non-probability types of samples.

In a probability sample, the subjects are chosen at random. Each subject in the population has an equal chance of being in the sample. Probability samples ensure mathematical representation of the population and a high degree of certainty in their results. Therefore, when researchers choose probability sampling techniques they ensure the results of the study can be generalised to the population and are able to tell whether their results occurred by chance.

Subjects in a non-probability sample are not chosen at random. There is no way to assess whether they are representative of the population. Therefore the results can only be applied to the sample and cannot be generalised to the population. It is very important for you to note the sampling method used when you read research studies, because it tells you whether you can confidently apply the study results to your own clinical situation as well as the specific setting of the study.

At this point you may be asking, 'If probability samples are so much better than non-probability samples, why would a researcher ever use a non-probability sample?' Good question! Non-probability sampling may be preferable for several reasons – it is less expensive and requires less time and

Box 5.5
Categories of samples

Probability sampling – random selection

1. A simple random sample is the most basic form of probability sampling in which all subjects in a population are numbered and a sample is selected randomly using a lottery or table of random numbers.
2. A stratified random sample is subdivided into groups according to some characteristic (e.g. gender – males and females; or ethnicity – those from an English-speaking background, those from a non-English-speaking background, Torres Strait Islander or Aboriginal). The subsets are then randomly sampled.
3. A cluster sample is a multistage sampling in which larger clusters (groups) are randomly selected first (e.g. hospitals) and then smaller clusters are randomly chosen (e.g. patients).
4. A systematic sample selects every *k*th (e.g. every fifth or seventh or twentieth) subject from a randomised list.

Non-probability sampling – no random selection

1. A convenience sample selects the most convenient subjects at hand.
2. A quota sample is conveniently selected according to pre-specified characteristic(s) (e.g. gender or ethnicity). A specific number from each characteristic is chosen.
3. A purposive sample uses subjects that are handpicked by the researcher, based on a set of defined criteria.
4. A non-random systematic sample selects every *k*th (e.g. every fifth or seventh or twentieth) subject from a non-randomised list or every *k*th subject as they become available (e.g. every third patient admitted to the unit).

fewer resources and, sometimes, generating a probability sample is not possible. For example, it may not be possible to generate a list of people in the population because no comprehensive source exists. At other times, generating such a list can be prohibitive in terms of time and expense. Think about compiling and numbering a list of 1000 or 10 000 or 100 000 subjects in a population. Access to certain subjects in a population may also be cost-prohibitive (e.g. subjects in another city, state or country). Access to certain subjects may be denied by the institutions or by the subjects themselves. Some populations are hidden and/or hard to access (e.g. stigmatised populations such as sex workers). You will find that many nursing and midwifery research studies take a pragmatic approach and use non-probability sampling techniques. Our ability to identify whole populations may change with the increases in population databases, research funding and support for nursing and midwifery, and as research studies and capabilities grow in sophistication and complexity.

The size of the sample is also important in ensuring the sample is representative of the population. As a general rule of thumb, the larger the sample, the more representative of the population. The researcher considers several factors when selecting a sample size. These include the size of the overall population, the availability of the population, the variation in characteristics of the population, the cost and time expended per subject, and the number of participants (power analysis) required to make sure the findings can be analysed to significance. The size of the sample also affects the statistical techniques that can be used. Statistics used to analyse several variables simultaneously (multivariate statistics) require larger sample sizes. When you read a research study, check the sample size. If a sample is small (under 30 subjects), particularly if it is a non-probability sample, the statistical strength of the study is limited and you should only use the study results with caution.

Calculation of sample sizes to allow for statistical testing of hypotheses is called 'power analysis'. Many research reports do not provide adequate justification for sample size; instead, it may seem that an arbitrary number is selected. Studies that provide power analysis will provide a justification for a sample size and ensure the size is neither too low nor too high. Low power is caused by having too few subjects in a study and where statistical analyses are limited. Low powered studies are not able to provide decisive results and the findings may be overlooked as inaccurate. High power enhances the level of statistical testing and also the accuracy and probability of obtaining significant results. However, there is still the risk of having too many subjects in a sample. Large sample sizes require increased resources and could result in insignificant results appearing to be significant purely because of how many participants are enrolled in the study (Type 2 Error as mentioned above). Power analysis will vary between studies and can be calculated according to the individual circumstances of each study. There are computer software packages and online interactive sites that can assist with power analysis.

There are also ethical implications associated with conducting studies with power that is either too low or too high; research should only be undertaken if the results are going to be relevant and applicable, using too small a sample or too large a sample influences the accuracy of the results.

Use study results with caution when the sample is small and sampling is non-probable.

Select data collection methods

To examine the proposed research questions or hypotheses, the researcher must be able to collect measurable information on the variables. These measurable bits of information are known as **data**. Quantitative data are collected using instruments. These instruments are classified by the type of data they are designed to collect and are generally physiological, behavioural or psychological in nature. Physiological data (for physiological variables) are generally measured using specialised biophysical instruments and specialised expertise by the user. You would be familiar with several of the biophysical measurements used in healthcare and healthcare research, for example: sphygmomanometers; thermometers; pulse oximeters; electrocardiograph machines; electroencephalograph machines and so on. We regularly use these instruments in clinical practice.

Behavioural data (observable actions of the subject) are generally collected through observation. In quantitative research these observations are evaluated and assigned numeric values. For example, degree of uncooperative behaviour (Box 5.3) was observed and rated in the study of young children who were being sutured for a laceration. The nurse observed the child's behaviour and assigned ratings at several predetermined intervals during the suturing procedure (the scale is presented in Table 5.1).

Table 5.1
Uncooperative behaviour scale

Score	Behaviour
0	No crying or physical protest
1	Mild verbal protest (e.g. ouch) or quiet crying
2	More prominent verbal protest/crying with movement of body parts; still complies with physician's request
3	Protest and movement make the procedure difficult
4	Protest stops the procedure and behaviour is addressed before procedure can be reinitiated
5	General prolonged verbal protest and body movement with no compliance

Adapted from Venham, L.L., Gaulin-Kramer, E., Munster, E., et al: Interval rating scales for children's dental anxiety and uncooperative behaviour. *Pediatric Dentistry*, 2(3): 195–202, 1980.

Psychological measurements are used to collect data about knowledge, feelings and attitudes. As these variables cannot be directly observed, an instrument is used that asks the subject to self-report on these variables. Such instruments include questionnaires and interviews. Questionnaires pose a series of questions for the subject to answer. In a quantitative study, the questions are usually closed-ended. This means that the subject is asked to select from a range of choices. Box 5.6 contains several closed-ended questions that might appear on a questionnaire. Questionnaires are: easy to administer; relatively inexpensive; can be mailed to a large, widely dispersed sample; and offer anonymity to the respondent.

Questionnaires used in research generally contain some type of scale designed to measure a certain psychological variable. Scales are instruments that assign numerical values to a set of responses on a series of questions or statements. These numbers are then added together for a score. This score is used as a measurement of the variable. The most common scale type is the

Box 5.6
Sample questions on a questionnaire

Please circle the answer that best describes you.

1. Are you:
    - Male
    - Female
2. Are you currently:
    - Single (never married)
    - Married
    - Separated
    - Divorced
    - Widowed
    - Co-habiting

Likert scale. Subjects are given a series of statements and several ranges of agreement or disagreement to choose from (agree through to strongly disagree with statements), frequency (very frequently through to never or not at all), importance (very important through to unimportant), or quality (high-quality through to low-quality). Box 5.7 gives an example of a few items from a Likert scale measuring attitudes to continuing education for nurses and midwives. The response to each item is assigned a number and the numbers from all the items are added to reflect the overall degree of agreement with the concept being measured.

One factor that will influence the efficacy of a questionnaire is the response rate. In particular, many mailed questionnaires have a low response rate, meaning that a lot of money can be wasted on postage and printing if the questionnaire is not filled out accurately and returned. For this reason it is very important to ensure optimal questionnaire design. An effective questionnaire is well laid out, easy to read with appropriate colours and font, not too onerous (not too long or too many questions), in plain language and accompanied by accurate instructions in language that is simple and easy to understand. Another issue to consider when mailing out questionnaires is that there is no guarantee the respondent will be the intended target. For example, a questionnaire about a women's health issue could be mailed out with the intent that a woman will complete it. However, the woman's husband or male partner could fill it out and the researcher would have no way of knowing this. Nor would the researcher be aware of group answers where a person answers the questions a certain way after being pressured or

Box 5.7
Sample Likert scale

SA	Strongly agree	**D**	Disagree
A	Agree	**SD**	Strongly disagree
U	Uncertain		

Please circle your degree of agreement or disagreement with the following statements:

1. Continuing education should be compulsory for nurses and midwives.
   SA A U D SD
2. Nurses and midwives should be able to demonstrate their clinical competency every year.
   SA A U D SD
3. Nurses and midwives should be encouraged to undertake postgraduate studies.
   SA A U D SD
4. Continuing education is only necessary for nurses and midwives if they are seeking promotion.
   SA A U D SD
5. Continuing education should be part of career planning for every nurse and midwife.
   SA A U D SD

influenced by others; for example, a group of teenagers completing a questionnaire in a magazine.

Interviews used to collect data in a quantitative study usually consist of a series of highly structured questions with the responses assigned numbers for statistical analysis. A structured interview is much like an oral questionnaire in which the investigator reads the questions and asks the respondent to provide their chosen response. Interviews do offer the advantage of allowing the interviewer to clarify responses and to ensure that all questions are answered. It also ensures the person who answers the questions is the one for whom the question was intended and that there is a reduced possibility of outside influences for responses given. The chief disadvantages are the added time and expense involved in the interview process.

Appropriate instruments must be selected to measure each variable being studied. This includes desired descriptive variables (e.g. gender, education level, and marital status), independent and dependent variables and important extraneous variables (e.g. variables that must be controlled using statistics).

Choices are made based on criteria such as the category of data (e.g. physiological, behavioural, psychological), cost, availability and the skill required to administer the instrument. It is important that the instrument chosen is appropriate for the data category, research question and is the best quality instrument the researcher can access.

Evaluate instrument quality

Instrument quality plays a big role in the selection of an appropriate instrument. The researcher is looking for 'good' instruments to measure the variables in the study. What is a 'good' instrument? A good instrument is one that is valid and reliable – validity and reliability are important concepts because a valid instrument measures what it is supposed to measure. A reliable instrument measures the variable consistently, dependably and accurately, across settings and with repeated use by different people. If an instrument is not reliable it cannot be considered valid, as you cannot rely on the accuracy of the results. There are various ways that researchers can establish the validity and reliability of instruments. Box 5.8 lists some frequently used ways of establishing validity and reliability. Familiarise yourself with these terms.

Instruments used in research studies should be evaluated for reliability and validity before use in the study. When you are reading research papers look for comments from the authors in relation to how they have ensured validity and reliability of the techniques they have used. These should all be reported. In the paper by Morris et al (2014), for example, the authors reported they used exploratory factor analysis and path analysis to establish construct validity and reliability of the survey instrument (Irish Nursing Minimum Data Set for General Nursing).

Biophysical measurements are generally accepted as valid measures of the variable; that is, we accept that they measure what they say they measure. However, reliability is an issue; that is, how consistently, dependably and accurately these can measure across different settings and be used by different people. Reliability can be addressed by ensuring these instruments are calibrated and the operators have sufficient and equivalent expertise. Questionnaires, scales, interviews and observations all need to be assessed for some form of reliability and validity to ensure the quality and credibility of the data collected. Negative implications could include the researcher's time, effort, financial costs and costs to the participant if instruments cannot be trusted to produce the desired results. A lack of reliability weakens the study findings so, no matter how meticulous a researcher has been with all other aspects in the conduct of the study, using untested instruments can defeat the purpose of the research and in some cases the findings are not reliable for use in practice. If the data are suspect, then the study results are suspect.

Now we have covered what is involved in phase 2 of a research study, take some time to complete the following student challenge.

Box 5.8
Types of validity and reliability

Validity

Validity is the extent to which an instrument measures what it says it measures.

Content validity

Content validity is assessed by a logical evaluation and judgment of whether the instrument adequately reflects the content of the concept. A blueprint may be used to construct the instrument, or a panel of judges may be asked to evaluate the instrument. This is a weak form of validity.

Criterion validity

Criterion validity is assessed using statistical measures. Instrument scores are correlated to scores on measures of selected external criteria. Also called concurrent or predictive validity, this is a stronger form of validity.

Construct validity

Construct validity is assessed using a combination of logic and statistical measures. It looks for the underlying meaning of the construct being measured. This is the strongest form of validity.

Reliability

Reliability is the degree of consistency or dependability of an instrument.

Internal consistency

Internal consistency uses correlation statistics (e.g. Spearman's, Cronbach's alpha, or Kuder–Richardson) to measure whether the subparts of an instrument all measure the same thing. Reliability values range from 0 to 1. The closer the value gets to 1, the more reliable the instrument.

Equivalence

Equivalence correlates two different forms of the same instrument (also called parallel forms) or the scores of two or more raters (also called interrater reliability). Reliability is reported as an r-value, with values ranging from 0 to 1. The closer the value gets to 1, the more reliable the instrument.

Stability

Stability correlates the scores obtained when an instrument is administered twice to the same group of subjects over a period of time. Reliability or r-values range from 0 to 1. The closer the value gets to 1, the more reliable the instrument.

Interrater reliability

Interrater reliability refers to the degree to which two or more raters independently score the same ratings or values for that feature that is being observed or measured.

STUDENT CHALLENGE

Scrutinising Phase 2

Look again at the quantitative nursing or midwifery research studies you examined for phase 1. Scan these studies and see if you can identify each of the elements we have discussed in phase 2.

1. Can you identify the research design as experimental or non-experimental? Remember that experimental studies use terms such as experimental, quasiexperimental, treatment group, control group, treatment, intervention or random assignment. Non-experimental studies use terms or phrases such as retrospective, ex post facto, correlational, 'purpose is to describe …' or 'purpose is to explore …'.
2. Can you identify the sample? Can you determine what the population was? (This is harder, because it is often inferred rather than directly stated.)
3. Can you determine whether a probability or non-probability sampling technique was used? Look for cue words such as 'random' for probability samples and words such as 'convenience' for non-probability samples. If the technique is not specified, the chances are it is a non-probability sample. What was the size of the sample in the studies you chose?
4. Was the setting described?
5. What instruments were used to measure the variables? Could you tell if the instruments were reliable and valid?

Once all of the decisions have been made in relation to methodology, it is important to develop a realistic timeline. Some elements of a research project take longer than others. For example, gaining ethics approval can take a long time so it is best to begin the ethics process as soon as possible. Other elements such as gathering of literature may continue throughout the life of the project. When applying for funding for research and for ethics approval, researchers are asked to indicate a timeframe for the study; an example of a timeframe is provided in Table 5.2.

Developing a budget

Research is a labour-intensive activity and requires adequate resources. Increasingly stretched funding for healthcare and healthcare research requires researchers to provide clear and strong justification for all items listed in the budget. Funding sources will scrutinise the budget closely and will reject an application if the budget is inflated, or unrealistically low. Designing the resource use and budget in a study is a crucial part of a proposal and attention to detail and accuracy are essential. Research budgets are organised into four main sections: personnel, equipment, consumables and travel.

Table 5.2
Timeframe table

	Jan	Feb	March	April	May	June	July	Aug
Design study								
Literature review								
Ethics approvals								
Recruit participants								
Collect data								
Analyse data								
Preparation of report and dissemination of findings								

- Personnel: this part of the budget should cover costs such as research assistants, statistician support, project officers, and transcription and data entry costs.
- Equipment: the budget can cover essential equipment including recording equipment and measuring devices (if, for example, a researcher wanted to measure blood sugar level, glucometer equipment would be essential), printing of questionnaires or data collection tables. It can also cover computer hardware and software, however this is increasingly the assumed responsibility of the investigating institution.
- Consumables: this covers items such as photocopying, postage and stationery.
- Travel: this may be required for multisite projects and in the dissemination of research at conferences.

Phase 3: conduct the study

Once the study has been conceived and designed, the planning phases are over and the researcher is ready to conduct the study. The researcher will now implement the study as outlined in the design and collect the data using the designated instruments and procedures. This is often an exciting time in the research process when all the preparatory work comes together so the study can begin.

Ethics approval and recruitment

When researchers use humans as subjects for study, they must protect them from harm. The first step in conducting a study is to obtain approval from an institutional Human Resources Ethics Committee (HREC) for the use of human subjects as described in detail in Chapter 4. Recruitment of participants within the sample is also guided by the process outlined in Chapter 4.

Collect data

At this point, the researcher puts the design into action and carries out the prescribed procedures for the study in the appropriate research setting. Treatments are conducted, instruments are administered and data are generated and recorded. After the data are collected, the researcher organises it into an appropriate form for analysis and phase 3 is brought to a close.

Phase 4: analyse the study

Data cannot be reported to research consumers in raw form as results would be too cumbersome and would not provide a very good picture of the sample or a clear answer to the research questions or hypotheses proposed. It is important that researchers analyse and summarise the data so others can understand and appreciate significant elements within it.

Research students are often apprehensive and uncertain about statistical analysis and interpretation of the data. However, like many things in research, there is a clear systematic approach to take in analysing quantitative data. Statistical analysis is just another approach to understand the meaning of the research findings, and is something you will develop greater skills in if you undertake further study.

Before we discuss the steps involved in the analysis phase, some background information is needed. To analyse variables statistically, they must be measurable. This means the variables must be represented in number form. There are four levels of measurement: nominal, ordinal, interval and ratio. The level of measurement guides you to what statistical analyses you can perform on each variable. Box 5.9 describes the four levels of measurement, which are also discussed below under the heading 'Describe the sample'. For statistical purposes, interval and ratio data are treated the same way and therefore can use the same statistical tests.

Describe the sample

When analysing the data, the researcher wants to build a picture or description of the sample. **Descriptive statistics** group the data in ways to make it easier to understand and is built on descriptive statistical tests and analyses. There are four common ways to describe data using statistics: (1) frequencies; (2) measures of central tendency; (3) measures of spread (dispersion of the data); and (4) measures of shape.

Frequency and central tendency: One simple thing we can do is to count the number of times (frequency) something occurs for a particular variable. Frequency counts can then be turned into percentages (number in a category divided by the number for the variable). Table 5.3 presents sample frequencies and percentages taken from a sample of 90 nursing students. We can see from this example that the majority of students in this sample were single females aged between 22–27, who were satisfied with school. Frequencies are most useful when reporting nominal and ordinal data as you can group several scores

Box 5.9
Levels of measurement

Nominal variables

Nominal variables are divided into two or more categories and assigned arbitrary numbers. These numbers have no rank order (i.e. no sense of one category being ranked at a higher level than another).

Example:

Gender: male 1, female 2

Marital status: single 1, married 2, separated 3, divorced 4, widowed 5

Ordinal measurement

Ordinal measurement reflects a rank order among the categories, but we do not know how much greater than or less than.

Example:

Pain: ranked on a scale of 1 to 10 with 10 being the worst pain and 1 being no pain.

Anxiety: ranked on a 5-point scale from low to high.

Job satisfaction: ranked on a 5-point scale from strongly agree to strongly disagree.

Interval categories

Interval categories are made up of 'real' numbers that allow us to order the numbers and to know the distance between those numbers. The intervals between the categories are equal.

Example:

Temperature: interval between the numerical values of 76 and 77 degrees is the same as the interval between the values of 44 and 45 degrees. A degree is a precise interval.

Time: hours, minutes and seconds are precise intervals.

Ratios

Ratios have the same properties as interval data, except that the measurement scale for the variable possesses a meaningful zero. This means that when zero is reached on the scale, the variable is absent.

Example:

Weight, height: zero means no weight or no height.

Blood alcohol level: zero means the lack of alcohol detected in the person's bloodstream.

Table 5.3
Frequencies and percentages ($n = 90$)

Variable	Frequency	Percentage
Gender		
Female	82	91%
Male	8	9%
Current marital status		
Single	46	51%
Married	34	38%
Separated	2	2%
Divorced	8	9%
Satisfaction with school		
Very dissatisfied	2	2%
Dissatisfied	9	10%
Uncertain	18	20%
Satisfied	45	50%
Very satisfied	16	18%
Age		
19–21	16	18%
22–24	27	30%
25–27	36	40%
28–30	11	12%

together and report the frequency and percentage of the groups as we did with the variable 'age' in Table 5.3. Frequencies for interval and ratio data can also be plotted on a graph to form a frequency distribution (Fig 5.3).

Measures of central tendency are statistical tests that describe how data for a variable tend to cluster together in a distribution. Central tendency is most commonly described using mode, median and mean, and again the measure you use is determined by the level of measurement. Mode and median are used for nominal and ordinal data, and mean or average are used for interval and ratio data (Box 5.10)

Measures of spread and shape: We can also use statistics to describe how data are distributed. We can describe how data clump or cluster together, how they spread apart and what shape the frequency distribution forms. These statistics are defined in Box 5.10. All these statistics let us reduce large amounts of data about a variable down to a manageable description whose meaning is commonly understood. Imagine if you tried to make sense of the

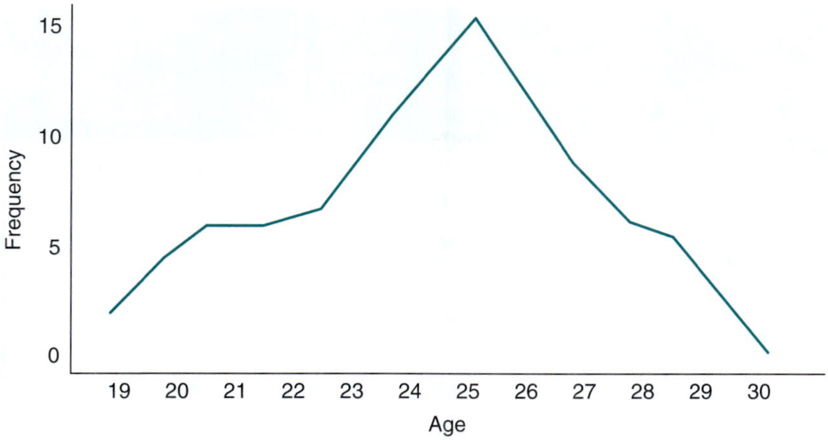

FIGURE 5.3
Example of a frequency distribution

reported ages for 5000 subjects if you had no precise way to count them, group them, or discuss how much the subjects were alike or different in age.

Most studies are conducted on a sample that is selected from a population. As such any statistics reported on that sample are estimates of the true population value (e.g. this could be a mean or proportion) and there will be some degree of error in the estimate. The confidence interval describes the range within which the supported value (i.e. size of the effect of an exposure) is expected to lie within a given degree of certainty (95% or 99%). Most health research uses a 95% confidence interval. Confidence intervals represent the probability of random errors, but not systematic errors (bias). Information on confidence intervals is readily available on the internet.

Answer the research questions

Once the researcher has described the sample, the next step is to analyse the data to answer the original research questions the study was designed to answer or to see whether the hypothesis was supported if this was the original aim of the study.

Descriptive analysis: In a descriptive study, the researcher can use the same descriptive statistics outlined above to describe the results from the variables set out in the research question; frequency, central tendency, spread and shape.

The research questions in example 1 in Box 5.3 regarding older people attending the emergency department were answered using descriptive statistics. The question 'What percentage of total emergency department visits are by older individuals over the age of 65?' was answered using frequencies and percentages. The question 'What are the primary reasons for presentation from older individuals over the age of 65?' was answered by categorising all the

Box 5.10
Descriptive statistical measures

Measures of central tendency are statistical tests that describe how data for a variable tend to cluster together in a distribution.

1. Mode (Mo) is the numerical value that occurs most often for a particular variable.
2. Median (Md) is the middle value in a frequency distribution of numbers.
3. Mean (M, X) is the average of all the scores.

Measures of dispersion are statistical tests that describe how data for a variable tend to spread out in a distribution.

1. Range is the distance between the highest and lowest scores for a variable.
2. Variance (V, s^2) is the average area of spread under a frequency distribution curve.
3. Standard deviation (SD, s) is the average distance of spread in a frequency distribution. It tells us how much, on average, the scores are spread out from the mean.
4. Confidence intervals (CI).

Measures of shape are statistical tests that describe the shape of the distribution for a variable.

1. Normal, where the curve or shape is bell-like.
2. Skewness reflects the degree of symmetry or asymmetry of the distribution curve (e.g. is the distribution symmetrical or asymmetrical?).
3. Kurtosis is the height of the distribution (e.g. how tall or flat is the distribution curve?).

primary reasons for presentation to an emergency department then reporting frequencies and percentages of each category.

Analysis of relationships or differences between variables: If the study asked questions or stated hypotheses that looked at the relationships or differences between variables, then the researchers need to use statistics that enable analysis of these relationships or differences. A wide variety of statistical tests are available for such analysis and the choice of each test depends on the number of variables, the level of data collected and the questions being asked. Increased access to personal computers and sophisticated statistical software has increased the complexity of statistical tests used. Many studies now identify and examine greater numbers of variables because analysis of multiple variables is now readily available. This means that reports of statistical analysis and study are increasingly complicated, making reading and understanding the results section of most studies difficult. At this stage it is not expected that you would recognise or understand why particular statistics were selected, or the precise meaning of the numbers generated by those tests.

Most hospitals and universities have statisticians who can help you to understand statistical issues if you are undertaking a research project. As a clinician, you will need a basic understanding of core concepts so that you can understand the researchers' interpretation of their results.

The following strategies and information will help you with this.

1. Different statistics have different requirements for use. Selection of the appropriate statistic is based on several factors, including the number of variables to be analysed, the level of measurement of the variables, the nature of the question asked (e.g. testing relationships or differences) and the sampling procedure used.
2. Research hypotheses may be translated into statistical hypotheses. This is merely a restatement of the research hypothesis in symbol form and is used to help researchers with decision making.
3. The results of statistical tests are reported as a number (e.g. $t = 4.26$, $F = 3.98$, $r = 0.68$). The letter gives a clue about the statistical test used (e.g. *t* is a *t*-test, *F* is an analysis of variance (ANOVA) test, *r* indicates a correlation). Many multivariate statistics generate a series of numbers that tell the researcher about several variables and how they vary as part of a multiple variable set.
4. The results from statistical tests (the numbers) are either significant or not significant. Significance is reported using a *P*-value (e.g. $P = 0.17$, $P = 0.03$, $P = 0.01$). A *P*-value of less than 0.05 is generally considered significant. Some researchers use a *P*-value of less than 0.01 to decide if a value is significant. Sometimes, non-significance is reported by using the letters NS.
5. A significant *P*-value (0.05) means there is a less than 5% possibility that the relationship or difference found between variables was caused by chance. In other words, you can have a high degree of certainty, 95% certain, that a difference or real relationship (correlation) exists between the variables tested. The lower the *P*-value, the more significant the result and the decreased likelihood of the result occurring by chance.
6. Statistical results are often displayed in table form.

When you read the results section, do not panic over the numbers and the discussion of those numbers. The researcher will explain and summarise the statistical results in text at some point in the presentation of results or the discussion. Look for this summary as you read and see if they answer the research questions or hypotheses that were first discussed. You are looking for information as to whether the variables are related or not. Or whether a particular group had different results from another group.

In example 2 in Box 5.3, the research question is: 'Will there be a difference between the anxiety levels and disruptive behaviours of young children whose parents are present during laceration repair versus those with no parental presence?' A Hotelling *t*-square test was used and the test found there was no significant difference (*P*-value was higher than 0.05) in behaviour or anxiety in those children who had their parents present when compared to those children whose parents were not present.

Remember we noted that the effects of extraneous variables (influences from sources outside the study) were sometimes controlled using statistics? In the study of children's anxiety and behaviour, age was identified as an extraneous variable that might influence whether parental presence made a difference. Another statistical test (analysis of covariance: ANCOVA) was used to look at differences between anxiety and behaviour when you controlled for the age of the children as an outside influence (extraneous variable). Using this statistical test the researchers could see that if you look at younger children only, there was a significant difference in both behaviour and anxiety when parents were present, with younger children being less anxious and more cooperative. As children became older, parental presence did not affect anxiety or behaviour. Researchers often look at the influence of particular aspects of a population to make sure they have not missed anything by analysing the group altogether.

In example 3 in Box 5.3, the **research hypothesis** is: 'Premature infants who receive extra tactile stimulation will have higher oxygen (Po_2) levels than those who do not.' In this study a *t*-test was used to compare the average (mean) Po_2 levels between those infants who received stimulation and those who did not. The resulting *t*-value was significant ($p < 0.05$), indicating there was a difference between the Po_2 levels between the two groups.

Interpret the results

Once the statistical analysis has been performed and the results have been examined, the researcher must interpret the results. This means making sense of the findings and how they fit into the existing research literature. Findings from descriptive studies are used to secure a tentative picture. There is very little to interpret because no relationships are tested among the described variables. Findings from exploratory studies that ask questions about relationships or differences among variables provide a starting point for the researcher to explain why relationships or differences were or were not present.

Findings from studies in which relationships or differences were predicted in the form of hypotheses allow for and require the most interpretation. An explanation of the findings is straightforward if the hypothesis was supported:

- The researcher would use the theoretical evidence to make a guess about variable relationships and whether this has been supported as was anticipated.

- The study would be interpreted to lend more proof to the underlying theoretical foundations.

However, if the hypotheses are not supported, the researcher must try to explain whether the negative result was due to a problem in the theoretical structure or the design of the study? Answers to these questions are usually presented in a discussion section and lead to the final phase of the process.

STUDENT CHALLENGE

Seeking Statistics

Examine your chosen research studies for the analyses used and the results of the analyses.

1. Can you locate a description of the sample? (Some studies include the description when discussing the sample and sampling techniques in the methods or research design section of the study.)
2. Can you find the answers to the research questions or hypotheses that were posed?
3. Can you locate where the findings were tied to the literature?

Phase 5: use the study

One important phase remains after the researcher discovers the answers to the questions posed in a study. It is important that the research findings are used to make recommendations for further research, to advise on the implications of this research for current practice and to share the findings with a broad audience so that others can learn from this knowledge. This phase completes the research process, emphasises its circular nature and ensures results are shared with the research consumer.

Recommend further research

Once the findings are stated and discussed, the researcher must decide what the findings mean for future research, what the next research study might look like and recommendations for further research to ensure the circular nature of the process. That researcher or another researcher can accelerate the advancement of nursing or midwifery knowledge and the usefulness of the current study by building a new study on the one just completed.

The researcher also examines and discusses any problems encountered while doing the study, known as 'limitations', to allow future researchers to correct error that might occur when repeating or extending a similar study. Examples of limitations might include uncontrolled extraneous variables that interfered with study results, difficulties in data collection, and not having enough subjects to complete advanced statistical analysis; this reduces confidence in the credibility of the study.

State implications for practice

The researcher must also decide what implications, if any, the study results can provide for nursing or midwifery practice. This assists the research consumer (i.e. all of us) in making use of the study results to provide the most effective and safe patient care.

Disseminate results

The final obligation on the part of the researcher is to disseminate the results of the study. The most common forms of communication are through peer reviewed published articles in nursing or midwifery research or specialty journals or through presentations at conferences. Publishing research as an article in an internationally recognised, well read and cited journal, has the most widespread effect. The resources required to undertake research and the burden of research on participants, places a responsibility on the researcher to communicate what was found to the research consumer so that there is an opportunity for the research to influence future clinical practice and research. More about this important step in later chapters.

STUDENT CHALLENGE

Entertaining the End

1. Examine your chosen research studies for future research recommendations and implications for nursing or midwifery practice.
2. Rejoice in the fact you have now worked through the entire research process.
3. In an upcoming chapter, we talk more extensively about how to read and critique research articles, so don't worry if you still feel uncomfortable with the material you're reading.

Once the results have been communicated, the researcher's job is finished and the research consumer's job begins. Health professionals have an obligation to keep their practice current and grounded in a solid scientific knowledge base. Health professionals need to develop skills to easily access and interpret relevant research so that they can provide the most effective and safest practices for individuals in their care.

RESOURCES KIT

Want to know more about quantitative research?

- Try entering 'quantitative research' as a search phrase using a search engine on the internet. A variety of interesting websites are devoted to 'quantitative research'.
- If you want more details and guidelines for different types of quantitative research try looking at some established reporting guidelines that are available on the internet. See some of the sites listed below:
  - STROBE **St**rengthening the **R**eporting of **Ob**servational Studies in **E**pidemiology http://www.equator-network.org/reporting-guidelines/strobe
  - CONSORT – **Con**solidated **S**tandards **o**f **R**eporting **T**rials http://www.equator-network.org/reporting-guidelines/consort
  - PRISMA – **P**referred **R**eporting **I**tems for **S**ystematic Reviews and **M**eta-**A**nalyses http://www.equator-network.org/reporting-guidelines/prisma.
- Check out the National Health and Medical Research Council (NHMRC) 2009 levels of evidence and grades for recommendations for developers of guidelines. Online. Available: https://www.nhmrc.gov.au/guidelines/resources-guideline-developers. 25 November 2014.
- Visit the book's Evolve website at http://evolve.elsevier.com/AU/Borbasi/maze for further information.

References

Adhikari UR, et al: An Exploratory Study to Identify Factors Associated with Noncompliance of Medications and Recommended Lifestyle Behavior after Renal Transplantation–A Pilot Study, *International Journal of Nursing Education* 6(1):73–77, 2014.

Brettle A, Raynor M: Developing information literacy skills in pre-registration nurses: An experimental study of teaching methods, *Nurse Education Today* 33(2):103–109, 2013.

Cho E, et al: Factors associated with needlestick and sharp injuries among hospital nurses: A cross-sectional questionnaire survey, *International Journal of Nursing Studies* 50(8):1025–1032, 2013.

Gray LC, et al: Profiles of older patients in the emergency department: Findings from the interrai multinational emergency department study, *Annals of Emergency Medicine* 62(5):467–474, 2013.

Hayes B, Douglas C, Bonner A: Predicting emotional exhaustion among haemodialysis nurses: a structural equation model using Kanter's structural empowerment theory, *Journal of Advanced Nursing* 70(12):2014.

Hickman LD, Rolley JX, Davidson PM: Can principles of the Chronic Care Model be used to improve care of the older person in the acute care sector?, *Collegian (Royal College of Nursing, Australia)* 17(2):63–69, 2010.

Losa Iglesias, ME, Becerro de Bengoa Vallejo R: Prevalence and relationship between burnout, job satisfaction, stress, and clinical manifestations in Spanish critical care nurses, *Dimensions of Critical Care Nursing* 32(3):130–137, 2013.

Morris R, Matthews A, Scott AP: Validity, reliability and utility of the Irish Nursing Minimum Data Set for General Nursing in investigating the effectiveness of nursing interventions in a general nursing setting: A repeated measures design, *International Journal of Nursing Studies* 51(4):562–571, 2014.

National Health and Medical Research Council (NH&MRC): *NHMRC levels of evidence and grades for recommendations for developers of guidelines*, 2009. Online. Available: https://www.nhmrc.gov.au/guidelines/resources-guideline-developers. 25 November 2014.

Papastavrou E, et al: Rationing of nursing care within professional environmental constraints: a correlational study, *Clinical Nursing Research* 23(3):314–335, 2014 Jun.

Shelton A, et al: Survey of attitudes of nurses and junior doctors to co-management of high risk surgical patients, *Contemporary Nurse* 44(2):189–195, 2013.

Song JE, et al: Empirical test of an explanatory theory of postpartum fatigue in Korea, *Journal of Advanced Nursing* 66(12):2627–2639, 2010.

Spoelstra SL, et al: An intervention to improve adherence and management of symptoms for patients prescribed oral chemotherapy agents: an exploratory study, *Cancer Nursing* 36(1):18–28, 2013.

Tsai HM, et al: The relationship of individual characteristics, perceived worksite support and perceived creativity to clinical nurses' innovative outcome, *Journal of Clinical Nursing* 22(17–18):2648–2657, 2013.

van der Riet P, et al: Are traditional Thai therapies better than conventional treatment for stroke rehabilitation? A quasi-experimental study, *European Journal of Integrative Medicine* 2014. doi:10.1016/j.eujim.2014.01.011.

Venham LL, Gaulin-Kramer E, Munster E, et al: Interval rating scales for children's dental anxiety and uncooperative behaviour, *Pediatric Dentistry* 2(3):195–202, 1980.

Wan XJ, et al: Disease stigma and its mediating effect on the relationship between symptom severity and quality of life among community-dwelling women with stress urinary incontinence: a study from a Chinese city, *Journal of Clinical Nursing* 23:2170–2180, 2014.

Williams KT: An Exploratory Study: Reducing Nursing Students Stress Levels Facilitate Perceived Quality of Patient Care, *Open Journal of Nursing* 4:512–519, 2014.

Wu SFV, et al: Differences in the perceptions of self-care, health education barriers and educational needs between diabetes patients and nurses, *Contemporary Nurse* 46(2):187–196, 2014.

CHAPTER 6

QUALITATIVE RESEARCH

Debra Jackson, Sally Borbasi and Tamara Power

CHAPTER OUTLINE

KEY TERMS

action research
case study
credibility
critical theory
data immersion
ethnography
findings
grounded theory
historical method
inductive reasoning
methodology
phenomenology
qualitative analysis
qualitative research
research design
setting or field
theoretical perspective/framework

LEARNING OBJECTIVES

After reading this chapter and following critical reflection the student will be able to:

1. Define qualitative research
2. Describe qualitative research classifications
3. Discuss conceptualisation for various research designs
4. Describe processes involved in conducting a study
5. Identify methods used in analysing various types of studies
6. Describe the reporting of study results and conclusions
7. Compare and contrast qualitative and quantitative research.

STUDENT QUOTE

When I read the qualitative study we were assigned about nurses' work in the ICU, I felt like I was right there living the experience. I could really identify with what was happening.

ABSTRACT

Qualitative research is used to examine subjective human experiences by using non-statistical methods of analysis. Research can be classified by the underlying theoretical perspective (paradigm) which is the researchers understanding of the nature of reality. For example, a constructivist approach subscribes to the idea that there are multiple subjective realities. A critical approach aims to critique existing ideologies, empower research participants and challenge political and social issues. Whereas, an interpretative approach will aim to explore, describe and make meaning of phenomena.

Qualitative research can otherwise be classified by research design (methodology) and the type of design chosen depends upon the question being asked. Research design classifications include phenomenology, ethnography, grounded theory, historical method and case study. Qualitative research processes vary across research methodologies. For example, a research question may ask, 'What is the experience of growing up without a father?' This question would be best answered by a phenomenological design.

The research aim (what the researcher wants to learn) provides a broad boundary that guides the conduct of the study. Data collection occurs predominantly through observation and in-depth interview, though other methods are also used. Analysis of the information or data generated by the research takes place using various methodologies to manage, interpret and synthesise it. With some qualitative approaches, analysis even dictates the direction and course of further data collection. Qualitative researchers search for patterns of meaning in the collected narrative, observational or other data. Findings are presented in a descriptive narrative format with excerpts of data used to illustrate key patterns and themes.

What is qualitative research?

In order to engage with the nursing and midwifery literature and effectively explore questions in those domains, an understanding of qualitative approaches as well as quantitative approaches is necessary. This chapter defines qualitative research, compares qualitative and quantitative approaches, explores various ways in which qualitative research can be classified and identifies and discusses phases of qualitative research processes.

Nurses and midwives have an interest in questions and issues that involve human subjectivity and in developing holistic understandings of people and their experiences. Understanding patient and family experiences can lead to changes in practice, education or management to improve healthcare delivery. These interests mean that nurses and midwives have embraced qualitative methods because these approaches provide methodical and rigorous pathways to exploring and drawing meaning from life experiences. As mentioned in chapter one, qualitative researchers draw on **inductive reasoning** processes and seek to examine and understand the whole of the phenomenon of interest. The focus of the research is on the process by which concepts are attributed with meaning in a given context rather than on cause and effect, or measurement of the concepts and their relationships. Qualitative researchers view reality as a subjective, multifaceted experience rather than as a single, fixed, objective actuality. Therefore even though people may experience a similar event, the meaning they attach to it and the way it affects them is nuanced and subject to individual interpretation.

Complex phenomena closely tied to the human experience or subjects about which little is known are readily understood using a qualitative approach, for example: What is it like to be lonely? What is the experience of loss through unsuccessful reproductive technology or a spontaneous miscarriage? How does it feel to be the recipient of a donated organ for a life-threatening condition? What is it like to be an international student studying nursing or midwifery in an Australian university? Information gained from investigating these research questions provides nurses and midwives with insight into how people experience events. Understanding experience means that policies and practices can be tailored.

Qualitative research uses multiple data collection procedures that rely heavily on researcher involvement. Qualitative researchers may seek to examine: individual lives and their stories and behaviour; organisations and their functioning; role relationships and intercommunications; or cultures and their conduct, interactions and social movement. Qualitative research projects are generally characterised by small sample sizes and rich descriptive data. Qualitative projects generate findings using analytical procedures that are non-statistical in nature.

No singularly defined scientific approach

No singularly defined scientific approach governs qualitative research. It is driven by multiple methods across various disciplines. Therefore, many aspects of qualitative research are not as clear-cut as those for quantitative research. While traditional quantitative research has concentrated on trying to establish cause and effect relationships, qualitative research permits multiple ways to explore the depth, richness and complexity inherent in most phenomena. Table 6.1 presents some of the differences between the two approaches.

Qualitative researchers do not claim their findings are generalisable. Because the study **methodology** embraces the examination of subjective phenomena, **findings** are considered to be idiosyncratic to a particular situation. That means they are considered to be representative of a particular person (or people), in a particular context or setting and not necessarily reflective of the experiences of the entire population. However, qualitative findings may be transferable to other people in similar contexts or settings. For example, understanding the experiences of refugees from West African countries could resonate with experiences of refugees fleeing other areas of the world.

Bias is a concept that needs to be understood in research. There are differing connotations regarding the notion of bias in qualitative methodologies to those you saw in quantitative research where bias/ subjectivity is something to be avoided at all costs. The prejudices,

Table 6.1
Differences between quantitative and qualitative research

Quantitative	Qualitative
Focuses on a small number of specific concepts and their relationships and differences.	Attempts to understand the entirety or whole of some phenomenon within a prescribed context.
Set on a predefined theoretical foundation. 'Educated guesses' made about relationship of concepts and study outcomes.	No preconceived theoretical boundaries or preconceived notions about study outcomes.
Researcher controls and interprets data.	Focuses on people's interpretations of events and circumstances rather than researcher's.
Tends to use larger samples.	Uses smaller samples.
Describes people in the study as 'subjects'.	Describes people in the study as 'participants', 'informants' or sometimes 'co-investigators'.
Uses language in a way that implies neutrality, such as writing in the third person.	Can be written up using the first person.
Uses structured procedures and formal instruments to collect information.	Collects information without formal structured instruments.
Collects information under conditions of control and manipulation.	Doesn't attempt to control the context of research, but attempts to capture it in its entirety.
Emphasises objectivity in collection and analysis of information. Attempts to exclude all forms of subjective 'bias'.	Attempts to capitalise on the subjective as a means of understanding and interpreting human experiences. Is comfortable with the notion of 'bias'.
Uses 'objective' tools to collect data.	Researcher is the instrument of data collection.

predispositions and experiences of the researcher and the influence these may have on the research findings are often made explicit in qualitative research (reflexivity). It is important to understand the differing 'methodological takes' on the need to counteract bias in qualitative research.

Many people assume that qualitative research is easily performed and fail to undertake adequate education in qualitative methodologies before embarking on qualitative studies. Qualitative research methodologies are founded on philosophical traditions and influences, the basic tenets of which need to be understood prior to designing the study. Conducting qualitative research requires every bit as much expertise as conducting quantitative studies and may take longer because of the nature of recruitment, data collection and analysis and in writing up – often considered a craft in itself. Qualitative research methodologies are not fixed, they are constantly evolving and developing. As previously stated it is important that qualitative researchers have a good grasp of the tenets that underpin qualitative research – this will inform the continued development of qualitative methods.

How is qualitative research classified?

Several terms are used to describe or classify qualitative research. We explore some of the more common classifications and terms so they will be familiar to you when you encounter them in the literature. Qualitative research may be classified by **theoretical perspective** or by **research design** (Box 6.1).

Box 6.1
Classification systems for qualitative research

Theoretical perspective – paradigm

1. Postpositivist
2. Constructivist-interpretive/interpretative
3. **Critical theory**
4. Poststructural/postmodern

Research design – methodology

1. Phenomenology, ethnomethodology
2. Ethnography, participant observation
3. Grounded theory
4. Historical method
5. **Action and applied research***
6. Case study

Adapted from Denzin & Lincoln (2011).
*Due to the challenges inherent in using this kind of methodology we only define **action research** in the Glossary of this textbook. Once you have a better understanding of the more commonly used approaches you will be able to understand better the differing specifics of action research and can explore it at your leisure.

Theoretical perspective (paradigm)

When theoretical perspectives are used to classify qualitative research they indicate the underlying belief systems that inform the research. Postpositivist research grew out of disenchantment with the radical objectivity of the positivist tradition and led to the beginnings of qualitative or interpretative approaches to research. The interpretive tradition seeks understanding of the world through the perspective of people who have lived a particular experience phenomenon (e.g. women who have had a mastectomy), or who have a particular way of being in the world (such as those from a particular cultural or social background). On the other hand, critical theorists are agents of change. They are interested in the social construction of experience and the material resources, power dynamics and ideologies of societies and use research to develop transformative knowledge (knowledge to effect positive and empowering change). Poststructural and postmodern studies may also be concerned with concepts such as culture, gender, power and oppression, and how these are represented in everyday life through language and structures such as large institutions and other constructs of social governance, which are often ingrained with social stereotypes and prejudices. Postmodern researchers believe in multiple realities.

Research design (methodologies)

Classification by research design or methodology provides us with slightly more direction as to what a qualitative study might be all about. Although it is important to understand that each of these designs is underpinned by a theoretical perspective, these are the most common classifications you are likely to see in the nursing and midwifery literature.

Phenomenology

Phenomenology is the study of lived experiences. The researcher examines human experiences through interviews and descriptions that come from the people who have lived a particular experience (also called phenomena). Phenomenological research seeks to describe the 'essence' of an experience as it is lived and to understand the objectivised subjective meaning of an experience. It is based on the premise that the way individuals 'know' is through their perceptions. Therefore reality is perceived as subjective and unique to individuals based on their experience. However, phenomenology is objectivised because it seeks to get beneath the everyday taken-for-granted assumptions that society may hold about a particular phenomenon and reveal it in a fresh light to produce new understanding.

Types of general questions that might be asked in a phenomenological study are 'What is it like to experience ...?', 'How does or did it feel?', or 'Tell me about your experiences of ...'. For example, 'Tell me about your experiences of being a surrogate mother.' After asking a broad general question, phenomenological researchers may use more specific questioning to probe and clarify aspects of the experience. Interviews and observations are most frequently used to collect data. Analysis occurs by searching the data for themes and patterns. Reflections are drawn on the meaning of the whole of the experience.

Recent examples of published Australian phenomenological studies can be found in articles by Kelly and McAllister (2013), who adopted a phenomenological approach to explore Australian nursing students' experience of preceptorship as they transitioned to new graduates, and Sambrano and Cox (2013) who used phenomenology to explore how Indigenous Australians experienced seclusion for mental illness. If done well, phenomenology as a research approach can be an extremely powerful vehicle for portraying human experience. Because it is founded on deeply philosophical ideas, at first its concepts can be hard to grasp. The work of UK academic Linda Finlay makes phenomenology more understandable (http://lindafinlay.co.uk/phenomenology). Finlay's (2011) description of the phenomenological project is highly recommended for those seeking to better understand this research approach.

See also the *Indo-Pacific Journal of Phenomenology*. It's free online and can be found at: http://www.ipjp.org.

Max van Manen's Phenomenology Online is also a good starting point: http://www.phenomenologyonline.com.

Ethnography

Ethnography is the systematic study of cultures or subcultures. It has its roots in anthropology. 'Culture' is a broad term whose meaning could range from study of a community in Western Samoa, to examination of a neighbourhood in Melbourne or Auckland, or investigation of the culture of a hospital, or of a group of people such as those who are homeless. Ethnography focuses on the study of the symbols, rituals and customs of an identified cultural group. It provides a picture of that identified group through observation and documentation of interactions in their daily lives.

Research questions in ethnography focus on issues such as:

- What procedures does a person follow that makes that person part of a group?
- What practices do group members engage in that result in a particular end product?
- What kinds of work do members engage in to accomplish the goals of the group?
- What are the everyday rituals, norms and patterns of behaviour within a specified social setting?

Ethnography focuses on group interactions and activities rather than on individual behaviours. Researchers immerse themselves in the culture or group to be studied. Data are gathered through observation and interview and are analysed for cultural patterns in an attempt to grasp the lifeways of a particular group in a particular environment.

Leininger was a prominent nurse ethnographer who has conducted a lifetime of ethnographic studies to examine the phenomenon of 'caring' from various cultural perspectives. She viewed caring as the central and unifying theme for the practice of nursing (Leininger & McFarland 2006). Recent examples of ethnographical studies in nursing can be found in a study by Lin et al (2013) that drew on ethnographic techniques to explore the factors that contributed to risk for patients being discharged from an Australian intensive care unit. Rollans et al (2013) used an ethnographic lens to explore the way child and family health nurses approach, interact with and undertake psychosocial assessment and screening with families in the early postnatal period. Early classic ethnographies can be attributed to pioneers such as Bronislaw Malinowski and Margaret Mead – later Claude Lévi-Strauss and Clifford Geertz. As is the case with the other qualitative methodologies, the philosophical, paradigmatic and theoretical aspects of ethnography are in a continuous cycle of deconstruction and reconstruction. Classical ethnographic approaches have been highly contested and reshaped/transformed over the years. Critical approaches to ethnography seek to emancipate and change.

Grounded theory

In **grounded theory** research, data are collected, analysed and used to develop a theoretical explanation and generate hypotheses for further research. Thus, the theory is generated from and 'grounded' in the data. Grounded theory is used to examine basic social processes that occur in a given phenomenon. Core concepts and dominant processes occurring in interactions are identified. Then the researcher attempts to discover explanations for these concepts and processes.

Research questions revolve around the chief concern or problem of individuals in a defined area. Examples of research questions that might be asked in a grounded theory study are 'How do people prepare themselves emotionally for surgery?' or 'How do cancer patients achieve hopefulness?' Data are collected using observational and interview techniques. Coding helps the researcher conceptualise the underlying patterns of the pieces of data collected. Categories of data are then developed. A form of analysis known as constant comparison analysis is used, whereby each piece of data is compared to data already collected. Concepts are developed as data are blended into larger and larger categories. Relationships between concepts are examined and then linked into a conceptual framework. The literature is then consulted to determine whether any similar associations have already been uncovered.

A grounded theory approach was used to explore the experience of living with long-term multiple myeloma after the first relapse (Stephens et al 2014). Maher (2013) also used this approach to develop a theory of how nurses respond to pressure between work and family commitments.

Try an internet search for Glaser and Strauss to find out more.

Historical method

Historical method research examines social phenomena by studying their historical context or their past. An historical study analyses a defined event, identifies key concepts and relationships and draws inferences in an attempt to understand the impact of that event on the present. Historical research involves revisiting an historical event, viewing it from a fresh perspective and searching for new meaning. Historical research is used to investigate past similar events or phenomena and derive common theoretical explanations of those events. For example, an historical study might try to explain a nursing shortage by examining past cycles of nursing shortages.

Historical researchers look at what has been, what is and what should be. The researcher begins with an acknowledged philosophical or interpretive point of view. This is important because this point of view influences how information is gathered, read and interpreted. Thus different researchers with varying points of view could revisit the same set of historical events and interpret them quite differently.

Historical research is somewhat different from the other forms of qualitative research discussed thus far. Rather than observing or interviewing people in the present, the historical researcher relies on historical documents and past written records. These might include diaries, letters, newspapers, articles, books, audio or videotapes, government or professional records and archives. People might be interviewed, but it would be to elicit their recollections of a past event. This type of interview is generally known as an oral history.

Historical research is not nearly as prevalent in the qualitative nursing or midwifery research literature as some of the other classifications we have discussed. However, an excellent example can be found in a paper by Fealy et al (2010), which critically examined sanitary reform in 19th-century hospitals, and the effects of this on theories of infection. The researchers drew on published sources including hospital archives and public health records. From this historical account, the authors have been able to point to issues that can be adapted to present-day situations. Dickinson and colleagues (2012) used an historical approach to examine the experiences of patients 'treated' for homosexuality and transvestism in the UK (1949–1992).

Case study

A **case study** is an in-depth examination of certain phenomena in an individual or in small numbers of individuals. It has also been used to examine the workings of a group, organisation or institution. It is a study of the particular. Nursing and medicine have long used this approach to detail what happens when a person has a certain disease. Medicine focuses on the disease and its processes, whereas nursing focuses on how the individual responds to the disease, the treatment and the environment. Much of the early research reported in the nursing literature used a case study approach.

Mixed methods (use of both qualitative and quantitative data) approaches are often used to generate comprehensive understandings of the case. For example, if you study an illness and its effects on an individual, some characteristics of the illness can be quantified or measured (e.g. vital signs, frequency of signs and symptoms). However, other characteristics are better described in narrative fashion (e.g. the feelings associated with illness).

Remember, a case can be any social unit – an individual, a family, a street, a school, a town, a hospital ward or birthing centre and so on.

The case study is used to examine one entity in-depth and to study and analyse patterns occurring in that one case. When researchers study more than one unit (e.g. individual, group or institution) they are really doing what is termed a collective case study or a series of case studies. This is conducted to see if patterns carry over from one case to the next. Case studies provide a way to study and analyse phenomena that are relatively rare. Though case studies have not been seen as frequently in the nursing literature as they once were, the method has undergone something of a renaissance and is being seen more frequently in the literature. Case study was used to examine the experiences of nurses working night shifts in regional hospitals in Australia (Powell 2013). Luck et al (2008) used an instrumental case study design to explore the meanings that Emergency Department nurses ascribe to acts of violence from patients, their family and friends and how these meanings impacted on the nurses' responses to such acts. Do the following Student challenge to enhance your understanding of these concepts. See Table 6.5 in the Resources kit for additional information.

STUDENT CHALLENGE

Scrutinising Study Classifications

1. Go to the library and look up the research studies cited as examples in the previous paragraphs. Can you tell why they are classified as they are?
2. Now choose several other current qualitative nursing or midwifery research articles. See if you can locate one study in each of the five qualitative research design categories. (Use the design category as your search term and limit the results to one or two years.)
3. Observe the general look and feel of the articles you've located. Note how they differ from quantitative reports. Note how they differ from one another.

What is the qualitative research process?

As you have already observed, qualitative and quantitative research look different in final written report format. The conduct of research is also different, with the processes of qualitative research being less segmented and therefore providing more scope for creative, expressive and innovative dimensions. Several phases of a given process frequently occur simultaneously or are revisited numerous times during the course of a study. Many of the decisions about various aspects of the process are made or altered as data are collected and certain trends or patterns are noted. There is an artistry and responsiveness to qualitative research, with a much greater focus on writing and rewriting in order to create a text representative of the phenomenon under examination.

In quantitative research, the conception and design of the study form a detailed blueprint for conducting, analysing and interpreting the study. In qualitative research, conceptualisation and design form only a broad umbrella-like structure for the study. Data collection and analysis dictate detailed study decisions. We will use the broad research phases identified in the previous chapter as we discuss the qualitative research process. However, keep in mind the phases are more fluid and less distinct for qualitative research and that the process varies for the different research classifications we have identified. You will see there are common issues to be addressed for all classifications of qualitative research. This section discusses those common features using phases of the research process identified in Chapters 5 and 11.

Phase 1: conceive the study

Identify the problem

As with quantitative research, the first task a qualitative researcher faces is to make a decision about what to study. The activities in this phase focus on identifying the phenomenon to be studied. This means an identification of some 'whole' or 'whole process' the researcher is interested in studying. This differs from quantitative studies, in which specific measurable concepts are identified. Table 6.2 presents specific examples by research design.

The initial identification of the phenomenon to be studied is done in the broadest sense. Phenomenological studies identify a phenomenon to be explored and seek individuals with experience of the phenomenon to be interviewed. Examples are parents of children in an intensive care unit or people who have undergone heart transplant surgery. The ethnographer may choose a group of people or a field setting with a broad statement of what is to be investigated. For example, the health beliefs and practices of Vietnamese immigrants or older residents of a nursing home might be selected. Grounded theorists begin with a broad area of social interest with no specific problem

Table 6.2
Identification of phenomenon

Research design	Identification of phenomenon
Phenomenology	Lived experience
Ethnography	Issue(s) of interest within a defined culture
Grounded theory	Basic social process
Historical method	Past event
Case study	Broad area for case(s) selection

in mind. For example, the area of interest might be hopefulness and cancer. Historical research begins with a broadly defined historical event such as the influence of Nightingale's system of nurse education in Australia and New Zealand.

Although all researchers bring their own frame of reference and belief systems to their work, qualitative researchers acknowledge and accept the role of subjectivity and intersubjectivity. This means qualitative researchers may state their preconceived notions or ideas about the study at the outset, while others will attempt to 'bracket' them by taking steps to set them aside during the investigation. A hypothesis-driven design is not a feature of qualitative research. However, historical research is a possible exception and may propose broadly stated hypotheses about expected relationships among historical phenomena.

Review the literature

Most qualitative designs include a literature review at this point. The review serves various purposes depending on the study classification. For example, phenomenological researchers may conduct a literature review to ascertain whether the area of interest (i.e. the lived experience) has been previously researched and there is a demonstrated need for such a study. They may also do a literature review to see how other researchers have used phenomenological ideas in the design and conduct of research. Ethnographers may do a literature review to help identify a culture or to identify a particular aspect of a culture that has not been previously researched. When a culture has been selected, they may do an extensive literature review for any available information about that defined culture.

Literature review is an integral part of historical research and the selection of the event to be studied. Historical researchers often conduct extensive literature reviews to place limits on the final topic to be studied. In fact, the initial literature review and narrowing of the event and the historical time span often require a large investment of time. Some case studies do an extensive literature review for all information available on the identified area of interest (e.g. a disease process). Others may review the literature as data are collected. Grounded theory researchers make a point not to look at the literature before beginning the study. In grounded theory studies, the literature review occurs after data collection and analysis have begun and theory has emerged from the data. Then the literature is reviewed and related to the developing theory emerging from the data. This is done to avoid 'contamination' of the data with preconceived concepts and notions about what might be relevant.

Formulate the research questions

Once the phenomenon of interest is selected, a research aim is formulated. This might be expressed in the form of a research question, purpose or objective. The aim is generally broad and serves as a general focus or guide for the study. More defined focal areas of the research often emerge as data are collected and analysed. Table 6.3 presents sample research aims for each design using the previously cited articles in the discussion on design classification.

Table 6.3
Sample research aims

Research design	Sample purpose
Phenomenology	To explore Australian nurse leaders' experiences of mentoring relationships. To explore the experiences of people living with hepatitis C.
Ethnography	To explore nurses' role on a medical assessment unit. To explore how nurses care for women during early miscarriage in a hospital gynaecological unit.
Grounded theory	To review the perceptions and strategies of drug users and nurses with regard to pain management in acute care settings. To explore the illness experiences and processes in relation to women undergoing coronary artery bypass graft surgery.
Historical method	To examine critically hospital sanitary reform with reference to theories about infection and contagion in Dublin hospitals, 1858–98. To trace the movement to professionalise nursing and midwifery that emerged in the colony of Victoria during the late 19th and early 20th centuries.
Case study	To analyse and describe women's different perceptions and experiences of childbirth following prolonged or normal labour. To explore the meanings that Emergency Department nurses ascribe to acts of violence from patients, their family and friends and how these meanings impact upon how nurses respond to such acts.

Do the following student challenge and see if you can identify the research intent in some sample studies.

STUDENT CHALLENGE

Reading Research Aims

Use the studies you found in the previous student challenge and the studies listed in this chapter.

1. For the studies that were identified in this chapter, see if you can locate the research aims listed in Table 6.2.
2. Now look at the other studies you located. Can you determine the research aim for each of them?
3. Examine the literature reviews. Can you tell when these were done? Are the reviews more comprehensive in some studies than in others?

Phase 2: design the study

Once the phenomenon has been identified and the general aim of the study is determined, the next phase is to determine the methodology and design the study around it. The chosen design dictates the general structure of the study and includes initial decisions about setting, sample selection and data collection methods. Remember, the qualitative process is fluid and sampling and data collection methods may evolve during the course of data collection.

Setting

The **setting** in qualitative research is often referred to as the 'field' because the study is set 'in the field' (i.e. the natural setting where the phenomenon under investigation occurs). Settings vary by type of research design. The selected setting assumes more importance in some research designs than in others. The data collection method may also influence the selected setting. Phenomenological research settings are usually chosen based on convenience for the people who are being studied. Since most of the data is collected through a series of interviews with individual participants, setting is secondary.

Ethnographical studies take place in a setting where the researcher can readily observe and interact with a grouping of people of a particular culture. If the culture of interest is people in an institution, a prison or nursing home might be an appropriate setting. If the culture of interest is the critically ill, the setting might be an intensive care unit. It is important that the setting in ethnographical research allows the researcher to see and interact with the people within the setting collectively. Observation is a key ingredient of an ethnographic study.

Grounded theory research takes place in a setting that allows the researcher to observe the selected social processes in action. This means an ability to observe both the environment and the selected participants in the study. Case study settings allow the researcher to view and interact extensively with the chosen case. Historical studies have no real setting. Data are collected from records, relics and artefacts located, for example, in libraries, museums, personal collections, or boxes in storage. Table 6.4 lists possible settings for the studies we've been following.

Samples and sampling

Samples in qualitative research tend to be small and selected using purposive or convenience sampling techniques, which means the sample is purposefully or conveniently chosen. The researcher is concerned that the selected sample be what is termed 'information-rich' – people who have experienced or are experiencing the phenomenon of interest and are willing and able to articulate that experience. This means the selected sample participants are able to provide a powerful picture of the phenomenon under study. For example, if the researcher wants to understand the experiences of women who have had 'change of life babies' they will be seeking women over the age of forty, who have experienced a planned or unplanned pregnancy and are willing to discuss the experience with the researcher.

Table 6.4
Examples of research settings

Research design	Sample settings
Phenomenology	Work, home and social setting
Ethnography	Work, home and social setting
	Hospital – operating room
Grounded theory	Clinical interaction
	Hospital and community
Historical method	None listed
Case study	Labour ward/birthing clinic
	Rural health services
	Emergency Department

Several other sampling techniques can be used to help provide an 'information-rich' sample. These include snowball, extreme, intensity, maximum variety and critical case (Denzin & Lincoln 2011). Box 6.2 discusses these techniques.

Box 6.2
Qualitative sampling techniques

Samples of convenience and purposive sampling

As described previously, these are commonly seen in qualitative designs.

In addition, the following may be seen.

Snowball sampling

This method involves getting recruited participants to help identify and recruit additional participants.

Intensity sampling

Selection of participants who are experiential experts or authorities about the selected phenomena (e.g. in the pain study, intensity sampling might choose those who have chronic pain).

Maximum variety sampling

The deliberate selection of participants who are different, who come from different backgrounds, for the purpose of observing commonalties of experience. (This is particularly helpful when exploring abstract phenomena such as love, joy or hope.)

Box 6.2
Qualitative sampling techniques—cont'd

Critical case sampling

Selection of participants identified as demonstrating what has been identified as a 'critical incident' while collecting and analysing data. (Once critical cases have been identified, additional purposive sampling is conducted to find cases that confirm or refute the critical case.)

Theoretical sampling

This technique is used in grounded theory whereby sampling continues until the theory is sufficiently developed.

Extreme or deviant case

Including highly unusual cases of the phenomenon of interest to make sure both the usual and unusual are captured. Incorporating deviant accounts adds to the credibility of research findings.

Grounded theory studies use a sampling technique called theoretical sampling. In theoretical sampling, the researcher begins by collecting and analysing data on an initial sample. This sample is called an open sample because the sampling process is not guided by data analysis. As data are collected and analysed (coded), concepts begin to emerge that will help form an evolving theory. These concepts are called categories and are identified by their repeated presence or absence in the data. The researcher then samples again, looking for additional data to support identified categories. The researcher continues sampling data collection and analysis until all identified categories are fully explored or saturated.

Sample selection in historical research is slightly different because the sample comprises data sources rather than people. The sampling process occurs simultaneously with data collection and analysis and is ongoing as the researcher refines the study topic. As the topic becomes more clearly defined, the pertinent data sources become more readily identified. This sampling process can cover an extended period of time. Initially the needed data are known only generally. The researcher spends time collecting and reading data sources, which allows the researcher to add greater clarity and definition to the chosen historical topic, which in turn allows the researcher to identify additional required data sources more clearly. Sampling and data collection cease when no new information is uncovered from several successive sources.

Data collection methods

Data for qualitative studies are gathered chiefly by use of observation and interview. When a researcher desires to study behaviour, activity and sequences of interaction, or the context or environment in which these behaviours and actions take place, observation is used. Observations may be classified by several features, such as structure, participation of the researcher and visibility of the researcher. Box 6.3 presents a fuller description of these classifications. Ethnographic studies use an unstructured participant approach. Grounded theory uses a combination of observational approaches.

Box 6.3
Classification of observation features

Structure

1. Structured: specified behaviours are predetermined and listed on a checklist to be counted or checked off during an observation period.
2. Unstructured: behaviours are described and recorded as or after they occur using a journal, diary or field notes. A detailed descriptive picture is recorded.

Participation of the researcher

1. Participant: the researcher is an active part of the activities or behaviours engaged in by the participants being observed.
2. Non-participant: the researcher is a bystander or passive participant in the activities being observed.

Visibility of the researcher

1. Concealed: the non-participant observer is hidden from those being observed. The activities might be recorded on video for later viewing and analysis, or activities might be viewed from a concealed space such as behind a two-way mirror.
2. Non-concealed: the observer is in full view of the participants.

Interviews allow the researcher to tap into the opinions, experiences, attitudes and belief systems of participants. Interviews can be on a continuum from structured to unstructured. Highly structured and focused interviews are used primarily in quantitative research and were discussed in Chapter 5. In-depth semistructured or unstructured interviews are generally used in qualitative research. Unstructured interviews are guided by the methodology and general aim of the research and are largely conducted in a conversational, storytelling style. The researcher might begin with a very broad, open-ended request, such as, 'Tell me about …'. As the person being interviewed tells the story, the interviewer may ask additional questions to encourage elaboration on a certain aspect of the story. Different styles of interview are used to produce the best data for answering the research question. For example, an ethnographic interview will differ from a phenomenological interview because the researcher is not seeking to explore the same constructs.

The real instrument in a qualitative study is the researcher. This is because the amount, type and quality of data retrieved are due in large part to the skills and abilities of the researcher, who must be able to enter the field and gain the trust of the people in that environment. Qualitative interviewing requires considerable skill and particularly so because it is often about sensitive or potentially distressing topics. Participants are therefore vulnerable. Narrative is often the primary source of data and poor interviewing skills will compromise the quality of data and therefore the study itself. The researcher must have well-honed interviewing skills, with a good feel for the ebb and flow of conversation and be able to keep the interview flowing with well-placed responses and cues. Interviewing requires active listening and the ability to pick up and follow-up on subtle leads or clues dropped in the course of the interview. The researcher must be able to put the participant at ease and know how to elicit information that participants may find hard to express. The researcher must have an eye for detail and be attuned to variations and changes when observing. The researcher needs to be able to capture in-depth what has been seen and heard. Finally, the researcher must have a good grasp of self. This means being aware of and able to recognise and reflect on feelings and beliefs that may influence the data collection and analysis. In short, quality data collection in a qualitative study demands a very skilled researcher. Qualitative data collection demands specialised skills on the part of the researcher.

Researchers use several tools to record their observations or interview results. These include audio and video recordings and field notes. Audio and video recordings are later transcribed for closer analysis. Field notes are a written account of what the researcher sees, hears, experiences and thinks during the course of data collection. Field notes can be classified into four basic types. The first is a brief description of what has occurred. Notes of this type contain key phrases and major events and are often jotted down in the field. The second type of note is an expansion of the first type. These are recorded immediately after a data collection session and expand on the brief notes, adding detail. The third type of note keeping is a reflective journal, kept by many researchers and containing descriptions of personal thoughts, feelings and responses that occur during the process of data collection. Finally, any insights, analysis of observations, judgments and interpretations made in the field are recorded and kept.

Qualitative researchers are concerned with the 'accuracy' and comprehensiveness of the data they collect. They do not tend to speak in terms of reliability and validity but rather in terms of the 'confirmability' of the study. Confirmability comprises three attributes: credibility, auditability and transferability. **Credibility** is a term used in qualitative research to examine whether or not the explanation or interpretation of data matches what has been described or recorded. Credibility may be examined and crosschecked through the use of two techniques: member checks and audit trails (Jackson et al 2003). Though controversial (St Pierre 1999), member checks are made by having study participants review the material once it has been analysed and interpreted. Credibility then is a question of validity. Some might call this 'truth' but in qualitative research the notion of truth is a complex issue, as some people believe there may be many 'truths', each being grounded in 'its own context and personal perspective' (Shank 2002). Data are considered dependable when what is recorded matches what actually occurred. The use of audio and video recordings and multiple samplings helps ensure data are dependable.

Audit trails (decision trails) ensure that adequate documentation is available about the data collection and analysis processes. Enough detail should be provided to enable another researcher to repeat the study. This is known as auditability.

Fittingness or transferability relates to when the findings 'fit' into contexts outside the study situation. It is important to understand that the notion of validity or rigour in qualitative research is a contested space and theorists are constantly extending its agenda (Lincoln et al 2011). Look for a decision trail and authenticity in any research report and you should be halfway there.

STUDENT CHALLENGE

Scrutinising Phase 2

Look again at the qualitative nursing or midwifery research studies you examined earlier. Scan these studies and see if you can identify each of the elements we have discussed in phase 2.

1. Identify the settings.
2. Identify the sample and sample size.
3. Did any of the studies use snowball, intensity, maximum variety, critical sampling or extreme sampling techniques?
4. What data collection methods were used?
5. Did any of the studies address the issues of reliability and validity? (Look for key terms such as accuracy, credibility, member checks or audit trails.)

Phase 3: conduct the study

This phase receives a lot of time and attention in qualitative research. The conceptualisation and planning stages are usually preliminary and loosely defined, in order to lay a broad set of boundaries for data collection. As data collection begins, data analysis may occur simultaneously. Data collection and analysis can lead to ongoing conceptualisation and planning about further collection and analysis. So we again see the fluid and repetitive (iterative) nature of the qualitative research process.

From your reading of Chapter 4 you will understand that the issues of participant approval and informed consent as they apply to qualitative research differ from those of quantitative research. Most of the guidelines and procedures used by institutional ethics committees were designed for quantitative research methods. Although qualitative studies do not involve invasive, potentially risky procedures such as trialling drugs or treatments, there are still some key ethical considerations. Like other researchers, investigators using qualitative approaches have to be able to demonstrate that procedures of informed consent are addressed and also that participation is voluntary and that participants are able to withdraw from the study at any time. Frequently, the focus of qualitative research is on things that are intensely personal and even traumatic in nature, so participation in qualitative studies can involve participants being asked to recall (and therefore in a way relive) very traumatic life events. This means there is the potential for emotional distress. Institutional ethics committees will expect to see strategies for dealing with the possibility of emotional distress in participants.

Consent forms often do not contain a detailed description of the study or the risks and benefits because they are not known at the time of data collection. Permission is obtained for interviews and for the use of audio and video recording equipment. Confidentiality is assured. Consent may need to be renegotiated with participants as data collection progresses and information emerges that may send the collection process in a new direction.

Subjects of qualitative research studies are often called participants or informants rather than subjects. Many qualitative researchers see the term 'subject' as too closely associated with the concept of experimentation and the connotation that people are being experimented on like laboratory specimens. The term 'participant' or 'informant' is used to convey the sense of mutual participation and trust building that occurs between the researcher and the people being researched and is reflective of a qualitative world view.

Data collection is a lengthy process in most qualitative studies. Whereas data collection in typical quantitative studies might take from several minutes to several weeks, data collection in qualitative studies may last for months or even years. The process of data collection is often described in more detail in qualitative studies because the collection process is often used to make decisions about the credibility of the data. Take the following challenge.

STUDENT CHALLENGE

Study Conduct

Look again at the qualitative research studies you examined for phases 1 and 2. Look for evidence of the steps in phase 3.

1. Were the rights of human subjects protected in these studies? What evidence did you find to support this?
2. Is there evidence of approval by an institutional ethics committee?
3. Was informed consent obtained?
4. What information was provided about what occurred during data collection?

Phase 4: analysis

Analysis of data in qualitative studies is an inductive process and involves examining words, descriptions and processes. Analytical procedures vary according to the design, but all require the researcher to read and re-read field notes and transcripts, to ensure familiarity with the data. This is often called **data immersion** or dwelling with the data. It lets the researcher get in touch with not only the content but also the feeling, tone and emphasis being communicated.

Initial analysis efforts are directed at setting up a system to make large volumes of data more manageable. A system is needed that allows the researcher to file, code and easily retrieve needed data. Computer programs can assist in this management and analysis process. The researcher searches for themes, patterns and meaning in the data and arranges this information in some way that classifies or categorises it.

Methods of analysis

Several specific formats and methods have been developed to analyse the data collected for various types of qualitative research. Common techniques used in phenomenological research include methods by Giorgi (1970), Spiegelberg (1976), Colaizzi (1978), van Kaam (1984), Parse et al (1985), van Manen (1990) and, more recently, interpretative phenomenological analysis (Smith et al 2009). All these methods are similar, requiring qualitative researchers to immerse themselves in the data and use inductive reasoning to sort and make sense of, and to extract and synthesise meaning from, the data. Once the data is more manageable, the researcher begins to refine categories and to assign meaning. Data are compared and contrasted, similarities and differences noted and processes and relationships defined. Finally, descriptions are constructed that represent the synthesis of material. These descriptions may take the form of a metaphor or an analogy or may be presented as a common theme, or series of themes. Great care is taken in the synthesis of the research and several drafts may be required in order to portray the experience in a meaningful light. Art has increasingly become a medium through which to express qualitative work – see for example Willis, P (2000, 2002).

Grounded theory has a very well-defined method of data collection and analysis, described by Glaser and Strauss (1967), Strauss (1987) and Strauss and Corbin (1990). The key is the use of techniques known as theoretical sampling and the constant comparative method. Theoretical sampling was discussed earlier in the sampling section. In the constant comparative method of analysis, the researcher categorises units of meaning through a process that compares recorded incident to recorded incident until concepts and categories of concepts begin to emerge. As this occurs, theoretical constructs and relationships are developed and a theory emerges.

Ethnography uses several analytical methods such as ethnoscience, life history, network and event analysis and the natural history method to examine conceptual and structural patterns in an identified culture. Ethnoscience techniques are designed to explore the 'mental maps' that people use to navigate everyday life (Dobbert 1984). Examination takes place at four levels. Data are described, classified, compared and explained. Description occurs using a technique known as domain analysis; classifications are made through taxonomic analysis; and comparisons are made through componential analysis. Explanation occurs by using the information from the first three analytic steps to make sense of the cultural patterns that emerge. Spradley (1979, 1980) provides a good basic discussion of the four levels used in the ethnoscience approach. A life history gathers in-depth information about an informant's life and examines how similar or different individual patterns are from surrounding cultural patterns. Network and event analysis techniques are used to examine social structures. If you are interested in critical ethnography, try an internet search for Phil Carspecken.

Historical studies use analytical techniques that examine the documents gathered to determine their importance, reliability and validity. Initial importance may be judged in various ways, including a gross classification into three categories, such as: 'clearly valuable', 'mildly interesting' and 'not valuable'. Valuable documents are included in the write-up. Interesting documents are re-reviewed and non-valuable documents are deleted from the study.

Case studies use a content analysis methodology that allows the researcher to search for patterns or themes in the data using a specific set of rules governing coding and the formation of categories and category relationships.

Findings

The findings in most qualitative studies are presented in a way more immediately understandable to the novice reader of research than the results in most quantitative studies. This is because the language used is commonly in a descriptive narrative form. However, you will notice that many qualitative researchers have a very sophisticated use of language and you will see words used that you may not be familiar with. You will also notice many of these papers present very complex ideas that may require reading, reflection and rereading in order to grasp their meaning fully. Frequently, findings are illustrated with the use of excerpts of participants' narratives. A good qualitative presentation of findings leaves the reader with a clear, cohesive picture of the phenomena under study that is validated by snapshots/quotes from the participants themselves.

STUDENT CHALLENGE

Analysis and Results

Examine your chosen research studies for the analyses used and the results of the analyses.

1. Can you identify the specific analytic methods employed?
2. Were the results understandable? Did you get a sense of what had been uncovered in the study? Did they ring true?
3. Did you find the results easier to decipher than those in the quantitative studies you examined in Chapter 5?

Phase 5: use the study

Qualitative research is a powerful tool for getting the human face of health or midwifery care into the public domain and reminding health professionals of the centrality of the human experience in the provision of such care. Qualitative research is used to raise awareness/understanding of issues related to the human experience. It answers questions that cannot be reduced to statistical measurement. Qualitative research is a powerful tool that may persuade policy-makers and decision-takers to take heed of an issue. Qualitative research findings can change policy and inform practice and should lead to better care by nurses and midwives who, because of their increased insight, can modify their approaches. Because qualitative researchers are often studying hidden or poorly understood aspects of human existence they usually have recommendations for further work. Recommendations for further research may include ideas for both quantitative and qualitative studies, but do remember that ultimately it is the research question that drives the methodology.

Consumers of research (such as you, the reader) need to be able to satisfy themselves that the findings of qualitative research are credible and trustworthy. Ensuring the trustworthiness of the study and its findings is crucial if qualitative research is to be as equally valued by the scholarly community as rigorous quantitative research. Although the notion of rigour is contentious in qualitative work, as discussed, qualitative researchers have developed concepts such as adequacy and credibility to ensure that qualitative studies meet the criterion of scientific rigour.

The qualitative researcher is under the same obligation as the quantitative researcher to disseminate the results of the research study. The avenues for this dissemination are much the same for qualitative and quantitative researchers and include journal articles and conference presentations. However, qualitative studies may also be found in book form because of the length of presentation. These formats allow fuller description and use of a greater number and variety of example illustrations obtained from data collection.

STUDENT CHALLENGE

Examining Your Chosen Research Studies

1. What did you glean from the studies' conclusions?
2. What implications might stem from the studies that can be applied to:
   - your professional practice?
   - education and/or policy development?
3. How would you compare your overall experience of reading qualitative research studies with reading quantitative research studies? Did you find one type easier to read and understand than the other? Do you think there would be value in combining both approaches?

Using qualitative and quantitative research approaches together

One question students frequently raise is whether quantitative and qualitative methods can be used together. Some researchers do combine the two methodologies to study certain phenomena and this is referred to as mixed method research and is covered in the next chapter.

RESOURCES KIT

Table 6.5
Difference between paradigm; methodology and method

A **paradigm** is understood as a *lens or a way of looking at the world; a world view/a mindset*. It is made up of sets of perceptions, beliefs/ assumptions, values and practices, shared by communities of researchers that constitutes a way of viewing reality and determines how inquiry/discourse prevails within disciplines. 'The various paradigms are characterized by ontological, epistemological and methodological differences in their approaches to conceptualizing and conducting research, and in their contribution towards disciplinary knowledge construction' (Weaver & Olsen, 2006, p. 259). Each paradigm has specific perspectives on the nature of social reality and assumptions about human existence (ontology) and beliefs about the nature of knowledge; how we come to know things (epistemology). Realists, for example, believe there is a truth to be discovered out there in the world, that we come to know objectively, whereas relativists believe there are multiple perspectives of reality and therefore multiple truths and that we come to know the world subjectively and intersubjectively. The two dominant paradigms are qualitative (relativism/post positivist) and quantitative (realism/positivist), but in this book you will read about others, such as Indigenous paradigms (relativism, critical). In addition there are sub paradigms that sit within the dominant ones. These are the empirical paradigm (quant) and the interpretive and critical paradigms (qual).	**A methodology** fits within the traditions of the paradigm and is understood as the approach/frame of reference taken by the researcher *to guide the conduct of obtaining the information sought*; that is, doing the research. It is informed by theory; its philosophical underpinnings, which constitute assumptions about knowledge, values, reality and logic (McGregor et al 2010). Often called the basic tenets of the approach, these are the principles that determine how the methods are to be deployed and interpreted. Understanding and remaining true to the basic tenets of the methodology ensures the research is carried out as a rigorous form of inquiry. For example, while phenomenology and ethnography as methodologies both fall within the qualitative interpretive paradigm and are faithful to that mode of understanding they are influenced by different strains of philosophical thought that influence how the research will be conducted; including what counts as data and how that data will be analysed etc. Ethnography has its roots in symbolic interactionism and looks to exploring the inside shared views of the members of a culture in order to proffer a version of reality from the standpoint of the members of that culture as practised in a particular context (which may be within an institution or community of people). Phenomenology, based on the principles of phenomenological philosophy, which in itself has several theoretical and methodological extensions, has as its goal to understand human experience through the description of phenomena. Don't forget it is the research question itself that determines the methodology, so each of the above would have different research questions and goals.	**Methods** are determined by the methodology and are the techniques or processes used to sample, collect and analyse data and report the results, for example, writing field notes; administering a survey. The methods need to 'fit' the methodological approach taken. In the previous chapter you saw that an experimental study falls under the quantitative empirical paradigm and that data will usually be collected by instruments that have been carefully calibrated. On the other hand, the collection of qualitative data is usually undertaken by the researcher themselves. Open-ended interviews for example, may well be used as methods in both ethnography and a study that draws on the principles of phenomenology however the conduct of the interviews will be different because they stem from different methodologies and seek differing data. Should the ethnography fall under the methodology of critical ethnography (hence a critical paradigm) the interview will be different again.

Want to know more about qualitative research?

Check out the activities and links on the Evolve website.

Try entering 'qualitative research' as a search phrase using a search engine on the internet. A variety of interesting websites are devoted to qualitative research.

Visit the book's Evolve website at http://evolve.elsevier.com/AU/Borbasi/maze for further information.

References

Colaizzi P: Psychological research as a phenomenologist views it. In Vaille RS, King M, editors: *Existential phenomenological alternatives for psychology*, New York, 1978, Oxford University Press.

Denzin NK, Lincoln YS, editors: *The sage handbook of qualitative research*, ed 4, Thousand Oaks, California, 2011, SAGE Publications.

Dickinson T, Cook M, Playle J, et al: Queer' treatments: giving a voice to former patients who received treatments for their 'sexual deviations', *Journal of Clinical Nursing* 21:1345–1354, 2012. doi:10.1111/j.1365-2702.2011.03965.x.

Dobbert ML: *Ethnographic research: theory and application for modern schools and societies*, New York, 1984, Praeger.

Fealy GM, McNamara MS, Geraghty R: The health of hospitals and lessons from history: public health and sanitary reform in the Dublin hospitals, 1858–1898, *Journal of Clinical Nursing* 19:3468–3476, 2010.

Finlay L: *Phenomenology for therapists: researching the lived world*, Chichester, 2011, Wiley-Blackwell.

Giorgi A: *Psychology as a human science: a phenomenologically based approach*, New York, 1970, Harper and Row.

Glaser BG, Strauss AL: *The discovery of grounded theory: strategies for qualitative research*, Chicago, 1967, Aldine.

Jackson D, Daly J, Chang E: Qualitative methods. In Beanland C, Schneider Z, LoBiondo-Wood G, et al, editors: *Nursing research methods, critical, appraisal and utilisation*, ed 2, Melbourne, 2003, Harcourt Australia.

Kelly J, McAllister M: Lessons students and new graduates could teach: A phenomenological study that reveals insights on the essence of building a supportive learning culture through preceptorship, *Contemporary Nurse* 44:170–177, 2013.

Leininger MM, McFarland MR, editors: *Culture care: diversity and universality: a worldwide nursing theory*, ed 2, Boston, 2006, Jones and Bartlett.

Lin F, Chaboyer W, Wallis M, et al: Factors contributing to the process of intensive care patient discharge: An ethnographic study informed by activity theory, *International Journal of Nursing Studies* 50:1054–1066, 2013.

Lincoln YS, Lynham SA, Guba EG: Paradigmatic controversies, contradictions, and emerging confluences, Revisited. In Denzin NK, Lincoln YS, editors: *The sage handbook of qualitative research*, ed 4, Thousand Oaks, California, 2011, SAGE Publications, pp 97–128.

Luck L, Jackson D, Usher K: Innocent or culpable? Meanings that emergency department nurses ascribe to individual acts of violence, *Journal of Clinical Nursing* 17:1071–1078, 2008.

Maher J: Women's care/career changes as connection and resilience: Challenging discourses of breakdown and conflict, *Gender, Work & Organization* 20:172–183, 2013.

McGregor SLT, Murnane JA: Paradigm, methodology and method: Intellectual integrity in consumer scholarship, *International Journal of Consumer Studies* 34(4):419–427, 2010. Online. Available: http://www.consultmcgregor.com/documents/research/Methodological-paper-2010-for-web.pdf 28 February 2015.

Parse RR, Coyne AB, Smith MJ: *Nursing research qualitative methods*, Maryland, 1985, Brady Communications.

Powell I: Can you see me? Experiences of nurses working night shift in Australian regional hospitals, *Journal of Advanced Nursing* 69:2172–2184, 2013.

Rollans M, Schmied V, Kemp L, et al: Negotiating policy in practice: Child and family health nurses approach to the postnatal psychosocial assessment, *BMC Health Services Research* 13:133, 2013.

Sambrano R, Cox L: 'I sang "Amazing Grace" for about 3 hours that day': Understanding Indigenous Australians' experience of seclusion, *International Journal of Mental Health Nursing* 22:522–531, 2013.

Shank GD: *Qualitative research: a personal skills approach*, New Jersey, 2002, Merrill Prentice Hall.

Smith J, Flowers P, Larkin M: *Interpretative phenomenological analysis: theory, method and research*, London, 2009, SAGE Publications.

Spiegelberg H: *The phenomenological movement*, The Hague, 1976, Martinus Nijhoff.

Spradley JP: *The ethnography interview*, New York, 1979, Holt, Rinehart & Winston.

Spradley JP: *Participant observation*, New York, 1980, Holt, Rinehart & Winston.

St Pierre EA: The work of response in ethnography, *Journal of Contemporary Ethnography* 28:266–287, 1999.

Stephens M, McKenzie H, Jordens CFC: The work of living with a rare cancer: Multiple Myeloma, *Journal of Advanced Nursing* 2014.

Strauss AL: *Qualitative analysis for social scientists*, New York, 1987, Cambridge University Press.

Strauss AL, Corbin J: *Basics of qualitative research: grounded theory procedures and techniques*, London, 1990, SAGE Publications.

van Kaam A: *Existential foundation of psychology*, New York, 1984, Doubleday.

van Manen M: *Researching lived experience: human science for an action sensitive pedagogy*, New York, 1990, State University of New York Press.

Weaver K, Olson JK: Understanding paradigms used for nursing research, *Journal of Advanced Nursing* 53(4):459–469, 2006.

Willis P, Smith R, Collins E, editors: *Being, seeking, telling: expressive approaches to qualitative adult education research*, Flaxton (Queensland, Australia), 2000, Post Pressed.

Willis P: Poetry and poetics in phenomenological research, *Indo-Pacific Journal of Phenomenology* 3(1):1–19, 2002.

CHAPTER 7

MIXED METHODS RESEARCH

Elizabeth Halcomb and Sharon Andrew

CHAPTER OUTLINE

KEY TERMS

concurrent mixed methods
mixed methods research
multiple method research
sequential mixed methods
triangulation

LEARNING OBJECTIVES

After reading this chapter and following critical reflection the student will be able to:

1. Define mixed methods research
2. Outline the reasons for conducting mixed methods research
3. Identify and describe the various mixed methods research designs
4. Describe the practical considerations in undertaking mixed methods research
5. Discuss reliability, validity and rigour in mixed methods research.

STUDENT QUOTE

Mixed methods research captures both the art and science of practice. It recognises that not all nursing and midwifery research problems can be reduced to numbers, and that words do not always tell the complete picture either.

ABSTRACT

As a way of understanding the complexity of the world in which we live, a range of professions are turning to mixed methods research. Mixed methods designs use a combination of qualitative and quantitative data collection methods in a single study. In this way, mixed methods research seeks to build on the strengths and mitigate the limitations of both qualitative and quantitative approaches. Like pure qualitative and quantitative research, mixed methods studies need to be systematically planned. While mixed methods research follows many of the steps of the research process of pure qualitative and quantitative research, it also has some unique considerations that need to be understood by both the researcher and the research consumer. Mixed methods designs can be classified by the sequence in which the qualitative and quantitative data are collected, the relative priority given to each method, the stage at which the qualitative and quantitative data are integrated and whether an overall theoretical perspective will be used to guide the research process. Mixed methods research also allows the researcher to go beyond predetermined designs to creatively develop a research plan that will most effectively answer the specific research question.

What is mixed methods research?

In Chapters 5 and 6 you learnt about two very different approaches to gathering data to answer research questions. An alternative approach to either qualitative or quantitative research is to combine both qualitative and quantitative methods of data collection in a single study. This is called **mixed methods research**. As you discovered in the previous chapters, qualitative research is often useful to explore the experiences of individuals whereas quantitative research allows the researcher to form generalisable conclusions about a population (Hayes et al 2013). Used together in mixed methods research, the combination of qualitative and quantitative data collection provides a broad and flexible approach to address complex research problems. The depth of insight into a research problem made available by mixed methods research makes it suitable for studying many of the complex problems explored in nursing and midwifery research (Simons & Lathlean 2010; Andrew & Halcomb 2012).

Despite its advantages, the conduct of mixed methods research is not appropriate to provide answers for every research question. For example, a study seeking to identify the incidence of postoperative wound infections in mothers after a caesarean section would be best answered through purely quantitative data. Such a study would be much less resource-intensive and cost-effective than a mixed methods study on the same issue and yet still provide adequate information to answer the research question. However, if the study also sought to capture the impact of the postoperative wound infections on, say, quality of life or mothering, then adding a qualitative dimension would likely be justified. Care must be taken to rationalise clearly why a mixed methods design, rather than a purely qualitative or quantitative approach, is being used in the particular investigation. The scope of the research question should be the primary driver in the decision to use a particular methodological approach (Andrew & Halcomb 2009).

When reading reports of mixed methods studies, all of the principles you have learnt about qualitative and quantitative research design, data collection and reporting apply. A major difference in mixed methods research occurs in terms of mixing the qualitative and quantitative components (Simons & Lathlean 2010; Maudsley 2011). As you move through this chapter you will see that a well-designed mixed methods study is more than simply combining qualitative and quantitative data collection in a single research report. Mixing of qualitative and quantitative data collection is the key to mixed methods research. Mixing can be undertaken during the problem identification, data collection, data analysis and/or reporting phases of the study (Creswell & Plano Clark 2011; Glogowska 2011). This mixing involves tasks such as designing complementary data collection procedures, synthesis of datasets during analysis and evaluating conflicting and confirming findings. Issues related to mixing qualitative and quantitative methods will be discussed throughout this chapter.

The debate over mixing methods

The relative values of qualitative, quantitative and mixed methods research designs have long been a source of debate amongst nursing scholars (Risjord et al 2004; Halcomb & Andrew 2005; Ridenour & Newman 2008). There are those who believe that, because of the different epistemology, ontology, philosophy, and goals and purposes, qualitative and quantitative approaches cannot be mixed without causing a violation of these differences (Greene et al 1989; Thurmond 2001; Doyle et al 2009). For other scholars mixed methods has increasingly become an accepted research approach (McEvoy & Richards 2006; Simons & Lathlean 2010; Glogowska 2011; Maudsley 2011).

It is not the purpose of this chapter to provide in-depth analysis of the relative merits of qualitative and quantitative research. What we will do is demonstrate that a combination of qualitative and quantitative methods has the potential to provide greater insight into many complex nursing and midwifery issues than could be gained from using either method in isolation (Simons & Lathlean 2010; Andrew & Halcomb 2012).

Rationale for using mixed methods designs

Projects that use mixed methods designs should clearly articulate a rationale for the use of **multiple method research** and demonstrate the qualitative and quantitative dimensions of the study (Lavelle et al 2013; Halcomb & Hickman 2015). The decision to use a mixed methods design should be based on balancing the value of combining the qualitative and quantitative data collection against the increased resources and skills required (Halcomb & Hickman 2015).

Given the importance of demonstrating a rationale for undertaking a mixed methods study, rather than conducting a purely qualitative or quantitative investigation, it is useful to understand the goals to be achieved by using mixed methods designs. Whilst clearly research problems where multiple perspectives will provide a more detailed understanding of the issues are most suited to mixed methods approaches, there are a number of purposes described for using mixed methods designs. These are: (1) confirmation/corroboration; (2) complementarity; (3) initiation; (4) development; (5) expansion; and (6) enhancement of significant findings (Greene et al 1989; Bryman 2006; Halcomb & Andrew 2009; Wisdom et al 2012). Researchers are not limited to one reason for conducting mixed methods research but rather may have multiple motives for using a mixed methods design in their work. Table 7.1 outlines the purposes for which mixed methods designs can be used and provides examples from the published literature.

Confirmation/corroboration

The early social science, psychology and educational researchers saw the combination of qualitative and quantitative data as a means of confirming the

Table 7.1
Purposes of mixed methods research

Purpose	Definition	Example
Confirmation/ Corroboration	To corroborate results using data collected through different methods.	The use of interviews and quantitative methods (e.g. survey) to measure the same phenomenon. Njie-Carr (2014) compared (triangulated) interview and survey data to explore partner violence in women with HIV.
Complementarity	To seek elaboration, illustration or clarification of the results from one method with the data collected to the other method.	Gill et al (2012) initially administered surveys to paediatric nurses to collect information about medication administration and compliance with the hospital protocol around drug checking and administration. This identified areas where nurses might not be compliant. Three focus groups were held with nurses to understand the factors that influence why some nurses did not follow the protocol.
Initiation	Where one method is used to reveal the contradictions in findings from the other method.	Andrew et al (2011) investigated patient satisfaction using quantitative surveys and qualitative interviews. The results for the quantitative survey indicated that patients were highly satisfied with their care. Data integration allowed the researchers to examine the contradictions between the quantitative and qualitative findings as some patients had a suggestion for change even if they scored their care high on the survey.
Development	These studies are sequential designs where the data from the initial data collection inform the development of the subsequent method.	In their study to develop a nursing context index (NCI) following a literature review, focus groups with nurses were conducted to assist in the selection of the questions for the NCI instrument (Slater et al 2009). A pilot study was then conducted to test the reliability and validity of the instrument.
Expansion	These studies extend the depth and scope of the inquiry by using different measures to explore different inquiry components.	Interviews with patients and nurses and a pre-post survey of nurses was conducted to evaluate the introduction of a bedside handover in three rural hospitals in South Australia (Bradley & Mott 2013). In the final phase of the study nurses were interviewed to expand on the survey findings.

Adapted from: Andrew & Halcomb 2006; Halcomb & Hickman 2015

results of one method with those of the other (Campbell & Fiske 1959). This use of different data sets was also known as **triangulation** (Halcomb & Andrew 2005). Results and conclusions from the different data collection methods were expected to converge and this was seen as a way of confirming the study findings and increasing their validity (Denzin 1989).

Complementarity

Complementarity refers to the use of both quantitative and qualitative data to elaborate, enhance the meaningfulness of findings, provide illustrations and clarification of the results of one method with the findings of the complementary method (Greene et al 1989; Morgan 1998; Halcomb & Hickman 2015). In this way the mixed methods format uses the strengths and weaknesses of quantitative and qualitative data collection to complement each other and this can give the study more breadth and scope than either method could achieve if used in isolation (Andrew et al 2008; Andrew et al 2011).

Initiation

Researchers undertaking mixed methods research for the purposes of initiation seek to explore inconsistency and contradiction and take new perspectives on existing frameworks (Greene et al 1989; Shepard et al 2002). This can lead to reframing the research question to explore the research problem from a variety of perspectives (Onwuegbuzie & Leech 2004). By exploring the research problem from different perspectives, the breadth and depth of the results and interpretations are increased (Greene et al 1989). Thus, mixed methods research may reveal a unique characteristic of the phenomenon being studied that may be overlooked when using either qualitative or quantitative methods alone.

Development

Findings from one method of data collection may generate questions or a hypothesis that needs to be tested by another method (Greene et al 1989). A common type of mixed methods investigation is for the purpose of instrument development (Polit & Beck 2010). In this type of study, the investigation may start with qualitative interviews or focus groups whose findings are then used to develop a quantitative research instrument (Slater et al 2009). The newly developed instrument may then be piloted by a quantitative survey. Sometimes in-depth interviews may be conducted at the same time as the survey is administered to determine the effectiveness of the items in the instrument. Another example relates to sampling. In this strategy one method of data collection may be used to identify particular individuals or cases that then become the sample for the second method of data collection. For example, a survey could be used to explore health and wellbeing after an acute cardiac event. From this survey individuals who indicate depression could be approached to participate in interviews to explore their experiences.

Expansion

Studies undertaken for the purpose of expansion seek to broaden the scope of the investigation by using different methods of data collection to measure the various components of the research problem most appropriately (Greene et al 1989).

Enhance significant findings

Onwuegbuzie and Leech (2004) describe the final purpose of using mixed methods designs as the enhancement of significant findings. The significance of a study can be determined in terms of statistical, practical, clinical or economic significance (Onwuegbuzie & Leech 2004). The collection of both qualitative and quantitative data in a single study can assist in a more comprehensive evaluation of the significance of study findings in each of these areas. This may be particularly useful when an intervention may provide clinically, but not statistically, significant improvement in an outcome measure.

Philosophical approaches to mixed methods research

Mixed methods research has been increasingly described as the third methodological approach, in addition to the traditional qualitative and quantitative approaches to research (Tashakkori & Teddlie 2003; Johnson & Onwuegbuzie 2004). However, to consider mixed methods research as a methodological approach, its underlying philosophical basis must be identified and understood. A philosophical approach, sometimes described as a world view, is the lens through which someone sees the world (Halcomb & Hickman 2015). Mesel (2013) argues that a range of philosophical approaches can be used to underpin mixed methods research. These can include pragmatism, a transformative (emancipatory) approach or, more recently, critical realism (Andrew & Halcomb 2006; Creswell & Plano Clark 2011; Maudsley 2011; Andrew & Halcomb 2012; Walsh & Evans 2014).

Pragmatists argue that the researcher should use whatever techniques work to achieve the best answer for a specific research question (Creswell & Plano Clark 2011). They value both subjective and objective measures to reveal answers to the research question (Andrew & Halcomb 2006; Feilzer 2010; Creswell & Plano Clark 2011). From this perspective, it is justifiable to combine qualitative and quantitative data collection methods in a single study if this is the most appropriate means to answer the research question.

A transformative (emancipatory) approach seeks to recognise cultural differences and injustices throughout the entire research process (Mertens 2003; Creswell & Plano Clark 2011). Mixed methods designs provide a focused strategy by which multiple perspectives can be gathered and considered.

In contrast, critical realism accepts that considering multiple outlooks can facilitate the best understanding of reality (McEvoy & Richards 2006; Creswell & Plano Clark 2011; Maudsley 2011). Since mixed methods research provides a framework for gathering multiple outlooks it is well suited to a critical realist approach to research (McEvoy & Richards 2006).

Creswell and Plano Clark (2011) describe various models of adopting world views within mixed methods research that are beyond the scope of this introductory book. These models can involve employing a single or multiple world view within the study design. Whilst there is no right or wrong philosophical approach for a mixed methods study, the way in which the study is designed and undertaken should be consistent with its underlying philosophical approach.

Decisions in mixed methods designs

Researchers need to make several decisions that have an impact on the design of mixed methods research. Creswell and Plano Clark (2011) propose three questions that must be addressed by the researchers during the planning stage of mixed methods research:

1. In what sequence will the qualitative and quantitative data collection be implemented?
2. What relative weighting will be given to the qualitative and quantitative methods?
3. At what stage of the project will the qualitative and quantitative data be integrated?

Implementation sequence

The timing of the data collection within a mixed methods study may be simultaneous (concurrent or parallel) or sequential (Andrew & Halcomb 2009). In **concurrent mixed methods** studies, qualitative and quantitative data are collected at, or approximately at, the same time. Therefore, in concurrent studies, data integration must occur during either the data analysis or the interpretation phases. Concurrent studies have the advantage of being able to collect a large amount of data over a relatively short period of time (Creswell et al 2004). **Sequential mixed methods** studies involve at least two phases of data collection, one after the other. In sequential studies, the study duration is often much longer than a single qualitative or quantitative study, as the data collected during the first phase are usually used to inform the subsequent data collection. This may be problematic when the researcher is working within set time constraints, such as during a research degree (Halcomb & Andrew 2009).

Priority

The second consideration is the relative priority to be given to the qualitative and quantitative methods of data collection. This decision is guided primarily by the aims of the research. For example, in exploratory studies where there is a paucity of understanding, the qualitative method is often given the higher priority (Kroll et al 2005). In studies where there is unequal priority, one dataset are clearly secondary to a larger primary design (Creswell et al 2011).

Alternatively, researchers may collect comprehensive qualitative and quantitative data sets and give them equal emphasis in the analysis.

Integration

The integration of the qualitative and quantitative data refers to the 'point of interface' at which the researcher mixes the two datasets (Andrew & Halcomb 2009; Creswell et al 2011; Zhang & Creswell 2013). For obvious reasons, the researcher needs to consider the sequence in which data are collected when deciding at which point integration will occur. The purpose of integration is also to maximise the strengths of each method whilst at the same time minimising their weaknesses (Creswell et al 2011). In practical terms, the integration of qualitative and quantitative aspects can be undertaken at numerous stages throughout the research process. During data collection open and closed ended items can be included in the same survey tool, and during data analysis or interpretation qualitative and quantitative data can be compared (Creswell et al 2011). The three distinct strategies that have been proposed in the literature for combining data are described in Table 7.2 (Zhang & Creswell 2013).

Merging or integrating data can be achieved in various ways (Creswell et al 2011; Zhang & Creswell 2013). One example is when statistical survey findings are reported followed by interview quotes that either support or refute the statistical data. Another example is developing a table to compare the qualitative and quantitative findings including where they triangulate but also where one method might add expansion to the other method. Various strategies for undertaking this kind of integration have been reported in the literature (Andrew et al 2008; O'Cathain et al 2010; Bazeley & Kemp 2012).

Connecting data involves using one dataset to inform the second data collection (Creswell et al 2011; Zhang & Creswell 2013). For example, a survey may assist in identifying individuals with particular characteristics who are then interviewed.

The final strategy for integrating the datasets is embedding data (Creswell et al 2011; Zhang & Creswell 2013). In these designs a secondary data collection, usually qualitative, may be undertaken to explore the experience of participants and/or providers within an experimental study (Creswell et al 2011).

Regardless of the nature and timing of the integration, care must be taken to ensure the two methods, datasets or findings are truly integrated (Creswell 2011), rather than simply using one dataset to embellish the 'real' results (Foss & Ellefsen 2002).

Mixed methods research designs

Mixed methods research designs allow a degree of creative freedom that is not always available in other research designs. With this in mind the following

Table 7.2
Models of mixing

Model of mixing	Definition	Example
Integration	Qualitative and quantitative data are collected concurrently and analysed separately. Integration occurs during the interpretation.	Rickard et al (2011) conducted a study to explore the roles of research nurses and possible career pathways. Data were collected via a 104-item survey tool, which combined three previously validated instruments and a series of semi-structured interviews. The qualitative and quantitative data were collected separately and only integrated during the reporting phase.
Connection	One approach is built upon the findings of the other approach.	Meixner et al (2013) surveyed providers of brain injury services within a region about the barriers to accessing crisis intervention services. A second phase of the study involved a series of focus groups that investigated the survey findings to reveal greater levels of understanding.
Embedding	The analysis of one type of data is embedded within the other. Commonly this involves a small qualitative component nested within a quantitative study.	Zwar et al (2010) conducted a cluster randomised controlled trial to test the uptake and effectiveness of a package of smoking cessation support provided primarily by the practice nurse. Qualitative interviews were conducted with patients, nurses and general practitioners who participated in the trial to evaluate the implementation, feasibility and acceptability of the intervention.

Adapted from: Zhang & Creswell 2013
Reproduced with permission from Nursing Standard (Halcomb & Hickman 2015)

discussion provides an overview of some of the common types of mixed methods study designs. Broadly, there are three types of designs in mixed methods research, namely: (1) concurrent (or convergent/parallel) designs; (2) sequential designs; and (3) embedded (or nested) designs (Creswell et al 2011). The characteristics of each of these designs are summarised in Table 7.3 and discussed below.

Currently there is no agreed nomenclature of mixed methods research designs. Whilst the most popular design names have been used here, slightly different names may be found to describe these designs in the various literature. Additionally, many authors of mixed methods research do not explicitly identify the type of mixed methods design within their research report. Moreover, some research designs do not explicitly identify themselves as being mixed methods research, although they commonly use qualitative and quantitative data collection methods within their design. For example, case study, evaluation studies and participatory action research may use mixed methods designs. Case study research, for example, may use qualitative and quantitative methods with the design providing a 'bridge' or link between the

Table 7.3
Types of mixed methods designs

Research design	Process	Purpose	Level of interaction	Priority
Convergent parallel (concurrent)	Qual Quant	To obtain different but complementary data to answer a single research question.	Data collected and analysed independently.	Equal
Sequential explanatory	QUANT → qual	Qualitative data are collected to explain the quantitative findings.	Quant data frames qualitative data collection.	Quantitative dominant
Sequential exploratory	QUAL → quant	Quant data builds on qualitative findings to provide generalisability.	Qualitative data frames quant data collection.	Qualitative dominant
Embedded / Nested	Qual (quant) Or Quant (qual)	To obtain different data to answer a complementary research question.	Embedded dataset provides answers to a complementary research question.	Can be either Qualitative or Quantitative dominant

Reproduced with permission from Nursing Standard (Halcomb & Hickman 2015)

qualitative and quantitative data collections (Luck et al 2006). Evaluation studies may use qualitative and quantitative methods to determine the effectiveness of a clinical practice or a model of care or an educational program. In participatory action research, through critical reflection and action, both the researcher and the study participants may work together to perhaps evaluate and change a clinical practice or model of care. We emphasise that the research question must be the primary driver when choosing a research design and hence use of a particular methodological approach (Andrew & Halcomb 2009).

Concurrent designs

A concurrent, convergent or parallel design is implemented when the researcher uses quantitative and qualitative methods to confirm or corroborate findings (Andrew & Halcomb 2009; Creswell et al 2011). As integration occurs during the data analysis phase, data are collected concurrently. The process of data analysis involves merging and comparing the two sets of data (Creswell et al 2011). Although the relative priority of the datasets is ideally equal, priority may be given to either dataset (Andrew & Halcomb 2009). For example, in a study of Indigenous Australians' participation in pre-registration nursing courses, West et al (2013) concurrently collected statistical data about student numbers related to commencement, attrition, progression and completions for a sample of nursing schools and interviewed a purposive sample of academics and third year nursing students. This study reported the findings separately and then integrated them in a table. By doing this it was possible to compare (triangulate) the qualitative and quantitative findings to achieve a comprehensive understanding of the topic.

Sequential designs

Sequential designs are multiphase projects in which one data collection follows after the other is completed. Whilst often there are two phases, larger projects may involve additional phases.

Sequential explanatory

A sequential explanatory study involves a primarily quantitative study followed by qualitative data collection (Andrew & Halcomb 2009). This design is highly suitable for the detailed exploration of a problem where little is already known, or to explain the results of a quantitative study (Tashakkori & Teddlie 2003). The use of a sequential explanatory design can identify subjective meanings behind purely quantitative survey responses. For example, in their study about family resilience when a member of a family has chronic pain, West et al (2012) used four questionnaires to examine different components of family resilience. Subsequently, interviews were undertaken with two individuals from ten families to gain a richer understanding of the quantitative results (West et al 2012).

Sequential exploratory

Like the sequential explanatory design, the sequential exploratory design has two phases, with priority given to the initial data collection (Andrew & Halcomb 2009). However, in the sequential exploratory design, the first phase is comprised of qualitative data collection and analysis, followed by quantitative data collection and analysis (Andrew & Halcomb 2009). In this design, integration of the two data collection methods occurs during the interpretation phase of the study. Tashakkori and Teddlie (2003) assert the most common situations where this design is used include developing and testing research instruments, identification of the prevalence of a particular phenomenon with a population, or any problem where there is a need to interpret relationships.

An example of a sequential exploratory study can be found in the study reported by Hamshire, et al (2013) who explored nursing students' course experience. Initially, they undertook interviews with students to explore their experiences and expectations regarding their nursing course. The findings from these interviews informed the development of an online survey tool which was completed by 1080 nursing students from nine UK universities.

Embedded/nested

The embedded or nested design has a predominant method of data collection that guides the project and then a secondary method, of lesser priority, nested within the predominant method (Andrew & Halcomb 2009; Clark et al 2013). A nested approach can provide a broader perspective of the research problem by adding quantitative data to enrich the description of participants or collecting qualitative data to explore an aspect of the issue that cannot be quantified. The most common example of a nested study is the collection of qualitative data from participants or intervention providers in an experimental study to understand their experience of the intervention process (Clark et al 2013). In a nested design, mixing of the qualitative and quantitative data occurs during the analysis phase of the project (Teddlie & Tashakkori 2009).

An example of a nested design can be seen in the randomised controlled trial of a yoga intervention for women with major depression conducted by Kinser et al (2013). Quantitative outcomes from this trial included depression severity, stress, anxiety and rumination. In addition, participating women were asked to participate in interviews and maintain daily logs to collect data about the feasibility and acceptability of the intervention.

STUDENT CHALLENGE

Identifying Mixed Methods

Choose two journal articles that report mixed methods studies. Note that it can be challenging to locate articles reporting mixed methods designs. In addition to using 'mixed method' as a keyword in your search it may be necessary to look for articles that contain both 'qualitative' and 'quantitative' as keywords. Remember that 'multi method studies' is a subject heading in many databases. Although using this term will retrieve papers reporting mixed methods studies it may also locate studies that collect data using two or more data collection methods from the same research tradition, that is, within method triangulation studies (Halcomb & Andrew 2005).

Review each of the journal articles and identify the:

1. Type of mixed methods designs used
2. Sequence in which the qualitative and quantitative data were collected
3. Relative priority given to the qualitative and quantitative data collection and analysis
4. Stage of the project at which the qualitative and quantitative data were integrated.

Also consider the following questions:

1. If you were to replicate the study, would you have sufficient information about how integration was achieved by the researchers?
2. Was it clear how the two sets of data informed the development of the study results?
3. How does the format of these papers differ from purely qualitative and quantitative studies?

Practical considerations for mixed methods research

Meticulous planning and justifiable rationales are as vital when planning mixed methods research as in planning purely qualitative or quantitative projects (Halcomb & Andrew 2009; Creswell et al 2011). In addition to having a realistic research problem of sufficient interest and the capacity and resources required to gather the required data, the size and scope of data collected during mixed methods research needs to be considered (Halcomb & Andrew 2009; Creswell 2011). The use of two distinctly different methods of data collection requires a high level of resources and researcher time. For obvious reasons the process of data collection will likely take more time and be more expensive to conduct than a purely qualitative or quantitative study (Tashakkori & Teddlie 2003; Halcomb & Andrew 2009).

Additionally, researchers undertaking mixed methods research require a broad range of skills in both qualitative and quantitative data collection techniques, as well as skills relating to the mixing of datasets (Andrew et al 2008). For this reason, mixed methods research is often most effectively conducted by research teams, where several researchers can contribute different expertise to the conduct of the project (Creswell et al 2011).

The large amount of data that are often generated during the course of a mixed methods investigation is a clear limitation. For many researchers, reporting and presenting these data in a meaningful way can be difficult (Glogowska 2011). The increase in the number of mixed methods papers being submitted in recent years has helped to raise prominence of issues around dissemination. Wisdom et al (2012) identify that issues such as reviewers lack of expertise, audience expectations, journal word limits and the decision making around publishing in a mixed methods or clinical journal still face mixed methods researchers.

A further limitation of mixed methods research is that using two data collection methods may serve only to increase the magnitude of the inherent errors if a study has a design flaw or bias. For this reason the use of a mixed methods approach must be clearly justified in the planning phase of the study. Additionally, consideration must be given to employing strategies to enhance the validity, reliability and rigour of the investigation (O'Cathain et al 2008).

STUDENT CHALLENGE

The Advantages and Disadvantages of Mixed Methods Research

1. Referring to this chapter, discuss the advantages and disadvantages of using mixed methods research designs in nursing and midwifery research.
2. Considering one of the studies that was discussed in Chapters 5 and 6, think about the implications of undertaking this study as a mixed methods investigation. How would the study change? What might a researcher gain? What would be the advantages?
3. Try writing a research question/s that would lend itself to a mixed methods research design.

Establishing reliability, validity and rigour in mixed methods research

Critical analysis of the validity, reliability and rigour of mixed methods studies is as important as it is in purely qualitative or quantitative investigations. Despite advances in the literature around the use of mixed methods, many reports of mixed methods research continue to lack sufficient detail around the methods used (Wisdom et al 2012). Broadly, any critical appraisal of mixed methods research should consider both how well the work meets the qualitative and quantitative appraisal criteria and specific criteria around the application of mixed methods (Creswell et al 2011). In recent years a growing number of frameworks have been proposed to guide people in critically appraising mixed methods research (Heyvaert et al 2013). These various frameworks can either be generic or targeted to a specific mixed methods design. Whilst the specific aspects may vary slightly all frameworks have commonalities as outlined in Box 7.1 (Creswell et al 2011; Heyvaert et al 2013).

Conclusion

Mixed methods research designs provide the nursing and midwifery researcher with another means for creatively exploring the complexity of problems faced in contemporary health care. As researchers become increasingly skilled in the use of mixed methods techniques, a greater depth of understanding about phenomena of study than would be possible through the use of either qualitative or quantitative methods in isolation will be achievable. It is important to realise that a good understanding of the differences in the philosophical underpinnings of both approaches is essential to the successful use of mixed methods.

Box 7.1
Sample criteria for critical appraisal of mixed methods studies

- Are there clearly stated purposes or questions that the mixed methods data collection seeks to answer?
- Are the multiple purposes or research questions matched with appropriate methods of data collection? Are both the qualitative and quantitative methods justified?
- Has the researcher followed the quality criteria for qualitative data collection?
- Has the researcher followed the quality criteria for quantitative data collection?
- Have the limitations of the various data collection methods been identified?
- Is it clear when the qualitative and quantitative data were integrated during the course of the study? Has this integration provided a better understanding about the problem than either individual source?
- If there were conflicting results, were these adequately explained by the researcher?

RESOURCES KIT

Resources

Additional resources can be located on the internet by using keywords such as 'mixed method' in the search engine.

Check out the activities and links on the Evolve website.

International Journal of Multiple Research Approaches (Taylor & Francis) is a journal aimed at research, scholarship, educational, researcher and practitioner perspectives on multiple, hybrid, synergistic, integrated and cultural research approaches. This focus includes both multiple and mixed methods research: http://www.tandfonline.com/toc/rmra20/current.

The *Journal of Mixed Methods Research* (Sage Publications) is a journal devoted to publishing papers reporting mixed methods studies and methodological issues relating specifically to mixed methods research regardless of professional discipline: http://www.mmr.sagepub.com.

Recommended reading

Andrew S, Halcomb EJ, editors: *Mixed methods research for nursing and the health sciences*, London, England, 2009, Wiley-Blackwell.

Creswell JW, Klassen AC, Plano Clark VL, et al: *Best practices for mixed methods research in the health sciences*, 2011, In Office of Behavioral and Social Sciences Research: National Institute of Health.

Creswell JW, Plano Clark VL: *Designing and conducting mixed methods research*, ed 2, Thousand Oaks, California, 2011, SAGE Publications.

Halcomb EJ, Hickman L: Considerations in mixed methods research, *Nursing Standard* 29(32):37–43, 2015.

Hayes B, Bonner A, Douglas C: An introduction to mixed methods research for nephrology nurses, *Renal Society of Australasia Journal* 9(1):8–14, 2013.

References

Andrew S, Halcomb EJ: Mixed methods research is an effective method of enquiry for working with families and communities, *Advances in Contemporary Nursing* 23(2):145–153, 2006.

Andrew S, Halcomb EJ, editors: *Mixed methods research for nursing and the health sciences*, London, England, 2009, Wiley-Blackwell.

Andrew S, Halcomb EJ: Mixed Method Research. In Borbasi S, Jackson D, editors: *Navigating the maze of research: enhancing nursing & midwifery practice*, Marrickville, New South Wales, 2012, Elsevier, pp 147–166.

Andrew S, Salamonson Y, Everrett B, et al: Beyond the ceiling effect: using a mixed methods approach to measure patient satisfaction, *International Journal of Multiple Research Approaches* 5(1):52–63, 2011.

Andrew S, Salamonson Y, Halcomb EJ: Integrating mixed methods data analysis using NVivo©: An example examining attrition and persistence of nursing students, *International Journal of Multiple Research Approaches* 2(1):36–43, 2008.

Bazeley P, Kemp L: Mosaics, Triangles, and DNA Metaphors for Integrated Analysis in Mixed Methods Research, *Journal of Mixed Methods Research* 6(1):55–72, 2012.

Bradley S, Mott S: Adopting a patient-centred approach: an investigation into the introduction of bedside handover to three rural hospitals, *Journal of Clinical Nursing* 23(13–14):1927–1936, 2013.

Bryman A: Integrating quantitative and qualitative research: How is it done?, *Qualitative Research* 6(1):97–113, 2006.

Campbell DT, Fiske DW: Convergent and discriminant validation by the multitrait-multimethod matrix, *Psychological Bulletin* 56(2):81–105, 1959.

Clark VLP, Schumacher K, West C, et al: Practices for embedding an interpretive qualitative approach within a randomized clinical trial, *Journal of Mixed Methods Research* 7(3):219–242, 2013.

Creswell JW, Fetters MD, Ivankova NV: Designing a mixed methods study in primary care, *Annals of Family Medicine* 2(1):7–12, 2004.

Creswell JW, Klassen AC, Plano Clark VL, et al: *Best practices for mixed methods research in the health sciences*, 2011, Office of Behavioral and Social Sciences Research, National Institute of Health.

Creswell JW, Plano Clark VL: *Designing and conducting mixed methods research*, Thousand Oaks, California, 2011, SAGE Publications.

Denzin NK: *The research act: a theoretical introduction to sociological methods*, Englewood Cliffs, New Jersey, 1989, Prentice Hall.

Doyle L, Brady AM, Byrne G: An overview of mixed methods research, *Journal of Research in Nursing* 14(2):175–185, 2009.

Feilzer MY: Doing Mixed Methods Research Pragmatically: Implications for the Rediscovery of Pragmatism as a Research Paradigm, *Journal of Mixed Methods Research* 4(1):6–16, 2010.

Foss C, Ellefsen B: The value of combining qualitative and quantitative approaches in nursing research by means of method triangulation, *Journal of Advanced Nursing* 40(2):242–248, 2002.

Gill F, Corkish V, Robertson J, et al: An exploration of pediatric nurses' compliance with a medication checking and administration protocol, *Journal for Specialists in Pediatric Nursing* 17(2):136–146, 2012.

Glogowska M: Paradigms, pragmatism and possibilities: Mixed-methods research in speech and language therapy, *International Journal of Language & Communication Disorders* 46(3):251–260, 2011.

Greene JC, Caracelli VJ, Graham WF: Toward a Conceptual Framework for Mixed-method Evaluation Designs, *Educational Evaluation and Policy Analysis*, 1989.

Halcomb EJ, Andrew S: Triangulation as a method for contemporary nursing research, *Nurse Researcher* 13(2):71–82, 2005.

Halcomb EJ, Andrew S: Managing mixed methods projects. In Andrew S, Halcomb EJ, editors: *Mixed methods research for nursing and the health sciences*, London, England, 2009, Wiley-Blackwell, pp 50–64.

Halcomb EJ, Andrew S: Practical considerations for higher degree research students undertaking mixed methods projects, *International Journal of Multiple Research Approaches* 3(2):153–162, 2009.

Halcomb EJ, Hickman L: Considerations in mixed methods research, *Nursing Standard* 29(32):37–43, 2015.

Hamshire C, Willgoss TG, Wibberley C: What are reasonable expectations? Healthcare student perceptions of their programmes in the North West of England, *Nurse Education Today* 33(2):173–179, 2013.

Hayes B, Bonner A, Douglas C: An introduction to mixed methods research for nephrology nurses, *Renal Society of Australasia Journal* 9(1):8–14, 2013.

Heyvaert M, Hannes K, Maes B, et al: Critical Appraisal of Mixed Methods Studies, *Journal of Mixed Methods Research* 7(4):302–327, 2013.

Johnson BR, Onwuegbuzie AJ: Mixed methods research: A research paradigm whose time has come, *Educational Researcher* 33(7):14–26, 2004.

Kinser PA, Bourguignon C, Whaley D, et al: Feasibility, Acceptability and Effects of Gentle Hatha Yoga for Women With Major Depression: Findings From a Randomized Controlled Mixed-Methods Study, *Archives of Psychiatric Nursing* 27(3):137–147, 2013.

Kroll T, Neri MT, Miller K: Using mixed methods in disability and rehabilitation research, *Rehabilitation Nursing* 30(3):2005.

Lavelle E, Vuk J, Barber C: Twelve tips for getting started using mixed methods in medical education research, *Medical Teacher* 35(4):272–276, 2013.

Luck L, Jackson D, Usher K: Case study: a bridge across the paradigms, *Nursing Inquiry* 13(2):103–109, 2006.

Maudsley G: Mixing it but not mixed-up: Mixed methods research in medical education (a critical narrative review), *Medical Teacher* 33(2):e92–e104, 2011.

McEvoy P, Richards D: A critical realist rationale for using a combination of quantitative and qualitative methods, *Journal of Research in Nursing* 11(1):66–78, 2006.

Meixner C, O'Donoghue CR, Witt M: Accessing Crisis Intervention Services After Brain Injury: A Mixed Methods Study, *Rehabilitation Psychology* 58(4):377–385, 2013.

Mertens D: Mixed methods and the politics of human research: The transformative-emancipatory perspective. In Tashakkori A, Teddlie C, editors: *Handbook of mixed methods in social & behavioral research*, Thousand Oaks, California, 2003, SAGE Publications, pp 135–164.

Mesel T: The necessary distinction between methodology and philosophical assumptions in healthcare research, *Scandinavian Journal of Caring Sciences* 27(3):750–756, 2013.

Morgan DL: Practical strategies for combining qualitative and quantitative methods: Applications to health research, *Qualitative Health Research* 8(3):362–376, 1998.

Njie-Carr V: Violence Experiences Among HIV-Infected Women and Perceptions of Male Perpetrators' Roles: A Concurrent Mixed Method Study, *Journal of the Association of Nurses in AIDS Care* 25(5):376–391, 2014.

O'Cathain A, Murphy E, Nicholl J: The quality of mixed methods studies in health services research, *Journal of Health Services Research and Policy* 13(2):92–98, 2008.

O'Cathain A, Murphy E, Nicholl J: Three techniques for integrating data in mixed methods studies, *BMJ (Clinical Research Ed.)* 341(2010):2010.

Onwuegbuzie AJ, Leech NL: Enhancing the interpretation of significant findings: The role of mixed methods research, *Qualitative Report* 9(4):770–792, 2004.

Polit DF, Beck CT: Generalization in quantitative and qualitative research: Myths and strategies, *International Journal of Nursing Studies* 47(11):1451–1458, 2010.

Rickard CM, Williams G, Ray-Barruel G, et al: Towards improved organisational support for nurses working in research roles in the clinical setting: A mixed method investigation, *Collegian (Royal College of Nursing, Australia)* 18(4):165–176, 2011.

Ridenour CS, Newman I, editors: *Mixed methods research: exploring the interactive continuum*, Carbondale, 2008, Southern Illinois University Press.

Risjord MW, Dunbar SB, Moloney MF: A new foundation for methodological triangulation, *Journal of Nursing Scholarship* 34(3):269–275, 2004.

Shepard MP, Orsi AJ, Mahon MM, et al: Mixed-methods research with vulnerable families, *Journal of Family Nursing* 8(4):334–352, 2002.

Simons L, Lathlean J: Mixed Methods. In Gerrish K, Lacey A, editors: *The research process in nursing*, London, 2010, Wiley-Blackwell, pp 331–342.

Slater P, McCormack B, Bunting B: The development and pilot testing of an instrument to measure nurses' working environment: the Nursing Context Index, *Worldviews on Evidence-based Nursing* 6(3):173–182, 2009.

Tashakkori A, Teddlie C, editors: *Handbook of mixed methods in social and behavioural research*, Thousand Oaks, California, 2003, SAGE Publications.

Teddlie C, Tashakkori A, editors: *Foundations of mixed methods research: integrating quantitative and qualitative approaches in the social and behavioral sciences*, Thousand Oaks, California, 2009, SAGE Publications.

Thurmond VA: The point of triangulation, *Journal of Nursing Scholarship* 33(3):253–258, 2001.

Walsh D, Evans K: Critical realism: An important theoretical perspective for midwifery research, *Midwifery* 30(1):e1–e6, 2014.

West C, Buettner P, Stewart L, et al: Resilience in families with a member with chronic pain: a mixed methods study, *Journal of Clinical Nursing* 21(23–24):3532–3545, 2012.

West R, Usher K, Buettner PG, et al: Indigenous Australians' participation in pre-registration tertiary nursing courses: a mixed methods study, *Contemporary nurse* 46(1):123–134, 2013.

Wisdom JP, Cavaleri MA, Onwuegbuzie AJ, et al: Methodological reporting in qualitative, quantitative and mixed methods health services research articles, *Health Services Research* 47(2):721–745, 2012.

Zhang W, Creswell J: The use of 'mixing' procedure of mixed methods in health services research, *Medical Care* 51(8):e51–e57, 2013.

Zwar N, Richmond R, Halcomb E, et al: Quit in general practice: a cluster randomised trial of enhanced in-practice support for smoking cessation, *BMC Family Practice* 11:59, 2010.

CHAPTER 8

INDIGENOUS INSIGHTS INTO NURSING AND MIDWIFERY RESEARCH

Juanita Sherwood and Denise Wilson

CHAPTER OUTLINE

KEY TERMS

Aboriginal and Torres Strait Islander peoples
colonisation
culturally competent
Indigenous peoples
Māori peoples
sociohistorical context
world views

LEARNING OBJECTIVES

After reading this chapter and following critical reflection, the student will be able to:

1. Describe Indigenous world views and knowledge
2. Discuss relevant ethics, values and protocols for research with Indigenous people
3. Explain Indigenous sociohistorical contexts, and impacts of colonisation and racism on their access to determinants of health
4. Discuss considerations for decolonising Indigenous health
5. Explain the principles of social justice, equity and rights as they apply to research
6. Use research in a culturally competent way to inform practice with Indigenous people.

STUDENT QUOTE

I treated all my patients the same. I now realise that equality does not mean sameness and that Indigenous peoples suffer disparities. This must be a key principle that informs research, along with it being appropriate and acceptable to Indigenous peoples.

ABSTRACT

Indigenous peoples globally, while diverse, share similar colonising histories and stories of the subjugation of their knowledge forms. Understanding the historical events of imperialism and colonisation that have negatively influenced Indigenous knowledge systems and ways of knowing is crucial when looking at research, especially when using it to inform practice when working with Indigenous peoples. Indigenous peoples are best positioned to discover knowledge and strategies to resolve the many health challenges that they face, and of recent times have been actively involved in reclaiming and developing Indigenous health knowledges. Understanding world views, Indigenous knowledge systems and ethical processes can assist nursing and midwifery students to analyse research with Indigenous peoples.

Knowledge which makes sense in one particular cultural context cannot always be understood through the tools which govern the understanding of other belief systems and world views (Jahnke & Taiapa 1999).

Introduction

Indigenous peoples have established ways of viewing and understanding the world, and have been researching the world for centuries. Yet, until relatively recent times, their ways of knowing and research have been invisible. The above quote highlights the risk of producing flawed knowledge in cross-cultural research, on which non-Indigenous researchers create evidence about Indigenous cultural realities from a different cultural orientation. Best possible evidence must inform nursing and midwifery practice and health services given the health status and health outcome disparities and inequities with which Indigenous peoples live. Such evidence must not only be relevant and reflective of Indigenous peoples' lives, as determined by themselves, it must also provide an accurate interpretation of their cultural positioning and their sociocultural realities. In this chapter, we draw your attention to the historical and contemporary contexts of suboptimal research practices imposed on Indigenous peoples globally, and the subsequent interpretations of research findings that have not been beneficial and have often reinforced negative stereotypes and explanations that focus on their perceived deficits. Many Indigenous peoples no longer accept such approaches to research. They have become wary of research and researchers – Indigenous and non-Indigenous alike – and choose to only engage in research that aligns with their goals and that reflects their Indigenous realities and which ultimately benefits their communities.

So who are Indigenous peoples? The United Nations defines Indigenous peoples as having:

> *... populated areas before the arrival of others and often retain distinct cultural and political characteristics, including autonomous political and legal structures, as well as a common experience of domination by others, especially non-Indigenous groups, and a strong historical and ongoing connection to their lands, territories and resources, including when they practice nomadic lifestyles. While the legal status of Indigenous peoples is distinct from that of minorities, they are often, though not always, in the minority in the states in which they reside (United Nations 2013).*

The term 'Indigenous' is inclusive of those groups of peoples who:

- identify, and are recognised by their communities, as Indigenous
- are historically linked to their respective countries or tribal areas prior to their colonisation, and
- have continuing connections to their tribal regions and the natural resources within them.

In addition, Indigenous peoples have:

- distinct languages, cultural beliefs and practices, and
- their own established social, economic and political systems.

Today, Indigenous peoples are marginalised groups in their countries, but they resolve to maintain and restore their ancestral and traditional environments and systems as distinct peoples and communities. First peoples, first nations, aboriginal, ethnic groups, iwi (tribe), or hapū (sub-tribe) are the different terms Indigenous peoples prefer, and reflect the modern understanding of being 'Indigenous' (United Nations 2008; World Health Organization 2007).

The Indigenous peoples of Australia and New Zealand are the **Aboriginal and Torres Strait Islander peoples**, and **Māori peoples**, respectively. They are not homogenous groups, as implied by these broad titles. Instead, they often identify by their nation or country in Australia, and their hapū and iwi in New Zealand. Nevertheless, they share similar histories of **colonisation** resulting in historic injustices that brought about depopulation, socioeconomic and political disenfranchisement, and marginalisation that rendered them as powerless minority groups within their own countries. Through processes of colonisation, contemporary Indigenous peoples have lost their land, languages and their cultural practices. Notably they suffer ongoing contemporary injustices and inequities compared to other population groups living in their countries.

Within the context of research, those advocating Western scientific paradigms invalidated and trivialised Indigenous peoples' well-developed knowledge systems and ways of knowing. In this chapter, we will provide an overview of the **sociohistorical contexts** of Aboriginal and Torres Strait Islander and Māori peoples and will stress the relevance of these contexts when reading and interpreting research. We will then discuss and position Indigenous **world views**, ethics, values and protocols as different from dominant world views that generally inform health research. Following this will be an explanation of decolonising Indigenous health as a way to better understand and address the health inequities they suffer. We end by talking about using research-based evidence relating to Indigenous peoples in a **culturally competent** manner to inform nursing and midwifery practice.

Sociohistorical contexts

The initial settlement of Australia and New Zealand by people from other countries, predominately the United Kingdom, brought with it imperialism and colonisation. Imperialism, informed by Western knowledge and traditions, is a method of control. It facilitated an agenda for Indigenous peoples to be the 'same' (assimilation) as settlers and colonisers. At the same time it created them as 'others' (marginalisation) and disempowered them culturally, economically, politically and cognitively (Chilisa 2012; Smith 2012). This was aided by invasion, land acquisition and the destruction of Indigenous political, social, economic and cultural systems that ensured they thrived and prospered (Smith 2012). Colonisation assisted Europe's expansion throughout the world, including a number of the countries within the Pacific.

It is important to appreciate the ways Indigenous peoples were constructed and represented, based on western world views that viewed Aboriginal Australians and Māori alike, as inferior, and the darker the skin of the people, the greater their perceived inferiority. This was influenced by social Darwinism that classified Indigenous peoples as 'species' (Smith 2012). This gave rise to terms such as 'noble savages' to describe Māori, for instance, whereby they were seen as primitive 'savages' but were also seen as 'noble' when compared to peoples of darker races. Colonisers (driven by their western perspectives and beliefs of being superior to those of whose land they stole or took by devious methods) assumed settlers, missionaries and themselves brought civilisation to Indigenous people they believed were uncivilised and savages.

Indigenous peoples were usurped from their homes, ways of life and freedom. Colonisation significantly impacted Indigenous peoples globally, resulting in separation from their traditional lands, aided by western laws and policies that stripped them of their sovereignty, autonomy and status. Smith stated it left a '... legacy of suffering and destruction' (Smith 2012). Colonisers, using these western paradigms, determined what constituted knowledge and how it would be produced. However, it systematically demeaned and devalued Indigenous knowledge, and associated racial agendas protected settlers and cast Indigenous peoples in negative ways, for instance needing to be quarantined because they were 'riddled with disease' (Anderson 2002). Such actions and beliefs, often published, highlighted significant differences between superior and clean Europeans and the primitive, disease-ridden and declining Indigenous peoples (Anderson 2002).

Smith simply concluded, 'they came, they saw, they named, they claimed' (Smith 1999). Research was synonymous with being scientific and had profound consequences for Indigenous peoples and their ways of knowing. The positioning of Indigenous people as 'other' guaranteed their objectification and marginalisation. Not only did this silence them, it denied and invalidated their world views and knowledges. Instead, it became normal to measure, judge and interpret Indigenous peoples against western scientific world views and standards (Smith 2012; Chilisa 2012; Bishop 1996; Denzin et al 2008). Past research provided disparaging accounts of Indigenous peoples that contributed to the current assumptions that Indigenous peoples are problematic (Durie 1998; Thomas 2004).

Western ways of knowing silenced Indigenous peoples globally and subjugated their knowledges (Smith 2012; Ermine et al 2004; Battiste & Henderson 2000). According to Ladson-Billings (2000), 'The hegemony of the dominant paradigm makes it more than just one way to view the world – it claims to be the only legitimate way to view the world'. Significantly, the negative constructions of Indigenous peoples persisted and informed research and policy targeting these communities, even when evidence confirmed such constructions were false (Guba & Lincoln 1989).

Researchers, using western scientific research tools and approaches, have generally investigated contemporary Indigenous health issues perpetuating Indigenous peoples being framed as problematic. Since the 1970s, Indigenous peoples globally, concerned about the socioeconomic and health disparities they experience, have been reclaiming and developing their own approaches to research. This includes asserting their right to investigate health and social issues affecting their health using tools informed by their own world views. Such approaches enable strengths-based and outcome-focused research undertaken by Indigenous peoples themselves, rather than problem-oriented research.

World views

A world view is a system of knowledge that develops from birth and is shaped by the social and physical environment that you grow up in. It is shaped by your culture, the experiences you have and the belief systems you encounter (Ranzijn et al 2009). World views are frameworks for understanding and investigating the world we live in. They support the way we act and relate in the world (Phillips & Brown 1991). World views are knowledge or cognitive systems (Marglin 1990), and provide models and contexts for processing, understanding and explaining information and knowledge (Smith 2012; Aerts et al 2007). They can be considered the mental foundations for the way we perceive and live in the world (Hart 2010).

World views are generally monocultural conceptual frameworks for the way you see and think about the world (Kovach 2009). They guide and determine an entire mode of living, particularly with regard to how we interpret and order our realities in the world we live. A paradigm involves a methodological process informed by a philosophical framework about what constitutes knowledge and ways of knowing, and that identifies relevant ethics and values (Chilisa 2012). The 'truths' produced by world views are, therefore, biased by a particular cultural standpoint (Denzin & Lincoln 2000). What this means is that there are multiple ways for seeing and understanding the world we live in. It is important that we appreciate that our own world views are no more right or better than other people's world views, and that there is no right or wrong world view, just different ways of viewing the world (Ranzijn et al 2009).

Indigenous world views

Indigenous paradigms are informed by their knowledge system, ways of being, values and methods of generating knowledge (see Box 8.1). It is important to note that while there is great diversity among the world's Indigenous peoples there are a number of perspectives that we do share. Key features of Indigenous world views are that they generally are:

- holistic in nature
- ecologically and spiritually based
- collective and relational oriented, and
- integrate the past, present and future (contrasting with dominant western ways that view time in a linear way).

Box 8.1
Indigenous research paradigm

Axiology	Values	Respectful and ethical practices, grounded in Indigenous cultural beliefs and practices. Indigenous peoples determine the transfer of information and knowledge. Elders play an important role as holders of knowledge and determine who will and can have access to it.
Ontology	Ways of being	Social and relational construction of Indigenous ways of being.
Epistemology	Ways of knowing	Knowledge systems are relational.
Methodology	Ways of doing research	Oral transmission, storytelling, yarning, songs, ceremonies, symbols.

Indigenous peoples have special and enduring connections with their traditional lands – these places are the basis of their survival and spiritual wellbeing, are a place of nurturing, and, what Daes calls, a place for learning (Battiste & Henderson 2000). Indigenous world views are dynamic, ensuring continuous reinforming of ways of knowing and living in the world. Therefore, the many social and technological changes occurring in our world influence many contemporary Indigenous peoples' traditional world views.

A particular feature of Indigenous peoples is our collective and relational way of living with others that includes all living and non-living entities and spirits (Hart 2010). This promotes collective responsibilities and intrinsic obligations to others. This differs notably from dominant cultural groups that endorse the self and individual success over the collective group. Chilisa and Tsheko (2014) explain this:

> *Knowing is something that is socially constructed by people who have relationships and connections with each other, the living and the non-living, and the environment. Knowers are seen as beings with connections with other beings, the spirits of the ancestors and the world around them that informs what they know and how they can know it ...the challenge is on how to bring this cultural knowledge into the research process.*

Therefore, it is important that research reflect Indigenous peoples' views of health and wellbeing, which is holistic and inclusive of the emotional, social, physical and spiritual dimensions of individuals, and their relationships with their families and others within their communities.

Indigenous knowledge and ways of knowing

Indigenous ways of knowing are secular and relational. Creation stories and tribal lands are the foundations of knowledge that inform spiritual and cultural praxis (Battiste 2002; Burgess et al 2005; Wilson 2008b; Yunupingu 1997). Indigenous knowledge systems are regulated through tribal authorities with defined roles and responsibilities, and systems and processes for research (Health Research Council of New Zealand 2010; Smallacombe et al 2007). Thus, embedded within traditional Indigenous knowledge are the ways in which people understand and function in the world about them, and what they value. This is relevant for understanding why many Indigenous peoples struggle when using health services – their views, values and practices of health differ markedly, something generally ignored by health professionals. Ideally, Indigenous paradigms are best to research Indigenous peoples. Oral traditions transmit knowledge via storytelling, song, music, designs on visual art forms, for example. The following briefly introduces you to Aboriginal and Māori creation stories, and how traditional ways of knowing remain relevant today.

Aboriginal Dreaming

Customary law has always been in place in Australia since time immemorial, laid down by the creating spirits of the Dreaming. Indigenous Australians maintain that their creation and beginnings were founded by the Dreaming, an era of creation – marking the time that Aboriginal occupation commenced in Australia (Stanner 1979). This way of knowing is universal to all Australian Indigenous groups (Razani et al 2007; Pawu-kurlpurlurnu et al 2008). Aboriginal peoples were created through the life force of their Dreaming ancestors, along with their respective lands, flora and fauna. Each Aboriginal person, no matter where they are from, has metaphysical and geographical relationships with all of the living and non-living beings of their respective Dreaming creators (Hume 2002). This is an essential standpoint of Aboriginal

Australians' world view, and is distinctly different from a western way of knowing them and their history (Sherwood 2010).

Māori whakapapa (genealogy)

Whakapapa provides a way of understanding the Māori world. It links the origin of humankind from Te Kore (a void, state of potential), to Te Po (the realm of darkness) holding Ranginui (the sky father) and Papatūanuku (the Earth mother), to Te Ao Marama (the world of light) where Ranginui's and Papatūnuku's children were born. The womb (Te Po) and birthing (Te Ao Marama) symbolically explain aspects of the origins of humankind. Whakapapa explains the genealogy of humans along with other living things, and importantly prescribes the integral relationships humans have to each other, the environment and other living things. In this way, it links past, present and future, humans and atua (gods), tupuna (ancestors), Papatūanuku (tribal area) and the whenua (land), and living things. Māori will begin interactions with others by citing their pepeha (tribal links), sharing their connections to their whenua (land), maunga (mountain), river (awa), waka (canoe), iwi (tribe), hapū (sub-tribe) and whanau (extended family). Whakapapa also provides practical knowledge that aids survival and influences the behaviours, obligations and responsibilities that, as Indigenous peoples, they have to one another and the environment and all things within it (Mead 2003; Mikaere 2011).

STUDENT CHALLENGE

Differentiating Indigenous and Western Knowledge Systems

Identify the features of Indigenous knowledge systems using the following headings: Epistemology (ways of knowing), Ontology (ways of being), Axiology (values) and Methodology (ways of transmitting knowledge). Then compare these to western biomedical knowledge systems that inform nursing and midwifery knowledge systems. How may these differences influence how you will begin to analyse published research?

Ethical Indigenous research

> *Getting the story right, telling the story well (Smith 2012).*

Indigenous ethical principles and values differ from those of western researchers, and premised on shifting research agendas away from those with problematising conceptualisations (Shibaski & Stewart 2005). Central to ethical research is recognising the differences in world views, and ways of knowing (Smith 2012; Battiste 2008; Sherwood 2010). Indigenous ethics are about responding and upholding the rights and dignity of Indigenous people involved within a research project. Importantly, it is about complying with their cultural protocols (Sherwood 2010; Chilisa 2012; Wilson 2008b). Indigenous peoples assert their right to self-determination rather than their disenfranchisement in research. This has led to the development of ethical guidelines for undertaking research with Indigenous peoples. Wilson and Neville (2009) refer to this as 'creating a space for dialogue and negotiation'.

The utilisation of 'binding ethical guidelines' is a method to assist in transforming 'western intellectual approaches' (Humphery 2001). Ethical research means that Indigenous peoples and their communities must be included throughout the research process, from the start of research ideas to disseminating the findings. Researchers should involve their local Indigenous community in developing the research proposal and establishing their cultural expectations and processes. The process aims to respect and ensure the hearing of Indigenous people's voices, views, practices and knowledges.

Aboriginal Customary Law in Australia determines 'who can claim, use and adapt and disseminate Aboriginal and Torres Strait Islander peoples' cultural expression and knowledge' (Janke & Dawson 2012). However, this has been ignored by researchers and academics in the past, with harmful impacts for those who trusted that their knowledge would be valued and not disseminated. Just as there are many Aboriginal peoples and nations within Australia there are many ways of Indigenous knowing, being and doing. Aboriginal and Torres Strait Islander peoples' ethics are grounded in their world view that 'requires that protocols be set by the Aboriginal and Torres Strait Islander community' to be followed respectfully by researchers, be they Indigenous or non-Indigenous. Aboriginal communities' approaches are set within an agenda of self-determination and survival that requires that they actively participate 'as stakeholders, research participants and researchers' (Shibaski & Stewart 2005) in any research that focuses on their communities.

Tikanga (doing things right) underpins ethical research with Māori in New Zealand. The Health Research Council has expectations about research with Māori, and ethics committees require researchers to show consultation with the appropriate Māori iwi or community groups (Health Research Council of New Zealand 2010; Health Research Council & the Ministry of Health 2010). Researchers are required to demonstrate responsiveness to Māori. In practice, this involves researchers explaining the consultation undertaken throughout the research process, and the cultural advice and support sought to ensure practices observe the tikanga. Furthermore, Te Ara Tika outlines the ethical guidelines and expectations for research with Māori (Hudson et al 2010).

Any research and all findings involving Indigenous peoples must be in the hands of their community. Furthermore, research must make sure it benefits the community and involves Indigenous research capacity building and opportunities for employment (for instance, as research team members or research assistants). Research that uses appropriate methods and methodologies (i.e. the world view and theory informing how research is planned, undertaken and interpreted) assists in ensuring research is appropriate, acceptable and meaningful for Indigenous communities.

Decolonising Indigenous health

The process of colonisation took place in Australia, New Zealand, the United States, Canada and Africa. Universally, Indigenous peoples yearn to be reunited with their land and regain balance of their natural world (Royal 2002). This informs the basis for decolonisation as a strategy of, and for reclaiming, Indigenous sovereignty, dignity and wellbeing. Recognising Indigenous world views as distinct ontological and epistemological traditions is essential when using Indigenous health research, particularly as western research methodologies remain limited as they generally ignore their histories of colonisation and the plight of many contemporary Indigenous peoples – for instance, the unacceptable inequities in health status and health outcomes.

Decolonisation, according to Chilisa (2012 p. 14), is '... a process of conducting research in such a way that the world views of those who have suffered a long history of oppression and marginalisation are given space to communicate from their frames of reference'. Knowledge about Indigenous peoples, particularly with regard to health research, is defined by evidence generated from dominant cultural viewpoints that pathologises them. It is, therefore, important that when reviewing health literature and research you ask: through whose eyes and world view has this research been analysed or interpreted? For instance, researchers generally construct research about Māori and their use of health services as non-compliance (Smith 2012). This is at odds with Māori accounts of their experiences of health services (see for instance, Penney et al 2011; Wilson & Barton 2012).

In appreciating Indigenous world views and ways of knowing, it is important that nurses and midwives are aware of the way Indigenous peoples understand health. As we have discussed, the dominant biomedical model, driven by western science, has influenced what constitutes 'valid' knowledge and evidence, including the methods of producing knowledge via research within the health arena. This research by focusing mainly on people's physical health or illness, influences not only how health services are structured and delivered, but informs nursing and midwifery practice. Furthermore, research driven by a deficit approach ignores the social and economic problems that are determinants of health affecting Indigenous peoples' health and lives. Instead, it generally reports Indigenous peoples as the problem. Such 'deficit' accounts and victim blaming bypass the role those systems, structures and health professionals' behaviours and attitudes have in perpetuating Indigenous health inequities and that makes health services difficult for

Indigenous peoples to use. When considering published research, it is important to consider Indigenous world views and their cultural values, beliefs and practices.

Rights, social justice and equity

Underpinning ethical and decolonising activities are the concepts of social justice, equity and rights. In addition to basic human rights, the United Nations Declaration on the Rights of Indigenous Peoples affirms Indigenous people's 'equal right to the enjoyment of the highest attainable standard of physical and mental health' (Article 24:2) (United Nations 2008). Australia and New Zealand (along with the United States and Canada), slow to endorse this declaration, did so in 2009 and 2010, respectively. Moreover, the Geneva Declaration on the Health and Survival of Indigenous Peoples calls for 'access to quality and culturally appropriate healthcare ...without discrimination' (United Nations Economic and Social Council 2002). In order to realise these rights, research better reflecting Indigenous people's health experiences is required.

In New Zealand, Māori also have rights under the Treaty of Waitangi, which was an agreement, signed in 1840, that set out the obligations of the British monarchy (and later the New Zealand government) to Māori peoples. The Treaty articles set out Māori rights to self-determination and equality with others living in New Zealand, although in health the principles of partnership, participation and protection are ways that health providers honour their obligations under the Treaty of Waitangi. Nonetheless, there have been long periods of time when the obligations under this treaty to Māori have not been afforded, not assisted by the Māori and English language versions differing and it being subjected to the political tenor of the day.

A social justice perspective involves privileging the voices of the 'researched and moving from a deficit-based orientation' to uncover the practices that ensured their survival (Chilisa 2012). It is grounded in rights and the concepts of equality, equity and rights. It is important to understand that inequities and disparities are evident in communities when social structures and systems are in place that disadvantage minority and marginalised groups, such as Indigenous peoples. Disparities in social and health status are unjust and unfair. Far from choosing a 'lifestyle', disadvantaged groups have difficulties in accessing the necessary determinants of health because of structural discrimination, which is related to increased risks of morbidity and mortality (Braveman & Gruskin 2003; Reid & Robson 2006). Equal approaches based on the notions of 'sameness' are not effective. While in some circumstances inequalities are (a) expected and (b) are acceptable (for instance, the inequalities in breast cancer between men and women), equitable approaches, on the other hand, require greater levels of attention and intervention to reduce the morbidity and mortality Indigenous peoples suffer. This invariably requires doing things differently. While this is a brief overview of these concepts, they lay the foundation for culturally competent use of research.

STUDENT CHALLENGE

Social Justice

Identify how local and national health policies and procedures promote social justice for Indigenous peoples in your community.

Culturally competent use of research

Cultural competence requires nurses and midwives to comprehend their own world views and sociocultural positioning. It also requires practice that is informed by a critical analysis of the sociocultural contexts that impact the health of Indigenous peoples (and other minority groups), to act in a respectful and responsive manner and to integrate their cultural needs into their plans of care (Wilson 2008a). This means that we need to engage critically with, and question, the research literature. Linda Tuhiwai Smith signals a caution about research undertaken from non-Indigenous perspectives (Smith 2012), particularly as non-Indigenous researchers generally interpret research findings from narrow perspectives, and persist on focusing on Indigenous deficits and blaming them as the sole cause for their health status. Indigenous peoples often provide different perspectives on the difficulty they have engaging with and using health services (Wilson & Barton 2012).

This offers a place to begin thinking about how, as nurses and midwives, we use research to inform our practice and to advocate for health services that meet the needs of Indigenous peoples. Persisting with the same approaches and endorsing research that does not accurately reflect Indigenous peoples' experiences simply perpetuates the status quo. We are far from being in the 'post' colonisation era because the processes of colonisation persist, for example, in the ways in which evidence is used to inform health services structure and delivery, and the ways in which health professionals are prepared to work with Indigenous peoples (Chilisa 2012; Sherwood 2013).

At this point in your career you may not be in a position to influence the way in which research is planned, undertaken and interpreted, but you can begin by being more critical about the way in which you question the research that informs your practice. We argue that cultural competence extends to the way in which nurses and midwives use research findings for evidence-based practice. Box 8.2 provides you with a set of questions, adapted in part from those posed by Linda Tuhiwai Smith, which you can use to begin questioning the research you are reviewing about Indigenous peoples, particularly if you intend to use it to inform your practice.

Box 8.2
Guiding questions to review research with Indigenous peoples

- Did the research team include Indigenous researchers and/or an Indigenous cultural advisory group?
- Who defined the research problem? Was the relevant Indigenous community(ies) involved in developing the research questions and aims?
- For whom is the study beneficial and relevant? Who says so?
- What knowledge will the Indigenous community gain from this research?
- What knowledge did the researcher gain from this research?
- What are the positive outcomes from this research?
- What were potential negative outcomes? How were potential negative outcomes removed?
- In what ways were the research findings communicated? Do the findings reinforce deficit explanations or negative stereotypes associated with Indigenous health or do they highlight a more strengths-based approach?
- To whom was the researcher(s) accountable?
- What processes were in place to ensure cultural support for the research, researched and researcher(s)?

Note: adapted from Smith (2012)

STUDENT CHALLENGE

Health Literacy

Indigenous peoples are often referred to as lacking health literacy, despite never having received information about their health conditions and the management of these, or have been given information in a manner that is laced with jargon and difficult for them to understand. How do researchers portray health literacy for Indigenous peoples? How do they, or do they not, focus the lens on health professionals in undertaking this research? How can the concept of health literacy be problematic for Indigenous peoples?

STUDENT CHALLENGE

Hard to Reach

Often researchers frame Indigenous peoples as 'hard to reach', yet they do not consider in what ways health services may be 'hard to use'. Find some research interviews undertaken by Indigenous researchers of Indigenous people about their experiences of trying to access and use health services. Would you now consider Indigenous peoples as 'hard to reach' or health services as 'hard to use'? What is the rationale for the conclusions you have drawn?

RESOURCE KIT

The following documents are useful for getting a fuller and more specific understanding of the considerations in undertaking research with Indigenous peoples:

Chilisa B: *Indigenous research methodologies*, Thousand Oaks, California, 2012, SAGE Publications.

Smiths LT: *Decolonizing methodologies: Research and Indigenous peoples*, ed 2, London, 2012, Zed Books.

Australia: National Health and Medical Research Council (NHMRC)

Values and Ethics – Guidelines for Ethical Conduct in Aboriginal and Torres Strait Islander Health Research (2003). Online. Available: https://www.nhmrc.gov.au/guidelines/publications/e52.

Keeping research on track: a guide for Aboriginal and Torres Strait Island peoples about health research ethics (2006). Online. Available: https://www.nhmrc.gov.au/guidelines/publications/e65.

New Zealand: Health Research Council

Guidelines for Researchers on Health Research Involving Māori (2010). Online. Available: http://www.hrc.govt.nz/news-and-publications/publications/guidelines-researchers-health-research-involving-m%C4%81ori.

Te Ara Tika – Guidelines for Māori Research Ethics: A framework for researchers and ethics committee members (Hudson et al 2010). Online. Available: http://www.hrc.govt.nz/news-and-publications/publications/te-ara-tika-guidelines-m%C4%81ori-research-ethics-framework-researcher.

Examples of Research Using Indigenous Methodologies

Cram F, Kennedy V: *Researching with Whānau Collectives* MAI Review, 2010 (3). Online. Available: http://www.review.mai.ac.nz/index.php/MR/article/view/382/561.

Graham J: *Nā Rangi tāua, nā Tūānuku e takoto nei: Research methodology framed by whakapapa* MAI Review, 2009 (1) Article 3. Online. Available: http://review.mai.ac.nz/index.php/MR/article/viewFile/199/226.

Sherwood J: Colonisation – It's bad for your health: The context of Aboriginal health, *Contemporary Nurse* 46:28–40, 2013.

Sherwood J, Kendall S: Reframing spaces by building relationships: Community collaborative participatory action research with Aboriginal mothers in prison, *Contemporary Nurse* 46(1):84–95, 2013.

References

Aerts D, Apostel L, De Moor B, et al: *World views from fragmentation to integration*, Brussels, 2007, VUB Press.

Anderson W: *The cultivation of whiteness: Science, health and racial destiny in Australia*, Melbourne, 2002, Melbourne University Press.

Battiste M: *Indigenous knowledge and pedagogy in First Nations education: A literature review with recommendations*, Prepared for the National Working Group on Education and the Minister of Indian Affairs Ottawa: Indian and Northern Affairs Canada. 2002.

Battiste M: Research ethics for protecting Indigenous knowledge and heritage: Institutional and researcher responsibilities. In Denzin NK, Lincoln YS, Smit LT, editors: *Handbook of critical and indigeous methodologies*, Los Angeles, California, 2008, SAGE Publications.

Battiste M, Henderson JY: *Protecting Indigenous knowledge and heritage: A global challenge*, Saskatoon, Canada, 2000, Purich Publishing.

Bishop R: *Collaborative research stories: Whakawhanaungatanga*, Palmerston North, NZ, 1996, Dunmore.

Braveman P, Gruskin S: Defining equity in health, *Journal of Epidemiology and Community Health* 57:254–258, 2003.

Burgess CP, Johnston FH, Bowman DMJS, et al: Healthy country: Healthy people? Exploring the health benefits of Indigenous natural resource management, *Australian and New Zealand Journal of Public Health* 29:117–122, 2005.

Chilisa B: *Indigenous research methodologies*, Thousand Oaks, California, 2012, SAGE Publications.

Chilisa B, Tsheko GN: Mixed methods in Indigenous research: Building relationships for sustainable intervention outcomes, *Journal of Mixed Methods Research* 8:222–233, 2014.

Denzin NK, Lincoln YS: *The practices and politics of interpretation*, Thousand Oaks, California, 2000, SAGE Publications.

Denzin NK, Lincoln YS, Smith LT: *Handbook of critical and Indigenous methodologies*, Thousand Oaks, California, 2008, SAGE Publications.

Durie M: *Whaiora: Maori health development*, Auckland, New Zealand, 1998, Oxford University Press.

Ermine W, Sinclair R, Jeffery B, et al: *The Ethics of Research Involving Indigenous Peoples: Report of the Indigenous Peoples' Health Research Centre to the Interagency Advisory Panel on Research Ethics*, Saskatoon, SK, 2004, Indigenous People's Research Centre, Saskatoon.

Guba EG, Lincoln YS: *Fourth Generation Evaluation*, Newbury Park, California, 1989, SAGE Publications.

Hart MA: Indigenous world views, knowledge and research: The development of an Indigenous research paradigm, *Journal of Indigenous Voices in Social Work* 1:1–16, 2010.

Health Research Council of New Zealand: *Guidelines for Researchers on Health Research Involving Maori*, Auckland, NZ, 2010, Author.

Health Research Council of New Zealand and the Ministry of Health: *Maori Health Joint Venture*, Request for proposals. Maori health literacy and palliative care (2010). Auckland, NZ, 2010, Health Research Council.

Hudson M, Milne M, Reynolds P, et al: *Te Ara Tika Guidelines for Māori research ethics: A framework for researchers and ethics committee members*, Auckland, NZ, 2010, Health Research Council.

Hume L: *Ancestral Power: The Dreaming, Consciousness and Aboriginal Australians*, Melbourne, 2002, Melbourne University Press.

Humphery K: Dirty questions: Indigenous health and 'Western research', *Australian and New Zealand Journal of Public Health* 25:197–202, 2001.

Jahnke HT, Taiapa J: Maori research. In Davidson C, Tolich M, editors: *Social science research in New Zealand: Many paths to understanding*, Auckland, NZ, 1999, Longman Pearson Education.

Janke T, Dawson P: *New tracks: Indigenous knowledge and cultural expression and the Australian intellectual property system*, Roseberry, NSW, 2012, Terri Janke and Company IP Lawyers.

Kovach M: *Indigenous methodologies: Characteristic, conversations, and contexts*, Toronto, 2009, University of Toronto Press.

Ladson-Billings G, editor: *Racialized Discourses and Ethnic Epistemologies*, Thousand Oaks, California, 2000, SAGE Publications.

Marglin SA: Towards the Decolonization of the Mind. In Marglin F, Marglin SA, editors: *Dominating knowledge: Development, culture and resistance*, Oxford, 1990, Claredon Press.

Mead HM: *Tikanga Māori: Living by Māori values*, Wellington, New Zealand, 2003, Huia.

Mikaere A: *Colonising myths Māori realities: He rukuruku whakaaro*, Wellington, New Zealand, 2011, Huia.

Pawu-kurlpurlurnu WJ, Holmes M, Box LA: *Ngurra-kurlu: A way of working with Warlpiri people*, Alice Springs, 2008, Desert Knowledge CRC.

Penney L, Barnes HMB, McCreanor T: The blame game: Constructions of Māori medical compliance, *AlterNative: An International Journal of Indigenous Peoples* 7:73–86, 2011.

Phillips GW, Brown WE: *Making sense of your world*, Chicago, 1991, Moody Press.

Ranzijn R, McConnochie K, Nolan W: *Psychology and Indigenous Australians: Foundations of cutlural competence*, South Yarra, Victoria, 2009, Palgrave Macmillan.

Razani J, Burciaga J, Madore M, et al: Effects of acculturation on tests of attention and information processing in an ethnically diverse group, *Archives of Clinical Neuropsychology* 22:333–341, 2007.

Reid P, Robson B: The state of Maori health. In Mulholland M, editor: *State of the Maori nation: Twenty first-century issues in Aotearoa*, Auckland, NZ, 2006, Reed Publishing.

Royal TAC: *Indigenous world views: A comparative study*, Otaki, New Zealand, 2002, Te Wānanga o Raukawa.

Sherwood J: *Do no harm: Decolonising Aboriginal health research*, Doctoral PhD, 2010, University of New South Wales.

Sherwood J: Colonisation – it's bad for your health: The context of Aboriginal health, *Contemporary Nurse* 46:28–40, 2013.

Shibaski S, Stewart P: Workshop report: Aboriginal and Torres Strait Islander people involved in ethics. *Cooperative Research Centre for Aboriginal Health Workshop*. Yunggorendi Mande, First Nations Centre for Higher Education and Research at Flinders University, Adelaide, South Australia, 2005, Cooperative Research Centre for Aboriginal Health.

Smallacombe S, Davis M, Quiggan R: *Desert knowledge: Scoping project on Aboriginal traditional knowledge*, Report of a study for the Desert Knowledge Cooperative Research Centre. Alice Springs, 2007, Desert Knowledge Cooperative Research Centre.

Smith LT: *Decolonizing methodologies: Research and Indigenous peoples*, Dunedin, NZ, 1999, University of Otago Press.

Smith LT: *Decolonizing methodologies: Research and Indigenous peoples*, London, 2012, Zed Books.

Stanner WEH: *White man got no dreaming*, Essays 1938–1973. Canberra, ACT, 1979, Australian National University Press.

Thomas DP: *Reading doctors' writing: Race, politics and power in Indigenous health research 1870–1969*, Canberra, 2004, Aboriginal Studies Press for the Australian Institute of Aboriginal and Torres Strait Islander Studies.

United Nations: *Indigenous peoples and the United Nations human rights system*, Fact sheet No. 9, Rev 2. New York and Geneva, 2013, Author.

United Nations: *Declaration on the Rights of Indigenous Peoples*, Geneva, 2008, Author. Online. Available: http://www.un.org/esa/socdev/unpfii/documents/DRIPS_en.pdf 29 July 2015.

United Nations Economic and Social Council: *Geneva Declaration on the Health and Survival of Indigenous Peoples*, 2002. Online. Available: http://www.dialoguebetweennations.com/n2n/pfii/english/HealthAnnex1.htm 29 July 2015.

Wilson D: The significance of a culturally appropriate health service for Indigenous Maori women, *Contemporary Nurse* 28:173–188, 2008a.

Wilson D, Barton P: Indigenous hospital experiences: A New Zealand case study, *Journal of Clinical Nursing* 21:2316–2326, 2012.

Wilson D, Neville S: Culturally safe research with vulnerable populations, *Contemporary Nurse* 33:69–79, 2009.

Wilson S: *Research is ceremony: Indigenous research methods*, Nova Scotia, Canada, 2008b, Fernwood.

World Health Organization: *Health of Indigenous peoples*, 2007. Online. Available: http://www.who.int/mediacentre/factsheets/fs326/en 29 July 2015.

Yunupingu G, editor: *From the Bark petition to native title*, St Lucia, QLD, 1997, University of Queensland Press.

SECTION 3

Walking the walk

Now that you have learnt about the different research paradigms and some inherent methodologies it's time to know more about how to review reports of research using the different approaches critically and explore the application of useful research findings to practice. Being able to read and apply nursing and midwifery research requires that you become comfortable with your new skills in using research evidence. This means practising these skills. This can be done by consistently reviewing research articles from various sources across clinical practice situations relevant to you. This will make you more proficient at applying your preferred review techniques when reading different reports of research. This section is designed to enable you to practise and develop your skills as a research consumer by providing a framework for critique and application of research results. The concept of research utilisation is explored and you are presented with approaches, criteria and strategies to enhance your research utilisation capabilities. In your professional life as a nurse or midwife, the ability to access and use quality research evidence to underpin your clinical practice is a necessity and is indeed a matter of practise, practise, practise.

CHAPTER 9

READING AND APPRAISING RESEARCH

Marie Hutchinson and Leah East

CHAPTER OUTLINE

KEY TERMS

appraisal tool
bias
blinding
clinical significance
critical appraisal
evidence
methodology
statistical significance
trustworthiness

LEARNING OBJECTIVES

After reading this chapter the student will be able to:

1. Differentiate between various study designs and their capacity to answer different questions
2. Explain the importance of appraising research and identifying relevance to practice
3. Understand the difference between statistical significance and clinical significance
4. Perform a rapid appraisal to establish whether a study is suited to answer a clinical question
5. Detail the questions asked in performing a critical appraisal
6. Follow the steps to critically appraise a qualitative research study
7. Follow the steps to critically appraise a quantitative research study.

STUDENT QUOTE

When you first look at a paper it is overwhelming, but once you read the abstract you can determine the relevance.

ABSTRACT

Reading and critically appraising research can be a challenging task, particularly for beginners. If you are a newcomer to reading research it can be difficult to make sense of study designs and data analysis methods. At first glance you may also find scholarly papers difficult to read, full of confusing terminology, or too complex. The good news is that learning to master the steps in critically reading research is not as difficult as you may think. In this chapter we address the challenges of becoming an informed and critical consumer of research and provide a step-by-step guide to conducting a critical appraisal. With a little knowledge and persistence you will find that understanding how to read and critically appraise evidence and ideas is not as difficult as it first appears.

Becoming a critical reader: the first step in translating evidence into practice

Nurses and midwives are the largest group of healthcare professionals and have the potential to significantly impact standards of care and clinical outcomes. Within the clinical context, the processes of critical thinking and reflection are employed in decision making and care planning. An important component of this process is making the link between critical thinking, contemporary research and ideas and the integration of **evidence**, clinical expertise and patient preferences (Greenhalgh 2010). Even though many gains have been made in applying evidence in practice, there remains a substantial time lag between when new ideas and results are first published and their uptake into practice (Bjørk et al 2013). One of the factors that contribute to this gap is the capacity of clinicians to locate, understand and critically appraise research. This issue continues to contribute to ineffective, outdated or potentially harmful practices (Guidroz et al 2010).

Reading and appraising research can be exciting, particularly if you approach reading a paper with some confidence. The appraisal framework provided in this chapter has been developed to provide you with the confidence to know what questions to ask and to help make sense of what you read. A fundamental first step in reviewing evidence and ideas is to do so through a critical lens. The second task is to understand the underlying question that drives you to seek out answers. Learning to focus your question will guide where you look for answers and the types of answers you are seeking. Thirdly, as not all evidence is useful or even valid, and even valid and reliable evidence might not be able to answer a specific question, it is important to develop the skills to critically appraise what you read (Ubbink et al 2013).

Asking questions and looking for answers

Nurses and midwives are in a unique situation to translate evidence and new ideas into practice. A key element in this process is becoming a critical consumer of evidence. This requires that you are aware of your information needs, the clinical situation, can convert this into answerable questions and seek out and appraise the answers you find. To get you thinking about the types of questions asked in practice, Box 9.1 provides examples of types of focuses for clinical questions and how these translate into research questions.

Once you learn how to frame questions, the next challenge is to begin to critically engage with new ideas and systematically appraise the validity and applicability of what you read. Chapters 10 and 11 address in further detail the process of formulating answerable clinical questions and searching for evidence.

Box 9.1
Types of questions and examples of research questions

Question focus	Research question
For a given patient, what is the better form of treatment?	Is compression therapy in conjunction with prophylactic thrombolytic therapy more effective than prophylactic therapy alone in reducing the incidence of deep vein thrombosis following joint surgery?
What are the potential risks of missed treatment?	Are nursing home patients with a diagnosis of dementia at increased risk for inadequate pain management?
What is the nature of patient preferences?	What are the birthing preferences of pregnant women aged between 20 and 25 years?

STUDENT CHALLENGE

Take a moment to consider the example questions in Box 9.1.

1. Have you asked similar questions during your course of study or in the clinical setting?
2. Can you think of a clinical question that you have raised recently? Do you have an evidence-based answer?
3. How ready do you think you are to engage with new ideas and review evidence to answer your question/s?

Critical thinking and reflection

To think critically is a fundamental skill that clinicians engage in to determine and implement safe quality health care (Price & Harrington 2010). In practice, and in our individual lives, we make decisions on a daily basis with some decisions involving more thought and some being easier to make than others. As such, when you have been required to make a difficult decision, it is probable that you have engaged in critical thinking, although you may not have been aware of this. Critical thinking involves the process of questioning, interpreting, analysing, determining relevance and making judgments on, for example, information, knowledge, professional practice and research (Price & Harrington 2010; Scully 2012; Parker 2014). In addition to actively engaging in critical thinking, students and clinicians also engage in reflection or reflective practice. Similar to critical thinking, reflection is a conscious process that involves exploration of thoughts, knowledge and practices in order to recognise inconsistencies, strengths, limitations and, for example, identify where change and adjustments are required within ourselves, the healthcare environment and clinical practice (Usher & Holmes 2014).

In addition to engaging in critical thinking and reflection, to ensure safe quality healthcare practices, it is vital for both students and clinicians to engage with literature and research evidence. In order to determine the relevance and strength of research evidence, we examine the literature through a critical lens, as it is easy to read research and think it is credible, unbiased and significant, particularly when it is well written and convincing. As you learned in Chapter 3 with regard to information on the web, there are dangers in accepting what you read at face value rather than being more critical. As Greenhalgh (2010) points out, a large proportion of studies have significant limitations and methodological flaws, many of which are not always apparent without careful examination. Now that you have learnt something about research and research processes it is time to learn how to critically appraise it to determine its worth.

STUDENT CHALLENGE

Reflect on a skill you have recently practised on clinical placement.

1. Why did you carry out this skill and why did you perform the skill the way you did?
2. Has research influenced the skill you have recently practised?

Taking a structured approach: performing a critical appraisal

A **critical appraisal** is a structured and systematic process through which the strengths and limitations of research studies are appraised and its clinical relevance is established (Porritt et al 2014). Internationally a large number of structured **appraisal tools** are available, with the majority developed for experimental studies. For the purpose of this chapter we have developed a simple checklist to guide you through the foundations of critical appraisal. The checklist reflects the commonly identified features of appraisal tools identified from a systematic review of published tools (Katrak et al 2004). Before conducting an appraisal, an initial preliminary assessment is useful to establish whether the paper is relevant to your needs.

The preliminary assessment

There are a number of preliminary questions that will help focus your thinking and quickly identify whether the paper is useful or suited to answering your question (see Box 9.2). This should be evident from reading the abstract, which ought to summarise the aims or underlying question, study design, important results and conclusions drawn. After the preliminary appraisal, if you consider the study is poorly designed or does not answer your question, you may not proceed to a full appraisal.

Box 9.2

Nine questions to ask in performing a preliminary appraisal

1. Why was the study undertaken?
2. What is the underlying question: is it relevant to my question or interests?
3. What type of evidence is provided?
4. Is there a clear statement of aims?
5. What was the overall design of the study?
6. Is the study design appropriate for the research question and study objectives?
7. Is the study population relevant to my question or clinical situation?
8. What were the outcomes of the study?
9. Are the results and conclusions relevant?

What is the underlying question: is it relevant to my question or interests?

The first questions to ask are focused on why the study was undertaken and whether the topic is relevant to your interests. The abstract of a research paper should clearly state the question the study was attempting to answer or why the study was undertaken. This may be written along the following lines: 'This study aimed to establish whether the use of clean technique increases the risk of urinary tract infection in a patient requiring intermittent catheterisation'.

What type of evidence is provided?

Research evidence can either be presented as a primary source, in which the original study and findings are presented, or in a secondary or other processed form (such as a narrative or literature review, systematic review or clinical guideline). If you are interested in answering a clinical question about treatment or interventions, you need to locate well-designed primary studies or a systematic review or meta-analysis (Moher et al 2009). The usefulness of these studies will be improved if measures of clinical significance are reported; if not the study is of less clinical value (Greenhalgh 2010). If you want to understand how knowledge is evolving or contemporary challenges and issues, a well-written narrative review would meet your needs.

What is the overall study design?

Once you have decided the paper is relevant to your needs, the next step is to understand the study design and type of evidence provided. It is often tempting to skip past careful consideration of **methodology**, particularly if you do not feel confident about research. Be careful with this temptation. Regardless of whether a study addresses an important question or presents findings that are applicable or statistically significant, you need to be mindful that, if it is poorly designed, its usefulness is limited (Greenhalgh 2010).

Is the study design appropriate for the research question and study objectives?

Table 9.1 illustrates the types of questions addressed through different study designs. In evidence-based practice certain research designs are given greater value over others. This value is made explicit through predetermined levels of evidence. For example, a randomised controlled clinical trial is considered gold standard and practitioners are much more likely to change practice based on the results of randomised controlled trials (RCTs) as opposed to other research designs, which fall lower on the hierarchy. Have a quick look at the NHMRC evidence hierarchy for further detail.

Applying the hierarchy of design types, the evidence will be stronger when the design chosen is at the higher end of the hierarchy of suitable designs. If it is towards the lower end, you need to consider why the authors have chosen this design. Do not automatically dismiss a study that sits towards the lower end of the spectrum, as these studies can be suited to certain questions.

Although RCTs and meta-analysis sit at the top of the evidence hierarchy, they are not necessarily best suited to answering all clinical questions. In clinical settings it is not always feasible to blind treatment allocation or to randomise patients (Nelson & Ballman 2013). Furthermore, nurses and midwives often seek to answer highly contextualised questions that are suited to study designs towards the lower end of the evidence hierarchy in statistical terms (Hinchberger 2009). It is important to understand that when little is known about a problem or issue, studies are often more descriptive and at the 'lower' end of the evidence spectrum. As the body of knowledge grows, so does the capacity to refine a more tightly structured and rigorous design (Punch 2014). Importantly as you learnt in Chapter 6, experience and meaning cannot be revealed through controlled study designs such as an RCT. Similarly, for a phenomenon about which little is known, the design chosen should be suited to discovery or revealing novel or unexpected patterns in the data (Gunnarsdottir et al 2006).

Table 9.1
Examples of different question types and the hierarchy of study designs suited to answer the question

Type of question	Hierarchy of suitable study types
Effects of interventions or treatments	
In patients with type 2 diabetes and obesity, is a structured exercise program more effective than standard medical treatment in improving diabetic control?	Meta-analysis>RCT>prospective cohort study>retrospective cohort study>case control>case series> qualitative study
How do women experience mothering a pre-term infant in a neonatal unit?	In-depth qualitative interview>cohort study>cross-sectional study>case study
Do oral nutritional supplements reduce the risk of decubitus ulcers in older hospitalised patients?	Meta-analysis>RCT>cohort >case control>case series
Experience of treatment	
How do patients with type 2 diabetes and obesity experience participation in a group exercise program?	In-depth qualitative interview>qualitative focus group >cohort study>cross-sectional study>case study
Aetiology or causality	
Are people with hypertension who have a difference in systolic blood pressure between arms at increased risk of cardiovascular events compared to those without hypertension?	Prospective cohort study>case control>case series
What were the characteristics of disease presentation of children diagnosed with measles during a specific outbreak?	Retrospective case series>case study
Establishing risk in a specific group – prognosis or prediction	
Are nursing home patients with a diagnosis of dementia at increased risk for inadequate pain management?	Meta-analysis>RCT>cohort study>case control>retrospective case series
Frequency or rate of disease or illness	
Are older persons in hospitals at increased risk of malnutrition?	Cohort study>cross-sectional study>retrospective case series>case study>qualitative study
Prognosis	
What is the illness progression of pneumonia when left untreated in adult women?	Prospective cohort study>retrospective cohort study>cross-sectional study>qualitative study>case study
Diagnosis	
Is tachypnoea a strong predictor of clinical deterioration in adult emergency department patients?	Prospective cohort study>prospective cross-sectional study>retrospective cohort study> retrospective cross-sectional study>case study

The detailed appraisal

Even if a paper reports statistically significant findings or the authors mount a convincing argument to substantiate their findings, in appraising the evidence a little detective work is required to ensure validity and reliability and that the findings drawn are relevant and credible.

Assessing methodological strength

In performing a more detailed appraisal of methodology careful consideration needs to be given to assessing features such as the sample and approach to recruitment, as well as issues of internal validity and reliability in quantitative research or trustworthiness in qualitative research (see Box 9.3).

Box 9.3
Questions to ask in appraising methodology

1. For quantitative studies, is the sample size adequate and does it have sufficient power? What was the response rate?
2. For qualitative studies, are participants the most appropriate to provide access to the type of information sought?
3. What was the source of the sample or participants and are they representative of the broader population to whom the research might apply?
4. For quantitative studies, is sufficient detail provided on recruitment and inclusion/exclusion criteria for the study (such as, disease stage, age, comorbidity)?
5. For quantitative studies, what was the sampling method? How were participants selected? Could the sampling method have introduced bias?
6. For quantitative studies, are the groups identical except for difference in exposure to the treatment or variable under investigation?
7. For experimental designs, are participants and investigators 'blinded' to treatment allocation?
8. Is there a clear description of how data were collected?
9. For quantitative studies, are the data collection methods and tools valid and reliable? Was the instrument used previously validated?
10. For qualitative studies, how does the researcher/s account for their own presence in the data collection and analysis? Have the authors provided detail as to how trustworthiness was achieved?
11. Were there any distorting, extraneous or contaminating influences that might have influenced the data collected? If methods change during the study are these adequately accounted for?

Sample size and design

For quantitative studies, a first consideration is the size of the sample and whether it has sufficient power to detect differences or establish causal relationships (LoBiondo-Wood & Haber 2014). Establish whether the authors have reported power, usually a power of 90% will give you confidence in the sample size (Polit & Beck 2012). Also check that the sample size at the end of the study, and in all groups, is sufficient in size to meet the initial power calculations. For the research to be applicable to other similar study populations, it is also important to establish whether subjects are representative of the group from which they are drawn and the wider population to whom the findings might be applied (Punch 2014). The authors should also provide sufficient detail for you to be confident that the treatment or comparison groups are similar.

The sample size for qualitative studies can be more difficult to appraise as often these studies are exploratory in nature, are focused on subjective experience and do not aim to be generalisable. Qualitative studies will often continue to recruit and collect data from participants until analysis of the data is not producing anymore 'new' knowledge or themes (data saturation). Generally, it is acceptable to have a small sample of participants in qualitative research (e.g. less than 25) (Wood & Ross-Kerr 2011). Similar to quantitative studies, it is also important to determine whether the sample was representative in answering the research question.

Measurement in quantitative research

In considering validity, you are aiming to establish the extent to which the measurement undertaken is accurate and measures what it intends to (Hulley et al 2013). Some forms of measurement are particularly inaccurate, for example, asking people to recall events over extended periods of time. You should also be mindful of whether or not the measurement tool employed is reproducible and reliable. The reliability or sensitivity of any measures employed should be reported, along with details on whether the measurement is sensitive enough to detect change (Jordan et al 2011). In addition, if multiple individuals are taking measures, it is important to establish whether the results would be the same between these people and what steps have been taken to ensure consistency (LoBiondo-Wood & Haber 2014). Also consider variance in equipment or the influence of time on measurement (Macnee & McCabe 2008). To improve confidence in reliability, studies may test for reliability between assessors, calibrate instruments between measurements or perform random spot checks to identify any errors or inconsistencies in data collection (Macnee & McCabe 2008).

Representation in qualitative research

As previously stated, in qualitative studies rigour is described and determined by trustworthiness. **Trustworthiness** refers to the extent to which the data truly represents, for example, participants' experiences and encapsulates the concepts of credibility (the accuracy of the presented data), transferability (the ability of the data to be transferable and be representative of other settings), confirmability, the objectivity of the data (Liamputtong 2013), and dependability (could the study be replicated and the same conclusions be drawn), (Burns & Grove 2009; Liamputtong 2013). To determine rigour when critically appraising qualitative research it is important to ask questions such as have the researchers developed an audit trail for the study to be replicated? Are participants' voices presented in the findings to reflect credibility? How many researchers were involved in data analysis? Were findings confirmed by more than one researcher? And could these findings be relevant to other participants in other healthcare contexts?

Identifying bias in quantitative research

As you read a paper you also need to think about whether there is evidence of **bias** in participant selection, data analysis and/or data collection methods that may influence the results in favour of the outcome or intervention under investigation (Liamputtong 2013). Bias can occur when there are differences between study subjects or study groups, which is poorly controlled or not accounted for in the analysis. In many studies, randomisation, stratification of the sample and **blinding** of treatment and allocation to groups are common strategies to limit bias. Additionally, if allocation to treatment is not blinded, there may be the possibility of bias (Polit & Beck 2012). Missing data is another factor that should be considered when you review study findings for bias. A study may commence with a balanced design, or the same number of subjects in each arm of the study, and due to loss of subjects to follow up or incomplete data (missing data) bias can be introduced into the study (Liamputtong 2013). In cohort studies or controlled trials, deaths and drop outs can occur; you need to not only consider how many dropped out, but also whether there are any clues to bias in the reasons for drop out.

Data analysis and findings

The next step in the appraisal is to establish whether the statistical tests or data analysis methods are appropriate for the data and whether the conclusions drawn are relevant to the findings presented (Box 9.4). Having worked through the questions on method you will have a good understanding of why and how the study was performed and this should make the results easier to understand and evaluate.

Data analysis methods

In reporting quantitative data analysis, the authors should report the test used and the findings. For example, were paired *t* tests used to analyse and compare two measurements of a dependent variable, was a measure of variance such as ANOVA used to compare differences among more than two groups (three or

Box 9.4
Questions to ask in appraising data analysis and findings

1. Is the type of analysis appropriate for the type of data collected?
2. For qualitative studies, is there sufficient in-depth description of the analysis method?
3. Is the data clearly presented?
4. Are drop out or missing data accounted for sufficiently?
5. For qualitative studies, are the results credible and trustworthy?
6. Are measures of clinical significance presented?
7. Are the conclusions drawn relevant to the findings?

more), or were correlation coefficients determined to report the association and strength of relationship between two variables (Plichta Kellar & Kelvin 2013)?

Qualitative studies use narrative rather than numbers to present the findings of the research. When appraising the findings of qualitative research it is important to assess the data collection methods and analysis techniques used in order to determine whether these were congruent with the research methodology design. For example, if the research used a grounded theory approach, ideally data collection and analysis should occur simultaneously, and data analysis occurs through open and focused coding, or if for example the study was ethnographic, data collection methods should include participant observation, informants and fieldwork (Lapan et al 2011). Additionally, although qualitative research does not generally use the term 'significant' as does quantitative research, ideally findings from qualitative studies should be new and of use and/or importance to the target audience.

Identifying statistical and clinical significance

When you read the results of statistical analysis you can be confident the findings are significant (not due to chance) when the p-value is below 0.05 (Polit & Beck 2012). The lower the p-value, the more confident you can be that chance has not influenced the results. To understand the clinical benefit of a study it is important to look beyond **statistical significance** and establish **clinical significance**, as tests such as the p-value do not necessarily provide evidence of clinical benefit (Neuhauser & Provost 2012) (see Box 9.5). In clinical trials measures of clinical significance are often calculated in terms of effect size, ratios of hazard or risk, risk reduction and numbers needed to treat (NNT) to gain a benefit. From the data of study findings presented in papers it

Box 9.5
Examples of questions relevant to establishing clinical significance

- How confident am I that I could use this treatment or intervention in practice?
- How many patients would need to be treated for one to benefit?
- What are the odds a patient will benefit?
- Might there be a risk of harm associated with the treatment?
- How many patients might be treated before one is harmed?

is possible to calculate many of these measures. At the end of this chapter there are a number of additional resources that provide further guidance on interpreting or calculating measures of clinical significance.

A commonly reported measure of effect is the confidence interval (CI). This measure provides the limits for the true effect size of the treatment or intervention in the population of interest. The CI is expressed as a range between two numbers, with the true but unknown effect value falling within this range. A 95% CI means that you can be 95% certain the level of effect for the study population falls within the calculated range (Macnee & McCabe 2008). The CI also provides insight into how precise the study results are and whether the same results would occur if the study was replicated. When appraising a study look for a CI value of 95% or above and a small gap in the interval. A wide gap between the upper and lower confidence intervals (e.g. 0.48–0.93) indicates poor precision (Macnee & McCabe 2008). Another important aspect of the CI is whether the range contains the value for 'no effect' for the test performed as this indicates a non-significant result. For absolute measures of clinical significance such as NNT and measures of risk difference the value for no effect is 0, while for ratio measures (such as the odds ratio or relative risk) 1 is the value for no effect. Therefore, a CI range of 0.8–2.1 for a test of relative risk is not statistically significant as the value for no effect (1) lies within the CI range (Greenhalgh 2010).

Putting it all together: two appraisal examples

To help you put the appraisal checklist outlined into practice, the following section provides two worked examples of an appraisal. Once you have read these through you should find it fairly straightforward to start using the checklist to conduct your own appraisals.

Example appraisal for a quantitative study

In this first example (Moore et al 2006), the authors employed a RCT design to compare clean and sterile intermittent catheterisation technique in a rehabilitation setting and establish time to symptomatic urinary tract infection in the two groups. This is an appropriate design for establishing aetiology or the effectiveness of treatment (refer back to Table 9.1). From the initial screening of the abstract the study appears to be well designed and the results presented are interesting and statistically significant (see Box 9.6).

Box 9.6
Results of preliminary appraisal

Aims: Compare the effect of clean versus sterile intermittent catheterisation technique in a patient group.

Design: Randomised control trial.

Ethics: No detail provided in the abstract.

Sample and setting: 36 patients with recent quadriplegia due to spinal cord injury.

Intervention/outcome: Rate and time to onset of symptomatic urinary tract infection (UTI).

Relevance of results and conclusion: 43% of subjects developed UTI; 37% from the clean group and 45% from the sterile group ($p > 0.05$).

Conclusion drawn: Clean intermittent catheterisation in the rehabilitation setting for this group of patients does not appear to increase risk of symptomatic UTI.

If you look no further than the abstract of this study, you would miss findings that need to be considered in translating this study into practice. A more detailed analysis (see Box 9.7) identifies a number of potential limitations with the study. For example, the sample size appears to have been half that required for sufficient power; the two groups appear to be unbalanced with regards to gender, which could have influenced the outcome; and, there is some uncertainty about accurate identification of asymptomatic UTIs. These factors need to be taken into consideration when interpreting the clinical significance of the study findings. Often more information needs to be sought from the researchers themselves before further determination can be made.

Box 9.7
Results of detailed appraisal

1. Sample and recruitment – might there be bias?

Is the sample representative? It is not possible to determine from the data presented whether the sample is representative of the broader population of patients.

Was group allocation randomised? Patients were randomised to groups by concealed numbers after signing consent to participate in the study. There is no detail on whether randomisation was blinded to study team.

Is the sample size large enough to minimise chance? There were 36 participants (16 in clean group and 20 in sterile group). Authors report this sample was sufficient for power of 0.80 and an alpha of 0.05. With this alpha the authors have accepted a type 1 error rate of 5%, meaning 5% of results might be due to chance (Stevens 2002).

2. Internal validity and reliability – is data collection valid and reliable?

Was group allocation blinded? The allocation of participants to the intervention or control group could not be blinded as staff performing the procedure and patients would be aware of group allocation. Laboratory staff and data manager were blinded to group allocation.

Were the groups similar at the start and who was excluded from the study? Groups appeared similar with regard to urinary history and health history prior to injury. Not possible to tell if groups were matched on demographic variables (i.e. gender and age). The sterile group was 90% male, the clean 63% male. This difference between groups might have influenced the study outcomes.

Are the data collection methods and tools valid and reliable? Weekly urine specimens were collected using sterile catheter. Night staff collected samples at the same time of the day and samples were analysed in a laboratory.

Were there any factors that might have influenced the data collected? Criteria were provided for identifying symptomatic urinary tract infections. No detail is provided as to how symptomatic UTI was identified, who recorded symptoms, or how frequently these assessments were performed or recorded. It is not possible to establish whether cases of asymptomatic UTI were missed or how reliable this assessment was.

Are interventions sufficiently controlled? Staff watched videos on sterile technique and standardised sterile equipment was employed. There was no determination made as to whether the techniques performed were sterile.

Continued

Box 9.7
Results of detailed appraisal—cont'd

Were there any distorting, extraneous or contaminating influences that might have influenced the data collected? The study appears to have been conducted over a two-year period. It is unclear how consistency in data collection and interventions were controlled for this period of time.

3. Data analysis methods

Is the analysis appropriate for the data? Analysis included chi-square and t-tests, which are appropriate for the type of data collected. The authors do not report whether the data was normally distributed.

4. Findings presented

Is statistical significance reported? The number and percentage of subjects that acquired symptomatic and asymptomatic UTI was reported, however the statistical significance of this was not reported.

Is drop out or missing data accounted for sufficiently? Importantly data collection was discontinued for more than half of the subjects before conclusion of the study. The authors give no consideration to the power of the remaining sample. It is likely to be very poor.

5. Conclusions

Are measures of clinical significance presented? Hazard ratios were calculated to establish time of onset of symptomatic UTI.

STUDENT CHALLENGE

Refer back to Table 9.1.

Can you identify a study design that might have been less problematic than an RCT for this study?

Example appraisal for a qualitative study

In this second example (Vermeire et al 2003) the authors aimed to explore the opinions and perceptions of people with diabetes about their illness and its treatment and what kind of problems they encountered in adhering to prescribed therapeutic regimens. The study employed focus group discussion, with content analysis performed on the recorded transcripts. The preliminary screening (see Box 9.8) indicated that the aims of this study were clear, the

Box 9.8
Results of preliminary appraisal

Aim: Determine diabetic type 2 patients' health beliefs, communication with healthcare providers and issues encountered with adhering to treatment within the context of their illness.

Design: Qualitative research design.

Is the study design appropriate for the research question and study objectives? The qualitative research design was suited for the data collection methods of focus groups and data analysis method of content analysis.

Did the study meet expected standards of ethics? The relevant ethics committee granted ethics approval.

Sample and setting: Forty-six patients participated in seven semi-structured focus groups.

Outcome: Several findings highlighted the difficulties patients experienced with information deficits relating to their illness and adhering to their diabetic treatment.

Relevance of results and conclusion: The findings from this study identify several areas that could be improved in regards to the healthcare treatment provided to patients with diabetes type 2.

Conclusion drawn: Patients who have a diagnosis of diabetes type 2 may be not receiving information and care that are tailored to meet their needs.

research design was congruent with the analysis and data collection methods used, and the findings of the study are relevant to the healthcare requirements and provision of patients who have been diagnosed with diabetes type 2.

However, on further appraisal some weaknesses can be identified. These limit the relevance of the findings. As summarised in Box 9.9, the sample was selected by pharmacists, which provides a limited population, as those not attending the pharmacy or attending other healthcare settings were not accessed. Further, although forty-six participants participated in this study and were involved in seven focus groups, only twelve participant extracts are provided. This raises the issue of whether participants and their voices are adequately represented and may limit the transferability of the research (see Chapter 6 for further discussion on credibility and trustworthiness in qualitative research).

Conclusion

This chapter has provided an introduction to how to critically read research. As a clinician it may be daunting at first to apply a critical lens to published

Box 9.9
Results of detailed appraisal

1. Sample and recruitment

What was the source of the sample or participants, and are they representative of the broader population to whom the research might apply? Participants were recruited via pharmacists, which limited the sample to those attending the healthcare settings in which the pharmacists were working.

What was the sampling method? This study used a convenience sampling method, which is suitable for qualitative studies. An inclusion and exclusion criteria was not provided and initially the study recruited 70 participants, yet the authors have not detailed why only forty-six participated. The authors have stated that data saturation was achieved.

2. Credibility and trustworthiness

Is there a clear description of how data were collected? Yes, seven focus groups were run by the same researcher and observer.

For qualitative studies, how does the researcher/s account for their own presence in the data collection and analysis? The authors have not provided detail on potential author bias within the data collection methods and analysis, although the authors do state that focus groups were 'non-directional' and analysis was undertaken by two researchers independently.

3. Data analysis methods

Are the data analysis methods appropriate for the type of data being measured? Data collected from the focus groups underwent content analysis; an appropriate data analysis method used in qualitative research.

For qualitative studies is there sufficient in-depth description of the analysis method chosen? The authors report that two researchers independently analysed the data with clarification of ideas achieved through computer software, however, no further detail was provided on whether the other authors confirmed the findings or how the software actually assisted in establishing congruity in the data analysis.

4. Findings presented

Is the data clearly presented? Findings from this study are clearly identified through themes.

For qualitative studies are the results credible and trustworthy? Due to the sampling methods, transferability is limited.

5. Conclusions drawn

Are the conclusions drawn relevant to the findings? The conclusions drawn from this study are relevant to the findings and may be useful in determining the healthcare needs of people with diabetes type 2.

research. When you have had a little practice at using the checklists provided in this chapter, you will find it is only a short step to reading and considering the utility of research for practice on a regular basis.

RESOURCE KIT

Alliance for Useful Evidence: http://www.alliance4usefulevidence.org.

The Joanna Briggs Institute: http://joannabriggs.org.

Agency for Healthcare Research and Quality: Advancing Excellence in Health Care: http://www.ahrq.gov/index.html.

The Cochrane Library: Independent high-quality evidence for healthcare decision making: http://www.thecochranelibrary.com.

Critical appraisal skills program: making sense of evidence tools and checklists: http://www.casp-uk.net/#!casp-tools-checklists/c18f8.

The University of Oxford, Centre for Evidence Based Medicine:

http://www.cebm.net/critical-appraisal.

NHMRC evidence hierarchy:

http://www.nhmrc.gov.au/_files_nhmrc/file/guidelines/developers/nhmrc_levels_grades_evidence_120423.pdf.

References

Bjørk IT, Lomborg K, Nielsen CM, et al: From theoretical model to practical use: an example of knowledge translation, *Journal of Advanced Nursing* 69(10):1365–2648, 2013.

Burns N, Grove SK: Qualitative research methodology. In *The practice of nursing research: appraisal, synthesis, and generation of evidence*, St Louis, 2009, Saunders Elsevier, pp 507–551.

Greenhalgh T: *How to read a paper. The basics of evidence-based medicine*, ed 4, West Sussex, 2010, Wiley-Blackwell.

Guidroz AM, Burnfield-Geimer JL, Schwetschenau HM, et al: The nursing incivility scale: Development and validation of an occupation-specific measure, *Journal of Nursing Management* 18(3):176–200, 2010.

Gunnarsdottir HK, Sveinsdottir H, Bernburg JG, et al: Lifestyle, harassment at work and self-assessed health of female flight attendants, nurses and teachers, *Work (Reading, Mass.)* 27:165–172, 2006.

Hinchberger PA: Violence against female student nurses in the workplace, *Nursing Forum* 44(1):37–46, 2009.

Hulley SB, Newman TB, Cummings SR: Planning the measurements: Precision, accuracy, and validity. In Hulley SB, Cummings SR, Browner WS, et al, editors: *Designing clinical research*, Philadelphia, 2013, Lippincott Williams & Wilkins, Wolters Kluwer, pp 32–42.

Jordan JE, Osborne RH, Buchbinder R: Critical appraisal of health literacy indices revealed variable underlying constructs, narrow content and psychometric weaknesses, *Journal of Clinical Epidemiology* 64(4):366–379, 2011.

Katrak P, Bialocerkowski A, Massy-Westropp N, et al: A systematic review of the content of critical appraisal tools, *BMC Medical Research Methodology* 4(1):22, 2004.

Lapan SD, Quartaroli MT, Riemer FJ, editors: *Qualitative research: an introduction to methods and designs*, San Francisco, 2011, Jossey-Bass.

Liamputtong P, editor: *Research methods in health: foundations for evidence-based practice*, South Melbourne, 2013, Oxford University Press.
LoBiondo-Wood G, Haber J: Reliability and validity. In *Nursing research: methods and critical appraisal for evidence-based practice*, Missouri, 2014, Elselvier Mosby, pp 289–309.
Macnee CL, McCabe S: *Understanding nursing research: using research in evidence-based practice*, Philadelphia, 2008, Lippincott William & Wilkins.
Moher D, Liberati A, Tetzlaff J, et al: Preferred Reporting Items for Systematic Reviews and Meta-Analyses: the PRISMA Statement, *PLoS Medicine* 6(7):2009.
Moore K, Burt J, Voaklander D: Intermittent catheterization in the rehabilitation setting: a comparison of clean and sterile technique, *Clinical Rehabilitation* 20:461–468, 2006.
Nelson H, Ballman K: Achieving the right volume of randomized controlled trials, *Annals of Surgery* 258(2):208–209, 2013.
Neuhauser D, Provost L: Why do we worship P < .05?, *Quality Management in Health Care* 21(1):4–8, 2012.
Parker S: Becoming a critical thinker. In Daly J, Speedy S, Jackson D, editors: *Contexts of nursing: preparing for professional practice*, Australia, 2014, Elsevier, Churchill Livingstone, pp 101–116.
Plichta Kellar S, Kelvin EA: *Munro's statistical methods for health care research*, Philadelphia, 2013, Lippincott Williams & Wilkins, Wolters Kluwer.
Polit DF, Beck CT: Quantitative research design. In *Nursing research: generating and assessing evidence for nursing practice*, Philadelphia, 2012, Wolters Kluwer Health, Lippincott Williams & Wilkins, pp 201–235.
Porritt K, Gomersall J, Lockwood C: JBI's systematic reviews: study selection and critical appraisal, *American Journal of Nursing* 114(6):47–52, 2014.
Price B, Harrington A: *Critical thinking and writing for nursing students*, Exeter, 2010, Learning matters.
Punch KF: *Introduction to social research: quantitative and qualitative approaches*, London, 2014, Sage.
Scully N: Critical thinking and the nursing process. In Kozier B, Erb G, Berman A, et al, editors: *Kozier and Erb's fundamentals of nursing*, French Forest, 2012, Pearson, 1, pp 196–210.
Stevens J: *Applied multivariate statistics for the social sciences*, Mahwah, New Jersey, 2002, Lawrence Erlbaum Associates.
Ubbink DT, Guyatt GH, Vermeulen H: Framework of policy recommendations for implementation of evidence-based practice: a systematic scoping review, *BMJ Open* 3:e001881, 2013. doi: 001810.001136/bmjopen-002012-001881.
Usher K, Holmes C: Reflective practice: What, why and how. In Daly J, Speedy S, Jackson D, editors: *Contexts of nursing: preparing for professional practice*, Chatswood, 2014, Churchill Livingstone, Elsevier, pp 117–135.
Vermeire E, Van Royen P, Coenen S, et al: The adherence of type 2 diabetes patients to their therapeutic regimens: a qualitative study from the patient's perspective, *Practical Diabetes International* 20(6):209–214, 2003.
Wood MJ, Ross-Kerr JC: The research design: Blueprint for action. In *Basic steps in planning nursing research: from question to proposal*, Massachusetts, 2011, Jones and Bartlett Publishers, pp 113–149.

CHAPTER 10

KNOWLEDGE TRANSLATION OF RESEARCH FINDINGS: CHALLENGES AND STRATEGIES

Anne Hofmeyer and Terri Gibson

CHAPTER OUTLINE

KEY TERMS

barriers and facilitators
evidence-based practice
evidence-informed decision making (EIDM)
knowledge translation
research literacy

LEARNING OBJECTIVES

After reading this chapter and critical reflection, the student will be able to:

1. Discuss the relationship between professional practice and evidence-based practice
2. Describe the link between research literacy and evidence-based practice
3. Discuss knowledge translation and explain how the concept is important
4. Identify individual and organisational challenges to translating evidence into practice
5. Use five key questions to discuss the knowledge translation planning process
6. Describe strategies to improve the use of research evidence in decision making
7. Develop research literacy.

STUDENT QUOTE

The link between research, knowledge and evidence-based practice is making sense. I can't wait to put the PICOT framework into action.

ABSTRACT

In order to meet professional standards, nurses and midwives must develop their research literacy skills to critically appraise, translate and apply research evidence in diverse contexts and practice settings. Possibly you are aware that research-based and contextualised practices are essential to address problems in health systems and care provision. But in reality, you might be unclear about how these concepts link with your professional practice and how best to develop your research literacy to meet these professional expectations.

The purpose of this chapter is to draw links with professional practice and build your understanding about how the knowledge translation (KT) process can enhance your capacity to implement research-based and contextualised practices to address health problems. In addition, we present a range of strategies to develop individual research literacy and improve organisational readiness for KT in healthcare systems.

The key message is that developing competence in research literacy is as critical to quality patient care as developing competence in clinical skills.

Introduction

We begin this chapter with a 'hypothetical but all-too-common real-world scenario' by Pravikoff and colleagues (2005, p. 41):

Nancy Adams is a 52-year-old RN in charge of a medical–surgical unit in a midsize acute care facility in Southern California. One of her patients, an 82-year-old woman with cancer and dementia, recently died from asphyxiation when her head became trapped between the side rails and the mattress on her bed. Ms Adams had learned in nursing school to make sure the side rails were always up on her patients' beds, and she has emphasised that to the nurses who work with her. Now she wonders whether that's the right intervention and how to find out. She asks several of her peers how they know that this intervention is best for patients. No one is able to provide actual evidence. It's just what they've always been taught to do. There is a small locked medical library in her facility – used mostly by a few physicians – and no one has ever told her where the key is. She'd heard about the CINAHL database and PubMed at a conference she'd attended recently, but her facility has no access to them. Besides, she has very limited computer skills. She has a computer in her office but uses it mostly for in-house email; the hospital administration doesn't allow internet access because it might be abused. She's at a loss as to how to find the information she needs.

STUDENT CHALLENGE

- Do you think much has changed in organisations in the decade since Pravikoff et al (2005) published their paper?
- Have nurses and midwives improved their understanding of research?
- Are nurses and midwives better educated in evidence-based practice?
- Do nurses and midwives demonstrate a greater readiness for evidence-based practice than indicated in the scenario?
- What advice would you give Nancy and her colleagues about accessing and implementing current evidence in their practice?

Evidence-based practice: your professional responsibility

In this chapter, we will use the term 'student' because you are a student of research. However we acknowledge that 'students' will have diversity of roles and experience in nursing and midwifery (i.e. nurse leaders, managers, clinicians or undergraduate students). This chapter underscores the importance of using current research evidence in clinical decision making and draws conceptual links with professional practice, **evidence-based practice** (EBP), and **knowledge translation** (KT). Research-based practice is a hallmark of professional nursing (ICN 2012). The professional responsibility of nurses and midwives is to provide relevant clinical care that is informed by current research evidence. In Australia and globally, key professional organisations have called for greater use of research evidence in decision making and the continuing professional development of nurses to build research literacy (ACN 2013; ICN 2012; Nursing and Midwifery Board of Australia 2006; STTI 2002; Council of Deans of Nursing and Midwifery [ANZ] 2006). In 2013, The Australian College of Nursing published the *Nursing Research Position Statement* that emphasised the 'importance of registered nurses being evidence-based practitioners, who are competent in practicing within an evidence-based framework to provide quality and safe nursing care' (ACN 2013, p. 2).

However, the lack of competent research skills is a major barrier to the provision of EBP (ACN 2013, p. 2). The Nursing and Midwifery Board of Australia (NMBA 2006) developed competency standards for the registered nurse. The NMBA (2006) argues that registered nurses must use current research knowledge to ensure their clinical decision making and practice is evidence-based. The relevant NMBA (2006, p. 4) national competency standards are 3.1 to 3.4 and are as follows:

- 3.1 Identifies the relevance of research to improving individual/group health outcomes,
- 3.2 Uses best available evidence, nursing expertise and respect for the values and beliefs of individuals/groups in the provision of nursing care,
- 3.3 Demonstrates analytical skills in accessing and evaluating health information and research evidence,
- 3.4 Supports and contributes to nursing and health care research.

In order to meet professional standards, nurses must develop their analytical skills to locate, critically appraise, understand and apply research findings in their clinical practice (Crookes & Davies 2004, p. xii). However, many nurses report feeling unprepared and uncertain about how to develop competent research skills to provide evidence-based care and thus meet professional expectations (Gerrish et al 2008; Fineout-Overholt & Johnston 2005a; Ellis 2013). Moreover, Pravikoff et al (2005, p. 40) highlight the lack of computer skills and note that 'many (nurses) don't understand or value research and have had little or no training to help them find evidence on which to base their practice'.

STUDENT CHALLENGE

1. Have you felt unprepared and uncertain about how to develop your computer skills and/or research skills?
2. On a scale of 1 (low) – 10 (high), how would you rate your current analytical skills in accessing and evaluating health information and research evidence? Why?
3. Provide an example of your EBP. What was the impact of using current research evidence in your decision making?

EBP can be understood as 'integrating individual clinical expertise with the best available external evidence from a systematic research' (Sackett 1996, p. 71), but must also incorporate the patient's preferences (Sackett et al 2000, p. 1). Notably, the haphazard use of current evidence by medical, nursing and allied health professionals in their decision making continues to be a global problem and is a significant barrier to the implementation of evidence-informed healthcare practice and policy (Scott et al 2012; Grimshaw et al 2012; Straus et al 2011). Extensive research has been conducted to identify individual and organisational facilitators (readiness) and barriers to the implementation of research-based decision making (Estabrooks et al 2006; Champagne et al 2014). Notably, out-dated personal beliefs can act as a barrier to the necessary behavioural change to enhance individual capacity in research-based decision making (Straus et al 2009).

Therefore, the purpose of this chapter is to draw links with professional practice and build your understanding about how the KT process can enhance your capacity to implement research-based and contextualised practices to address health problems. In addition, we present a range of strategies to develop individual research literacy and improve organisational readiness for KT in healthcare systems.

What is research literacy?

The term **research literacy** describes the process to develop skills and capacity to become 'evidence-based practitioners' who are capable of making evidence-informed decisions to provide relevant care (Halcomb & Peters 2009, p. 60). But many nurses and midwives have had minimal training to develop their computer skills and research literacy to support their EBP (Pravikoff et al 2005). The '4 *As* of research' were proposed by Crookes and Davies (2004, p. xiii) to explain how nurses can integrate research into their professional practice. Specifically, all nurses must: (1) demonstrate an **A**wareness of and access to research literature; (2) develop an **A**ppreciation (or ability) to understand and critique the language of research; and (3) develop competence in the **A**pplication of research findings to their local practice settings. Notably, the fourth 'A of research' is the **A**bility to conduct original (primary) research independently or in a team. Crookes and Davies (2004, p. xiii) acknowledge that fewer nurses will develop research literacy in the **A**bility to conduct original (primary) research. However, there is an expectation that all nurses must strive to build competence in **A**wareness, **A**ppreciation and **A**pplication.

STUDENT CHALLENGE

1. On a scale of 1 (low) - 10 (high), how would you rate your current research literacy in each of the '3 *As* of research' (**A**wareness, **A**ppreciation and **A**pplication)?
2. Consider which area/s you need to develop.
3. Draft a plan to develop your research literacy in the identified areas. What resources do you need to build your research literacy skills?

In order to build research literacy skills, nurses can adopt the five-step model designed to teach healthcare professionals EBP that originated from The Sicily Statement on EBP (Dawes et al 2005, p.1). The Sicily Statement declared:

> *Evidence-based practice (EBP) requires that decisions about health care are based on the best available, current, valid evidence. These decisions should be made by those receiving care, informed by the tacit and explicit knowledge of those providing care, within the context of available resources.*

This definition acknowledges multiple forms of knowledge are included in decision making for patients. So what other forms of knowledge count? Rycroft-Malone et al (2004, p. 81) outline the potential contribution of four types of evidence in the delivery of care, namely: 'research, clinical experience, patient experience and in addition, information from the local context'. Nurses must synthesise multiple sources of knowledge in their clinical decision making when planning quality care with patients and their families. Thus, a patient-centred model of quality care is informed by current research evidence, the preferences of the patient and family, and the knowledge and experiences of the healthcare providers. Johnston and Fineout-Overholt contextualised the five-step model (Dawes et al 2005) to teach nurses and midwives the key steps in EBP and developing research literacy. The five-step model is outlined below and equivalent references are juxtaposed:

1. **Translation of uncertainty to an answerable question** (Dawes et al 2005); Step 0 (Johnston & Fineout-Overholt 2005); Step 1 (Fineout-Overholt & Johnston 2005b).

2. **Search for and retrieval of evidence** (Dawes et al 2005); Step 2 (Fineout-Overholt et al 2005).
3. **Critical appraisal of evidence for validity, clinical relevance and applicability** (Dawes et al 2005); Step 3 (Johnston & Fineout-Overholt 2006); critical appraisal (Hill & Spittlehouse 2003); critique framework (Caldwell et al 2011); hierarchy of evidence for assessing qualitative health research (Daly et al 2007); levels of evidence (NHMRC 2009).
4. **Application of appraised evidence to practice, relevant implementation** (Dawes et al 2005); Step 4 (Fineout-Overholt & Johnston 2006); translation and implementation of research knowledge into practice and policy (Grimshaw et al 2012; Straus et al 2011; Straus et al 2009; Graham et al 2006; Lavis et al 2003).
5. **Evaluation of performance and effectiveness** (Dawes et al 2005); Step 5 (Fineout-Overholt & Johnston 2007); implementation and evaluation of evidence (Dogherty et al 2013; NCCMT 2012).

STUDENT CHALLENGE

Consider the following scenario: You are working in a surgical unit. There has been an unusually high incidence of wound infections that have been traced to poor hand hygiene by nursing and medical staff.

- Apply the five-step model to locate, appraise, implement and evaluate the best available evidence related to hand hygiene.

Historically, teaching research to nurses has focused on methods to generate primary evidence rather than teaching the steps of EBP to foster nurses' confidence and skills to search, retrieve, critique and implement relevant evidence in their clinical decision making (Fineout-Overholt & Johnson 2005a). Nurses and midwives have a professional responsibility to demonstrate a sound rationale for their decisions and utilise scientific research. We recall that Pravikoff and colleagues (2005, p. 40) asked a decade ago whether US nurses had the degree of readiness required to provide EBP. We suggest the notion of 'readiness' demonstrates an openness to change that is evident when we ask: 'what additional research evidence do we need to provide the best care for this patient?', 'how can we reduce the evidence-practice gap?' or 'how can we best answer this complex health care problem?'. As explained in greater depth in other chapters, a standardised format is used to guide the process of developing researchable questions. The PICOT framework can be used to guide this step. As Fineout-Overholt and Johnston (2005b, p. 158) describe:

P – Specific patient populations of interest,

I – Intervention of interest or issue of interest,

C – Comparison of interest (i.e. intervention or issue),

O – Outcome of interest,

T – Timeframe.

Timeframe may not always be relevant but is included in the PICOT format for consideration. Education in EBP is therefore imperative to prepare nurses and midwives to answer those questions (and others) by thinking systematically to identify problems, translate evidence/knowledge, and implement relevant evidence-based care to reduce the gap (Ellis 2013; Johnson et al 2010; Blenkinsop 2003; Laschinger et al 1990).

What is knowledge translation?

During the last 15 years there has been increasing attention on how to reduce the evidence-practice gap because 'one of the most consistent findings from clinical and health services research is the failure to translate research into practice and policy' (Grimshaw et al 2012, p. 1). The traditional modes of disseminating research findings (publications, conferences) and education do not have sufficient influence on policy or improve clinical care, despite the billions of dollars spent annually in evidence generation, research endeavours and training. Some argue the 'diversity and inconsistency of terminology is a potential barrier to synthesising, advancing and applying the findings' and inhibits communication and collaboration (Colquhoun et al 2014; Estabrooks et al 2006). Notably, researchers identified more than 100 terms to describe KT research, which impedes usefulness and potency of the topic (McKibbon et al 2010). Urgent work has been undertaken to clarify terminology for KT with the aim to improve the science of KT, advance common understandings and consistent utilisation (Colquhoun et al 2014) (Table 10.1). Put simply, if the field of KT remains confusing then the strategies developed by KT researchers to address the evidence-practice gap will be inaccessible to others so will not achieve its purpose. KT is defined by the Canadian Institutes of Health Research (CIHR 2010) as:

> *A dynamic and iterative process that includes the synthesis, dissemination, exchange and ethically sound application of knowledge to improve health, provide more effective health services and products, and strengthen the healthcare system. This process takes place within a complex system of interactions between researchers and knowledge users which may vary in intensity, complexity and level of engagement depending on the nature of the research and the findings as well as the needs of the particular knowledge user.*

Table 10.1
Knowledge translation terminology

Term	Used in	Definition
Implementation science	UK & Europe	Involves the most active transfer activities with the goal of creating a behaviour change. These activities include efforts to overcome barriers to implementing the research information through activities such as face-to-face contacts with experts and establishing audit and reminder systems to encourage users to change their behaviour or practice in the light of research findings (Johnson 2005, p. 11).
Research utilisation	UK & Europe	Research utilisation refers to the review and critique of scientific research, and then the application of the findings to clinical practice (Estabrooks 1998).
Dissemination	USA	Involves using intentional activities to share research findings strategically with particular stakeholders, such as mailing results to intended audiences and holding workshops and conferences to share findings. The goal is both to create awareness and change attitudes (Johnson 2005, p. 11).
Diffusion	USA	Is designed to promote awareness. Knowledge is made available via journals, newsletters, websites, mass media but is not directed toward a specific target. The goal is simply to *get the information out there* (Johnson 2005, p. 11).
Research use	USA	Use of evidence.
Knowledge transfer	USA	One-way flow of knowledge from researchers to potential users (Johnson 2005, p. 11).
Uptake	USA	Use of evidence.
Knowledge transfer and exchange	Canada	Researchers and decision-makers work together to build research questions relevant to their mutual needs and skills (Johnson 2005, p. 11).
Knowledge translation	Canada	A dynamic and iterative process that includes the synthesis, dissemination, exchange and ethically sound application of knowledge to improve health, provide more effective health services and products, and strengthen the healthcare system (CIHR 2010).
Knowledge translation	Australia	The creation of knowledge through research underpins improvement in Australia's health service delivery and intervention. However, it is widely acknowledged that there is a gap between discovery and implementation of knowledge from research. This gap slows the uptake of the benefits from research, for patients and for the operation of the health system. Closing this gap is a daunting task exacerbated by the volume of research that is available and the need to sometimes change commonly accepted beliefs and behaviours (Anderson 2012).

(table adapted from Johnson 2005, p. 11)

KT is an active response to increase the use of current, relevant research findings/evidence into practice. KT is the science of methods and interventions to integrate and simplify knowledge into usable formats and, secondly, the identification of **barriers and facilitators** to KT in individuals and organisational structures (Straus et al 2009; Graham et al 2006).

So in summary, the term KT includes all the steps between the creation of knowledge and its application in practice or policy. Therefore, collaboration is encouraged between researchers, clinicians, managers, policy makers, and healthcare users to identify vital research questions, and partner in the development and the implementation of evidence to answer complex problems (Johnson 2005). KT methods aim to move research evidence/knowledge into action, thus closing the gap between *knowing and doing* to address the knowledge-to-action gap (Straus et al 2009; Graham et al 2006). Deliberate and strategic actions to close the evidence-practice gap are urgently required. Collaborations between researchers and clinicians provide vital opportunities for communication and knowledge flow that is key to success because, as studies have shown, the generation of research evidence does not guarantee implementation or improvements to health services. Bridging the 'evidence-to-practice' gap necessitates change at multiple levels (individual, organisational structures, system) so barriers and incentives for change must be understood (Kitson 2011). The strategies must be tailored to bring about change in specific organisational contexts and with different professional groups (Grol & Wensing 2004) to implement contextualised practices that are relevant to the particular patient and their personal preferences and circumstances. Notably, EBP is a broader concept. When clinicians use the EBP approach, they go beyond the expertise and knowledge of clinicians and researchers, and consider the patient's preferences and values to develop a comprehensive plan of care (Rycroft-Malone et al 2004; Ingersoll 2000).

STUDENT CHALLENGE

1. Have the definitions of terms presented in Table 10.1 clarified your understanding of KT? What else do you need to study?
2. Write a paragraph that describes your current understanding of KT and relevance to your practice.
3. Describe when you used evidence in a specific context to plan relevant care for a patient (an example of your contextualised practice).

Why is knowledge translation important?

Globally, health systems are failing to provide quality healthcare services despite the billions of dollars assigned to fund them (Grimshaw et al 2012; Straus et al 2011). These trends of patients not benefiting from the latest evidence-based treatments were highlighted over a decade ago (Grol 2001) but remain widespread in contemporary healthcare systems. Further, 20% to 30% of patients may receive care that is not needed or could be potentially harmful to patients (Schuster et al 2005). Healthcare providers are not consistently meeting their goals of care so a failure to translate research evidence into practice and policy persists (Grimshaw et al 2012). The translation and implementation (utilisation) of recommended scientific evidence into routine healthcare and policy decisions is haphazzard, inconsistent and poorly coordinated (Eccles et al 2005; McGlynn et al 2003). Despite the existence of abundant clinical and health policy scientific evidence, gaps between best practice and actual clinical care persist due to the widespread failure to implement scientific evidence (Straus et al 2009; Grol & Wensing 2004). Therefore a better understanding of the individual and organisational readiness to translate research into **evidence-informed decision making (EIDM)** is urgently needed (Champagne et al 2014). This gap presents a major problem for managers who have the responsibility to support nurses, promote patient safety and increase research use in evidence-informed decision making in their organisations (Gifford et al 2014). 'EIDM depends on clinical expertise to integrate the best quality research evidence along with information about patient preferences, clinical context and resources' (Yost et al 2014, p. 156). Managers and clinical leaders identified barriers to their engagement in EIDM as 'not having enough time, knowledge, skills and confidence to find, appraise, and synthesise research findings for use in their decision making' (Gifford et al 2014, p. 399). This is interesting as these managers and clinical nurse leaders indicated they had deficits in the five steps of EBP (Johnston & Fineout-Overholt 2005).

It was noted that many of the barriers to nurses' use of research evidence in their decision making existed at the complex organisational level. Organisational level barriers include the 'existence of multiple initiatives and conflicting priorities' (Gifford et al 2014, p. 399), so a collaborative approach to problem-solving is a key to success. Researchers need to bridge the *knowledge to action gap* by planning strategies to address the barriers and facilitators in the context. Bridging the knowledge to action gap requires attitudinal and structural level change (individual, organisational, system). There is an urgent need for education in EBP to be available for all nurses in clinical practice to strengthen the use of EIDM (Melnyk & Fineout-Overholt 2002).

STUDENT CHALLENGE

Think about clinical settings where you have practiced.

1. Was there a focus on EIDM in clinical care? Describe how that focus was evident.
2. If not, what were the individual and organisational barriers to nurses and/or midwives engaging in EIDM? How might these barriers be overcome?
3. Thinking about the hand hygiene scenario presented earlier. What attitudinal and structural level change might be needed to improve hand hygiene in the unit?

What is the role of researchers in advancing knowledge translation?

The primary role of researchers has been the creation of knowledge and dissemination via traditional modes such as publishing in peer reviewed journals and delivering conference presentations. The field of KT science developed about two decades ago in response to widespread global concerns about the haphazard implementation of research evidence in health care (Straus et al 2009; Grol & Wensing 2004; Eccles et al 2005; McGlynn et al 2003). The responsibility is now on the researcher to change and to do more to engage the 'end user' of the research evidence. Researchers must plan new approaches to ensure their research evidence is understood and accessible in order to inform policy and clinical decision making. Increasingly, to facilitate the uptake of evidence, funding organisations are expecting researchers to include KT dissemination plans in grant proposals. The onus is now on the researcher to 'translate' their research knowledge into plain language formats that are easily accessible and appropriate for those who might apply the knowledge. Such individuals are referred to as 'end users' or 'specific/desired audiences' in the literature.

Five questions to build my understanding of the knowledge translation process

Lavis and colleagues (2003) identified five key questions to guide KT activities. In this next section, we will examine each question in order to develop your understanding, confidence and research literacy. The five questions are:

1. What should be transferred?
2. To whom should research knowledge be transferred?

3. By whom should the research knowledge be transferred?
4. How should research knowledge be transferred?
5. With what effect should research knowledge be transferred?

1. What should be transferred?

The answer to that question is the 'message'. The 'message' must be available in the form of dependable, accessible knowledge that can be understood and used with confidence by clinicians, managers and policy makers in their decision making. Creating the 'message' is a precursor to KT, but is a complex process involving knowledge synthesis. It is important that you understand this process and the best evidence to implement in your EIDM. The implementation of evidence from individual studies may be appropriate in specific contexts. However, there is a common view that individual studies 'rarely, by themselves, provide sufficient evidence for practice and policy change' (Grimshaw et al 2012, p. 2). There is broad agreement that KT must be informed by the replication and synthesis of global evidence and current systematic reviews (Grimshaw et al 2012; Brouwers et al 2009). The purpose of knowledge synthesis is to interpret results from systematic reviews within the context of all known evidence available globally (Brouwers et al 2009) (Table 10.2).

Straus et al (2009) note that *validity of the evidence* is the prime focus of systematic reviews rather than on the applicability of the evidence in various decision-making contexts. So researchers and individuals who work as knowledge translators must ensure the 'message' includes an applicability and implementation focus to support clinicians, managers and policy makers in their EIDM.

STUDENT CHALLENGE

Think back to the literature you accessed when you applied the five-step model in relation to the hand hygiene scenario.

1. Can you identify examples of first, second and third generation knowledge about hand hygiene from that literature?
2. Was there a clearly identifiable message being delivered in the third generation knowledge?
3. What message/s should be transferred to ensure best practice in hand hygiene?

2. To whom should research knowledge (the message) be transferred?

The answer is the 'target audience'. As we have read earlier, 'knowledge translation is defined as the use of knowledge in practice and decision making by the public, patients, health care professionals, managers and policy makers'

Table 10.2
Knowledge generation

Knowledge	Derived from	Knowledge related product
First-generation	Primary studies	Randomised trials
Second-generation	Knowledge synthesis	Systematic reviews
Third-generation	Tools and products such as decision aids and educational modules	User-friendly, implementable formats

(from Brouwers et al 2009, p. 1)

(Straus et al 2011, p. 6). KT involves the process of moving knowledge from research into practice to inform decision making (Graham et al 2006). Bridging the 'evidence-to-practice' gap requires change at multiple levels (individual, organisational structures, system) so potential barriers and facilitators for change can be identified and supported. The mechanisms and strategies must be tailored to bring about change in specific organisational contexts and with different professional groups (Grol & Wensing 2004) in order to facilitate a patient-centred model of care. This means researchers must firstly identify their 'target audience' – individuals (known as 'end users') they want to utilise the research findings in decision making.

Therefore researchers and knowledge translators must produce relevant documents and use appropriate language (i.e. plain language) to ensure their 'message' is understood by their intended 'target audience'. For example, researchers could collaborate with clinicians to produce a brochure of key facts and relevant messages to educate parents (target audience – end user) about a specific topic, rather than expecting parents to read a dense academic research article written in academic language and then correctly interpret relevant messages. This specific KT approach to disseminate research findings is a strategy to address a 'barrier' to the implementation of evidence. So in summary, researchers and knowledge translators need to firstly identify the different target audience/s and then disseminate knowledge in the form of relevant products, policy briefs, summaries and key messages and clinical practice guidelines. These efforts have the capacity to bridge the 'evidence-to-practice' gap, inform members of the target audience, and strengthen healthcare systems.

STUDENT CHALLENGE

1. With regard to the hand hygiene scenario, identify possible target audience/s.
2. What formats would be most appropriate to transmit the message/s to the target audience/s?

3. By whom should the research knowledge be transferred?

The answer to that question is 'the messenger'. Grimshaw et al (2012, p. 3) note the most suitable messenger will differ in relation to the 'target audience' and the nature of the message to be transferred. So 'the messenger' could be an individual working in an educational role (e.g. researcher, knowledge translator, healthcare professional), or a collective such as a group or organisation or larger system. Would you take direction from a nurse/midwife if you didn't think she/he was credible or competent? The extent to which an individual or organisation is deemed credible influences the ability to persuade others to adopt 'the message'. The term 'opinion leader' is used to describe individuals who are well connected, approachable and willing to answer questions to help others do their job (Lavis et al 2003; Grimshaw et al 2006). However, as shown in a study conducted by Hofmeyer and Scott (2007), the trait of approachability must be matched by sound research knowledge to ensure EIDM and safe care for patients. Two manager participants talked about nurses working in their units:

> *She's been here for quite a while. She has an opinion about everything and people will go to her because she does have a lot of good knowledge and good skills and she will teach. Now the down side is she also has a lot of opinions that aren't fact based. So staff are torn because she can be very nice and very approachable, but there's another side to her.*

'Opinion leaders are the informal leaders in the break room. When they talk everybody's listening to what they're saying. Those ones tend to be research driven ...' (Hofmeyer 2013, p. 786)

Building and maintaining effective, respectful relationships between opinion leaders and the users of knowledge is a key strategy to accelerate change to improve EBP and quality healthcare delivery (Estabrooks et al 2006; Valente & Davis 1999; Burt 1999). Relational capital (social capacity to get along with others) was confirmed in a national survey on utilisation of health research as key in knowledge transfer associated with quality patient outcomes (Landry et al 2002). At the individual level, the presence of research champions in organisations is considered to positively influence the use of research (Estabrooks 2003). Others argue that credible individuals working inside organisations can 'bridge' groups to exert influence and transmit knowledge as 'trusted aids'. Think about who you would ask for assistance to calculate medication dosages, or wound care, or teaching a woman about pain relief during labour. Would it be the same nurse/midwife? We suggest it is more likely you would ask different nurses/midwives (opinion leaders) for support because they had different clinical expertise in the areas that you needed help.

STUDENT CHALLENGE

1. Reflect on your clinical experiences. Can you identify any staff who you would consider to be opinion leaders as described above? What characteristics do they possess to make them influential?
2. Consider the hand hygiene scenario and identify who might be the best messenger/s to get the message across to the target audience? Why?

4. How should research knowledge be transferred?

The answer is to choose the appropriate KT strategy (from the numerous KT models available) to promote success. Planning for KT is more likely to be effective if the researchers or knowledge translators firstly assess the likely facilitators and barriers to success in the context. These insights will guide the choice of the most appropriate KT strategy to deliver the desired message and to whom (target audience). Time spent planning is crucial to success and will avoid wasted time and funding (Grimshaw et al 2012). The assessment to identify barriers and facilitators will inform the choice of KT strategies and tailor interventions to increase the effectiveness of professional behaviour change, facilitate decision making, and health system change. Barriers include the volume of evidence currently produced on a daily basis, access to the evidence and the required research literacy skills of individuals. Potential barriers can exist at the structural, organisational professional and consumer levels so need to be identified within the specific context (using relevant methods) and managed effectively.

Qualitative (interviews, focus groups) and quantitative methods (surveys) and observation could be used to identify potential barriers and relevant KT strategies to translate the knowledge to the target group and foster change (Grimshaw et al 2012; Grol & Wensing 2004). For example, if the aim was to improve nurse-patient communication on a specific health education topic, you could elicit views from individuals in both groups to identify barriers and potential interventions to support, inform, educate and support behaviour change.

STUDENT CHALLENGE

1. In relation to the hand hygiene scenario, what individual and organisational barriers might exist that could impede delivery of the evidence-based message/s?
2. What strategies could be used to overcome these barriers and ensure the message gets through to the relevant staff?

5. With what effect should research knowledge be transferred?

The answer is that the KT goal and evaluation would vary across target groups. For example, KT by clinicians would show the use of 'high-quality clinical practice guidelines' to improve the quality of clinical decision making (Brouwers et al 2009, p. 1), coupled with evaluating other organisational factors, barriers and facilitators. For policy makers, the aim may be to inform debate (Johnson 2005). Knowledge synthesis is the foundation for the development of clinical practice guidelines and decision aids to improve patients' participation in decision making about their health (Brouwers et al 2009). In order to enhance uptake (and use) of knowledge, researchers should also address the 'cultural gap' between themselves and the target group they wish to engage by using appropriate plain language and formats to communicate the message.

STUDENT CHALLENGE

1. Consider the hand hygiene scenario. What is the KT impact being sought?
2. How would you know if the hand hygiene messages have been implemented in clinical practice?

Following on from these broad strategies, we conclude the chapter with the following practical suggestions to develop individual and organisational readiness and competence in EIDM.

Strategies to develop individual and organisational readiness in EIDM

As stated earlier in this chapter, in order to meet the national competency standards, nurses and midwives must develop their analytical skills to locate, critically appraise, understand and apply research findings in their practice (research literacy). As discussed earlier in this chapter, Yost et al (2014, p. 156) eloquently explained that 'evidence-informed decision making (EIDM) depends on clinical expertise to integrate the best quality evidence along with information about patient preferences, clinical context and resources'. Importantly, Yost et al (2014, p. 162) identified two types of EIDM behaviours that provide a clear guide:

> *a) engaging in EIDM activities (i.e. searching for the best available evidence, critically appraising research evidence) in practice, and b) use of research evidence (i.e. an evidence-informed guideline, protocol, pathway) for practice change.*

In this section of the chapter, we will consider some practical ways that you, as an individual nurse or midwife, can demonstrate your research literacy through developing EIDM behaviours in your everyday practice. As a student reading the material in this book, you are developing your research literacy and demonstrating EIDM behaviours. Consider the following ideas:

- Recognise gaps in your research literacy; that is, generating a researchable question, PICOT, critical appraisal, interpreting and applying evidence in EIDM, evaluation.
- Set educational goals to build skills in required areas and access credible knowledge resources, highly skilled colleagues and opinion leaders.
- Understand the political, professional, organisational and patient-centred care context.
- Contribute to developing cultures that promote EIDM among clinicians, managers and students.
- Mentor the next generation of nurses in their research literacy and skills in EIDM.
- Learn to develop 'leading qualities', speak up to obtain the necessary resources for delivering evidence-based quality care for patients and thus meeting the goals of the healthcare organisation (Pravikoff et al 2005).

STUDENT CHALLENGE

Undergraduate student nurses and midwives are strongly encouraged to take responsibility for developing skills in research literacy and EIDM behaviours. Begin by considering how the following questions and strategies could develop your readiness to engage in this lifelong learning process:

1. What knowledge and skills do you have that will assist you to develop EIDM behaviours in your practice?

2. What further knowledge and skills do you need to equip you for EIDM?
3. How will you gain this additional knowledge and skills?
4. What about attitudes and behaviours?
5. Volunteer to participate in research activities and clinical audits in the practice setting.
6. Ask research-active academics if there are opportunities for you to observe them conducting focus groups and undertaking data analysis.
7. Apply for summer scholarships in research projects at the university or in a clinical research unit. These opportunities can offer 'hands on' mentoring and skill development in areas that build skills such as developing research questions, searching the literature, appraising and writing literature reviews, project teamwork, preparing ethics proposals, writing structured conference abstracts, developing conference presentations, designing conference posters and reporting research findings in plain language for specific target groups such as parents and children.

Strategies for becoming EIDM ready: adopt a culture of inquiry

A key factor in becoming EIDM ready is the adoption of a culture of inquiry in everyday clinical practice. Strategies for adopting a culture of inquiry include questioning clinical practices, engaging in professional development activities and joining relevant organisational and professional groups/committees.

Questioning clinical practices

You can do this by examining your practices and actions in the provision of client care and interrogating the evidence base underpinning those practices. Many routine nursing practices remain based on tradition rather than evidence (Flynn Makic, Martin et al 2013; Flynn Makic, Rauen et al 2014). For example, Flynn Makic et al (2013) identified four practices in critical care nursing that remain based on tradition, despite available research evidence supporting changes in those practices. Such traditional practices are often referred to as 'sacred cows' (Leake 2004; Flynn Makic, Martin et al 2013; Flynn Makic, Rauen et al 2014; Mick 2011). These are practices developed over time through 'trial and error', so are based on tradition rather than rigorous research. Suggestions for questioning practice include:

- Develop a list of the questions about the nursing/midwifery practices in your workplace.
- Listen to other colleagues in your unit/ward – are they questioning the same practices and why?

- Identify 'sacred cows' in your practice. Do this by questioning the practices that are the least logical, the most time consuming, and based on tradition.
- Read professional journals with a focus on identifying new research on traditional practices and consider how these ideas might be implemented in your unit/ward.
- Talk to other staff about 'sacred cows' they have identified. Ask what they did to try to change the practice and whether change was achieved. What barriers did they encounter in trying to change practice?
- Check the nursing/midwifery practice manual in your workplace and look up a specific nursing/midwifery practice guideline/procedure. Is the guideline/procedure referenced to current research evidence? How would you find out if it is based on the best currently available research evidence?
- Volunteer to participate in reviews of polices and guidelines on your ward/unit to gain experience in examining whether they are based on research evidence and professional standards of care (Leake 2004).

STUDENT CHALLENGE

Review a routine practice in your current clinical environment and examine the evidence base underpinning that practice.

1. Is there evidence to support the practice?
2. Did you find evidence to refute the practice?
3. Consider what you would do if you find evidence to refute the practice? Who will you discuss your finding with? What barriers might there be to changing the practice? How might those barriers be addressed?

Engage in professional development activities

As a health professional, you are required to engage in lifelong learning to be informed about the latest research evidence in your area of practice and ensure your practice is current. This includes engaging in formal and informal learning that is self-directed, provided by workplaces, or professional organisations. Approaches to engage include:

- Identify how to access evidence provided by your workplace; for example, through the intranet and library. Make the librarian your friend.
- Identify key electronic research resources such as quality websites and databases.

- Identify key quality peer reviewed journals that publish research relevant to your area of practice and set up email alerts for literature related to your area/s of practice – the librarian can assist with this.
- Make time on a weekly or fortnightly basis to read relevant literature and stay updated about latest research and developments in your practice area. Discuss and debate your findings with a colleague.
- Join and participate in a journal club in your workplace. If there isn't a journal club in your workplace, consider getting support to start a group.
- Join a relevant online discussion group – there are some excellent discussion groups where you can engage with clinicians and researchers around the world.
- Regularly attend professional development activities that will assist you to develop your skills in accessing, reading, critically appraising, implementing and evaluating research (Butz 2007; Fineout-Overholt and Johnston 2005a; Fineout-Overholt and Johnston 2005b). Such activities could include grand round research presentations, unit/ward-based education sessions, poster presentations, sessions at other health units or your local university.
- Attend conferences and actively engage and network with peers and leaders.

STUDENT CHALLENGE

Review your current strategies to lifelong learning and consider whether you would benefit from adopting any of the following ideas:

1. Identify five quality electronic research resources (e.g. quality websites and databases) that contain information relevant to your practice.
2. List five quality peer reviewed journals that publish research relevant to your practice.
3. Set up email alerts with relevant journals for literature related to your interests and area/s of practice. Remember, the librarian can assist with this.
4. Identify local, national or international online discussion groups that could be relevant to your interest and clinical practice. Join, participate and evaluate the benefits.

Join relevant organisational and professional groups/committees to influence change

Norms and networks form the basis of our social context and act as potential barriers or incentives to support learning, change and KT efforts. It doesn't matter what knowledge and understanding you have if you cannot influence change. Your ability to get along with others and integrate into the workplace culture and professional networks will enhance your effectiveness. A feature of lifelong learning is the ability to adjust to ever changing situations locally, nationally and globally. KT is a social process that occurs within relationships and across professional networks and teams (Estabrooks et al 2006). Therefore, social networks and norms (e.g. cooperation and trust) play a crucial role in facilitating learning and increased application of knowledge in your decision-making social context. Consider adopting the following strategies if relevant to your development:

- Join a relevant professional organisation linked to your area of practice. Most nursing/midwifery organisations provide a range of resources for members to access which may include journals and other online resources as well as workshops and other professional activities discounted to members. Membership of professional organisations also provides opportunities to contribute to review of clinical guidelines and standards in relevant areas of practice, often on a national scale.
- Identify/join relevant committees in your workplace where you will have exposure to development/review of practice guidelines, or clinical audit activities and outcomes.
- Find out if your organisation has a research or knowledge development/translation unit and identify opportunities to become involved in research activities undertaken by the unit and learn from the staff in the unit.
- Identify a mentor who can assist you to develop knowledge and skills related to EBP and support you to become involved in clinically focused projects (Gagliardi et al 2014).

STUDENT CHALLENGE

Review your current strategies to lifelong learning and consider whether you would benefit from adopting any of the following ideas:

1. Identify professional organisations relevant to your professional practice including one specialty focused organisation and identify the benefits and resources that come with membership of that organisation.
2. Identify the relevant committees within your workplace that focus on development/review of clinical practice guidelines and standards.
3. Does the organisation have a research/KT unit? What is the focus of the unit? Identify and make contact with the staff in the research unit and ask how you can learn from them/be involved in research-related activities?

Developing research literacy and EIDM in organisations

Culture change toward EIDM and delivery of safe, quality care remains a top priority for all healthcare organisations. We encourage managers and nurse/midwifery leaders in healthcare organisations to consider the following strategies to foster organisational readiness to provide health care that is patient-centred and informed by current evidence:

- Strengthen workplaces to support easy access to current evidence by ensuring computers linked to databases, libraries and evidence-based repositories (such as Cochrane and JBI) are readily available.
- Ensure current clinical practice guidelines are used in the organisation.
- Identify nurses/midwives who are viewed as 'opinion leaders' and provide opportunities to enhance their learning and skill development.
- Foster a culture of EIDM in the organisation.
- Establish strategies to build skills and confidence in searching and using current research evidence in problem-solving.

Conclusion

There is broad global agreement that the professional practice of nurses and midwives is demonstrated through their use of the best available research evidence in their clinical decision making. EBP and KT are key in achieving desired quality outcomes for patients. But in reality, students, nurses and midwives report being unclear about how best to prepare to respond to these professional expectations and develop EIDM behaviours. So the purpose of this chapter is to draw links with professional practice and develop understanding about how the KT process can enhance your capacity to implement research-based and contextualised practices to address health problems. We did this by using the hand hygiene scenario to illustrate the application of the KT process. We examined the KT debates in relation to individual practice and considered the barriers and facilitators in the workplace culture in healthcare organisations. The aim of KT is to address the evidence–practice gap and ultimately improve quality healthcare for patients. As Shea (2011, p. 4) reiterates, 'the touchstone of all KT research is an intent to change behaviour so that evidence-based interventions replace intuition and politics in the drive to improve the health of the community'.

In addition, we presented a range of strategies to develop individual research literacy, EIDM behaviours, and improve organisational readiness for KT in healthcare systems. The strategies could be adopted by managers and nurse leaders, clinicians (registered nurses and midwives), and undergraduate student nurses as well as midwives. This would strengthen organisational environments and facilitate individual research literacy. These are the key ingredients in EIDM and would provide the desired quality outcomes for patients.

The key message in this chapter is that developing competence in research literacy is as critical as developing competence in clinical skills. This means that you understand the relevance of aspiring to lifelong learning throughout your career as a healthcare professional in order to provide quality evidence-informed healthcare for patients and their families.

The next chapter provides an example of the research process including KT, in action.

RESOURCES KIT

Useful websites

Knowledge Translation Planning Template

Barwick, M. (2013). 'Knowledge Translation Planning Template-R', Hospital for Sick Children Toronto: http://www.sickkidsfoundation.com/grants/knowledge.asp.

http://www.sickkidsfoundation.com/grants/ktMethod/KT_Planning_Temp_Barwick.pdf.

Cochrane Collaboration

International organisation that conducts systematic reviews of health and medical research. Online. Available: http://www.cochrane.org 1 September 2014.

The Australian Government has funded the work of the Cochrane Collaboration in Australia through the National Health and Medical Research Council since 2001. Through a funded five-year agreement to 2017 the NHMRC has ensured access to the Cochrane Library. The Cochrane Library can be accessed at www.thecochranelibrary.com and access is free to all residents of Australia.

Systematic Reviews www.cochrane.org/cochrane-reviews.

Public Health Group http://ph.cochrane.org.

Database of Abstracts of Reviews of Effects (DARE). Online. Available: http://onlinelibrary.wiley.com/o/cochrane/cochrane_cldare_articles_fs.html 22 August 2014.

Agency for Healthcare Research and Quality (AHRQ): Translating Research Into Practice (TRIP) Program. Initiative focusing on implementation techniques and factors associated with successfully translating research findings into diverse applied settings. Online. Available http://www.ahrq.gov/research/trip2fac.htm 1 September 2014.

Campbell Collaboration (C2): International organisation that conducts systematic reviews of education, social welfare, social science research. Online. Available: http://www.campbellcollaboration.org 1 September 2014.

Canadian Institute for Health Research (CIHR): Federal agency responsible for funding health research in Canada for KT research, development, and dissemination. Online. Available: http://www.cihr-irsc.gc.ca/e/29529.html 1 September 2014.

Knowledge Translation Program (KTP) University of Toronto, Canada: Multidisciplinary academic program developed to address the gap between research evidence and clinical practice and the need to focus on the processes through which knowledge is effectively translated into changed practices. Online. Available: http://www.stmichaelshospital.com/research/kt.php 1 September 2014.

Knowledge Utilisation Studies Program, University of Alberta, Canada: Focus on nursing, social sciences and research utilisation in nursing. Online. Available: http://www.kusp.ualberta.ca 1 September 2014.

National Health Service (NHS) Centre for Reviews and Dissemination, University of York: Conducts systematic reviews of research and disseminates research-based information about the effects of interventions used in health and social care in UK. Online. Available: http://www.york.ac.uk/inst/crd/welcome.htm 1 September 2014.

Evidence-based websites

Academic Center for Evidence-Based Practice. University of Texas – Evidence-based presentation slides to advance evidence-based nursing practice, research and education within an interdisciplinary context (1 September 2014). Online. Available: http://www.acestar.uthscsa.edu 12 April 2015.

Evidence-Based Nursing. Centre for Evidence-Based Medicine, Toronto, Canada (1 September 2014). Online. Available: http://ktclearinghouse.ca/cebm/syllabi/nursing 12 April 2015.

Nursing Knowledge International. Evidence-based content: Sigma Theta Tau International (1 September 2014). Online. Available: http://www.nursingsociety.org/aboutus/PositionPapers/Pages/EBN_positionpaper.aspx 12 April 2015.

References

Anderson W: *New approach to identifying evidence-practice gaps and research priorities. NHMRC Research Translation Faculty*. Media Release NHMRC 17 August 2012. Online. Available: https://www.nhmrc.gov.au/_files_nhmrc/media_releases/release_120817_rtf.pdf 2012 19 May 2015.

Australian College of Nursing: *Nursing research position statement*, 2013, ACN Ltd Canberra. Online. Available: http://www.acn.edu.au 5 February 2014.

Barwick M: *Knowledge Translation Planning Template-R, Hospital for Sick Children Toronto*, 2013. Online. Available: http://www.sickkidsfoundation.com/grants/knowledge.asp 1 September 2014.

Blenkinsop C: Research: an essential skill of a graduate nurse? *Nurse Education Today* 23(2):83–88, 2003.

Brouwers M, Stacey D, O'Connor A: Knowledge creation: synthesis, tools and products, *Canadian Medical Association Journal* 2009. doi: 10.1503/cmaj.-081230.

Burt RS: The social capital of opinion leaders, ANNALS *AAPSS* 566 Nov:37–54, 1999.

Butz A: Evidence-based practice in nursing: bridging the gap between research and practice, *Journal of Pediatric Health Care* 21(1):53–56, 2007.

Caldwell K, Henshaw L, Taylor G: Developing a framework for critiquing health research: an early evaluation, *Nurse Education Today* 31(8):e1–e7, 2011.

Canadian Institutes of Health Research (CIHR): *More about knowledge translation at CIHR*, Ottawa, ON, 2010, Canadian Institutes of Health Research. Online. Available: http://www.cihr-irsc.gc.ca/e/39033.html 1 September 2014.

Champagne F, Lemieux-Charles L, Duranceau MF, et al: Organisational impact of evidence-informed decision making training initiatives: a case study comparison of two approaches, *Implementation Science* 9:53, 2014.
Colquhoun H, Leeman J, Michie S, et al: Towards a common terminology: a simplified framework of interventions to promote and integrate evidence into health practices, systems and policies, *Implementation Science* 9:51, 2014.
Council of Deans of Nursing and Midwifery (ANZ): www.cdnm.edu.au, 2006. 22 July 2014.
Crookes P, Davies S, editors: *Research into practice: essential skills for reading and applying research in nursing and health care*, Edinburgh, 2004, Baillière Tindall.
Daly J, Willis K, Small R, et al: A hierarchy of evidence for assessing qualitative health research, *Journal of Clinical Epidemiology* 60(1):43–49, 2007.
Dawes M, Davies P, Gray A, et al: *Evidence-based practice: A primer for health care professionals*, 2e Edinburgh, 2005, Elsevier Churchill Livingstone.
Dawes M, Summerskill W, Glasziou P, et al: Sicily statement on evidence-based practice, *BMC Medical Education* 2005. doi: 10.1186/1472-6920-5-1.
Dogherty E, Harrison M, Graham I, et al: Turning Knowledge into Action at the Point-of-Care: The Collective Experiment of Nurses Facilitating the Implementation of Evidence-Based Practice, *Worldviews on Evidence-based Nursing* 10(3):129–130, 2013.
Eccles M, Grimshaw J, Walker A, et al: Changing the behaviour of healthcare professionals: The use of theory in promoting the uptake of research findings, *Journal Clinical Epidemiology* 58(2):107–112, 2005.
Ellis P: *Understanding research for nursing students*, 2e, 2013, Matters UK Sage Learning.
Estabrooks CA, Thompson DS, Lovely JJE, et al: A Guide to Knowledge Translation Theory, *Journal of Continuing Education in the Health Professions* 26(1):25–36, 2006.
Estabrooks CA: Will Evidence-Based Nursing Practice Make Practice Perfect?, *Canadian Journal of Nursing Research* 30(1):15–36, 1998.
Estabrooks CA: Translating Research into Practice: Implications for Organizations and Administrators, *Canadian Journal of Nursing Research* 35(3):53–68, 2003.
Fineout-Overholt E, Johnston L: Teaching EBP: A Challenge for Educators in the 21st century, *Worldviews on Evidence-based Nursing* 2(1):37–39, 2005a.
Fineout-Overholt E, Johnston L: Teaching EBP: Asking Searchable, Answerable Clinical Questions, *Worldviews on Evidence-based Nursing* 2(3):157–160, 2005b.
Fineout-Overholt E, Hofstetter S, Shell L, et al: Teaching EBP: Getting to the Gold. How to Search for the Best Evidence, *Worldviews on Evidence-based Nursing* 2(4):207–211, 2005.
Fineout-Overholt E, Johnston L: Teaching EBP: Implementation of Evidence. Moving from Evidence to Action, *Worldviews on Evidence-based Nursing* 3(4):194–200, 2006.
Fineout-Overholt E, Johnston L: Evaluation: An Essential Step to the EBP Process, *Worldviews on Evidence-based Nursing* 4(1):54–59, 2007.
Flynn Makic MB, Martin SA, Burns S, et al: Putting evidence into nursing practice: four traditional practices not supported by evidence, *Critical Care Nurse* 33(2):28–44, 2013.
Flynn Makic MB, Rauen C, Watson R, et al: Examining the evidence to guide practice: Challenging practice habits, *Critical Care Nurse* 34(2):28–46, 2014.
Gagliardi A, Webster F, Perrier L, et al: Exploring mentorship as a strategy to build capacity for knowledge translation research and practice: A scoping systematic review, *Implementation Science* 9(1):1–19, 2014.
Gerrish K, Ashworth P, Lacey A, et al: Developing evidence-based practice: experiences of senior and junior clinical nurses, *Journal of Advanced Nursing* 62(1):62–73, 2008.
Gifford W, Lefebre N, Davies B: An Organisational Intervention to Influence Evidence-Informed Decision Making in Home Health Nursing, *JONA* 44(7/8):395–402, 2014.
Graham I, Logan J, Harrison M, et al: Lost in Knowledge Translation: Time for a map?, *The Journal of Continuing Education in the Health Professions* 36(1):13–24, 2006.
Grimshaw J, Eccles M, Greener J, et al: Is the involvement of opinion leaders in the implementation of research findings a feasible strategy? *Implementation Science* 1:3, 2006. doi: 10.1186/1748-5908-1-3.

Grimshaw J, Eccles M, Lavis J, et al: Knowledge Translation of Research Findings, *Implementation Science* 7:50, 2012.
Grol R: Successes and failures in the implementation of evidence-based guidelines for clinical practice, *Medical Care* 39(8):1146–1154, 2001.
Grol R, Wensing M: What drives changes? Barriers to and incentives for achieving evidence-based practice, *Medical Journal of Australia* 1806(6):S57–S60, 2004.
Halcomb EJ, Peters K: Nursing student feedback on undergraduate research education: Implications for teaching and learning, *Contemporary Nurse* 33(1):59–68, 2009.
Hill A, Spittlehouse C: What is critical appraisal?, *Evidence-based Medicine* 3(2):1–8, 2003.
Hofmeyer A: How can a social capital framework guide managers to develop positive nurse relationships and patient outcomes?, *Journal of Nursing Management* 21(5):782–789, 2013.
Hofmeyer A, Scott C: *Social Capital in Healthcare Services*. Final Report Faculty of Nursing, University of Alberta, Edmonton (Available from the first author), 2007.
Ingersoll GL: Evidence-based nursing: what it is and what it isn't, *Nursing Outlook* 48(4):151–152, 2000.
International Council of Nurses: *Closing the gap: From evidence to action*. 2012. Online. Available: http://www.icn.ch/publications/2012-closing-the-gap-from-evidence-to-action 30 July 2015.
Johnson LS: From knowledge transfer to knowledge translation: applying research to practice, *Occupational Therapy Now* July/August:11–14, 2005.
Johnson N, List-Ivankovic J, Eboh WO, et al: Research and evidence-based practice: Using a blended approach to teaching and learning in undergraduate nurse education, *Nurse Education in Practice* 10(1):43–47, 2010.
Johnston L, Fineout-Overholt E: Teaching EBP: 'Getting from zero to one'. Moving from recognizing and admitting uncertainties to asking searchable, answerable questions, *Worldviews on Evidence-based Nursing* 2(2):98–102, 2005.
Johnston L, Fineout-Overholt E: Teaching EBP: Critical Step of Critically Appraising Literature, *Worldviews on Evidence-based Nursing* 1(2):44–46, 2006.
Kitson A: Mechanics of knowledge translation, *International Journal of Evidence-Based Healthcare* 9(2):79–80, 2011.
Landry R, Amara N, Lamari M: Does social capital determine innovation? To what extent?, *Technological Forecasting & Social Change* 69:681–701, 2002.
Laschinger HS, Johnson G, Kohr R: Building undergraduate nursing students' knowledge of the research process in nursing, *Journal of Nursing Education* 29(3):114–117, 1990.
Lavis JN, Robertson D, Woodside JM, et al: How can research organizations more effectively transfer research knowledge to decision makers?, *Milbank Quarterly* 81:221–222, 2003.
Leake P: Teaming with students and a sacred cow contest to make changes in nursing practice, *The Journal of Continuing Education in Nursing* 35(6):271–277, 2004.
McGlynn EA, Asch SM, Adams J, et al: The quality of health care delivered to adults in the United States, *New England Journal of Medicine* 348(26):2635–2645, 2003.
McKibbon KA, Lokker C, Wilczynski NL, et al: A cross-sectional study of the number and frequency of terms used to refer to knowledge translation in a body of health literature in 2006: a Tower of Babel?, *Implementation Science* 5:16, 2010.
Melnyk B, Fineout-Overholt E: Putting research into practice, *Reflections on Leadership* 28(2):22–25, 45, 2002.
Mick J: Promoting clinical inquiry and EBP: the sacred cow contest strategy, *Journal of Nursing Administration* 41(6):280–284, 2011.
National Collaborating Centre for Methods and Tools (NCCMT): *Knowledge translation planning tool*, Hamilton, ON, 2012, McMaster University. Online. Available: http://www.nccmt.ca/registry/view/eng/131.html 30 July 2015.
National Health and Medical Research Council (NHMRC): *NHMRC levels of evidence and grades for recommendations for developers of guidelines*, NHMRC, 2009, Australian Government. Online. Available: https://www.nhmrc.gov.au/guidelines-publications/information-guideline-developers/resources-guideline-developers 22 July 2014.
Nursing and Midwifery Board of Australia: *National competency standards for the registered nurse*, Victoria, 2006, Nursing and Midwifery Board of Australia. Online. Available:

http://www.nursingmidwiferyboard.gov.au/Codes-Guidelines-Statements/Codes-Guidelines.aspx 22 July 2014.

Pravikoff D, Tanner A, Pierce S: Readiness of U.S. Nurses for Evidence-Based Practice, *American Journal of Nursing* 105(9):40–51, 2005.

Rycroft-Malone J, Seer K, Titchen A, et al: What counts as evidence in evidence-based practice?, *Journal of Advanced Nursing* 47(1):81–90, 2004.

Sackett DL: Evidence-based medicine: what it is and what it isn't, *British Medical Journal* 312(7023):71–72, 1996.

Sackett DL, Straus SE, Richardson WS, et al: *Evidence-based medicine: how to practice and teach EBM*, Edinburgh, 2000, Churchill Livingstone.

Schuster MA, McGlynn EA, Brook RH: How good is the quality of health care in the United States? (1998), *Milbank Quarterly* 83:843–895, 2005.

Scott SD, Albrecht L, O'Leary K, et al: Results from a Systematic Review of Knowledge Translation Strategies in the Allied Health Professions, *Implementation Science* 7:70, 2012. doi: 10.1186/1748-5908-7-70.

Shea B: A decade of knowledge translation research – what has changed?, *Journal of Clinical Epidemiology* 64:3–5, 2011.

Sigma Theta Tau International (STTI): *Evidence-based nursing position statement*, USA, 2002, Board of Directors.

Straus SE, Tetroe J, Graham I: Defining Knowledge translation, *Canadian Medical Association Journal* 181(3–4):165–168, 2009.

Straus SE, Tetroe J, Graham I: Knowledge translation is the use of knowledge in health care decision making, *Journal of Clinical Epidemiology* 64:6–10, 2011.

Valente TW, Davis RL: Accelerating the diffusion of innovations using opinion leaders, ANNALS, *AAPSS* 566:55–67, 1999.

Yost J, Thompson D, Ganann R, et al: Knowledge Translation Strategies for Enhancing Nurses' Evidence-Informed Decision Making: A Scoping Review, *Worldviews on Evidence-based Nursing* 11(3):156–167, 2014.

CHAPTER 11

BRINGING IT ALL TOGETHER: AN APPLICATION OF THE RESEARCH PROCESS

Hannah Dahlen, Virginia Schmied and Sally Tracy

CHAPTER OUTLINE

KEY TERMS

data
data collection
evidence-based practice
findings
hypothesis
research design
research question
sample

LEARNING OBJECTIVES

After reading this chapter and following critical reflection the student will be able to:

1. Understand the initial steps in designing a research study
2. Develop a research question using the acronym PICO
3. Understand further the importance of, and process of, undertaking a literature review
4. Understand and be able to discuss the difference between aims and objectives
5. Know whether a qualitative or quantitative design would work best to answer a question
6. Discuss the importance of ethical considerations in research
7. Identify the principles of good supervision/support for undertaking research
8. Discuss the different considerations in developing a research budget.

Don't wait for the light to appear at the end of the tunnel – stride down there and light the bloody thing yourself (Sara Henderson 1993).

STUDENT QUOTE

OK, I have an idea, but how do I start?

ABSTRACT

Now that you have been introduced to some basic principles surrounding research and the processes involved in conducting research, hopefully you are feeling inspired to one day take your own journey. Hopefully it all does not seem so mysterious to you now. In this chapter we bring some of what you have read to life. Using an example of a piece of research already completed we take you through the research process step by step. We begin where all good research begins – with the question, and how to develop a concise question and then use this question to search the literature. We explore the difference between aims and objectives and give you some guidance on how a research proposal should be written. Briefly we will walk you through the different designs you might want to use (remember qualitative and quantitative?). Important considerations such as ethics, timelines, budgets and finding a good supervisor or support for undertaking research are also discussed. While some of this material has been covered in previous chapters, here it is repeated and applied in a way that should consolidate what you have previously learnt and make it more meaningful. Even if you do not wish to conduct research yourself, or will not do so for a while, having good insight into how good research is conducted will stand you in great stead for critical appraisal and evidence-based practice. In illustrating the approach we took we hope the research process becomes clearer to you. Perhaps you might even consider an Honours year at some point. Talk to the academic staff; they will be able to provide advice on how to go about this.

It all begins with a question

As you have learnt, the ultimate aim of research is to enable us as nurses and midwives to provide evidence-based care. We want to make sure that we minimise harm and maximise benefit to our clients. **Evidence-based practice** has been described as 'the conscientious, explicit and judicious use of current best evidence in making decisions about the care of individual patients' (Sackett et al 2000). We undertake research in order to be able to provide our clients with the best possible care supported by the current best available evidence, whilst always keeping their individual needs central.

Research involves four components: (1) asking a question; (2) systematically collecting information in order to answer the question; (3) sorting, analysing and interpreting the information; and (4) communicating the findings to others (Asmundson et al 2002; Horsfall et al 2007). In order to undertake research, we need to begin with a question that needs answering.

Conceiving the study: identifying the problem

All good research begins with a question you want to answer. Most worthwhile ideas for research come from difficulties or confusion in clinical practice (Dobratz 2003; Horsfall et al 2007). Your question is the key to everything in research. Your question will shape the method you choose and the answers you get (Weaver & Olson 2006). Your question might be very specific or quite broad or exploratory, depending on how much knowledge is already out there about the area you are interested in. **Research questions** should be clear and unambiguous and it is important not to fall into the trap of trying to do too much within a given study (Asmundson et al 2002). A well-focused research question can contribute to better clinical decision-making (Thompson et al 2004). Someone else's research may have raised a question that you would like to answer through your own study or possibly through replication of an existing study in your own setting. Or the question may come to you during your daily work as a nurse or midwife. Questions often come to us from our practice, from our observations and the questions we are asked by our clients.

When the first author was a student midwife in the UK, she observed something that triggered a question in her mind. Years later she set out to undertake research in order to get an answer to that question.

Whilst caring for Lisa (not her real name) who was in the late second stage of labour, the first author noticed that Lisa seemed to be terrified every time a contraction came and the baby's head pushed against her perineum. She kept trying to draw the baby's head back into her body, at one point crossing her legs in desperation. Quietly the midwife who was helping left the room, returning minutes later with a bowl of steaming water. The midwife placed a warm cloth on Lisa's perineum and crooned softly, 'that will help, love.' Lisa's eyelids flickered momentarily and her gasping, sucking shrieks eased. She began to push, tentatively at first and then in a focused but amazingly relaxed way. Her distress visibly lifted. Lisa's perineum seemed to glide over the baby's head as all the tension was released and her newborn almost oozed into an amazed student midwife's waiting hands. Later, when the first author quizzed the midwife about the effect of the warm pack, she said, 'It soothes the ring of fire' (burning sensation in the perineum). This later became the title of a publication resulting from the research the first author undertook (Dahlen et al 2009).

There was a clear and sudden realisation that there was something very effective about this simple method. It was later on that more information came to hand about warm packs and the claim that they reduce perineal trauma. What was observed in Lisa's changed behaviour was that her pain was eased and she was able to give birth to her baby without holding back.

The first author became an avid user of warm packs from then on. This is often what happens when we observe something that seems to work well. Then as we use it and see benefits in other people our practice is reinforced and we become convinced about the benefits. The problem with this is we are not evaluating the effect of the care in a scientific and systematic way and we could be biased and unaware of the harm we are causing or the reality that in fact it makes no difference.

The answer became clear. This method of second-stage care needed scientific validation either to prove or disprove its effect. The first author became determined that this ancient midwifery knowledge not be lost and devalued in the medicalised world in which birth now occurred (Dahlen et al 2010). A question began to be formed that needed to be answered. Could the application of a warm pack to the perineum in the second stage of labour reduce perineal trauma and improve perineal comfort during and after birth? The idea for the warm pack trial was born but it took a further seven years to complete the research and have it published.

Turning your idea into a searchable question

Once you have an idea in your mind that you would like to explore, the idea needs to be phrased into a specific question, which is searchable. Use the acronym PICO; as described in Chapter 10 it is commonly used to help make a question more specific for search purposes.

P: What is the patient or problem? The question being considered above was the problem of perineal trauma and pain during the second stage of labour. The population or patients for whom the issue is relevant is women giving birth.

I: What is the intervention of interest? The intervention will be a perineal warm pack.

C: What is being compared? We want to compare women who have a warm pack applied to their perineum in the second stage of labour to women who don't.

O: What is the outcome? We are interested, as described in the story above, to find out if applying a warm pack to the perineum in second-stage labour will reduce perineal trauma and improve comfort for women.

When assessing qualitative research however, the PICO method may not be so easy to apply. Figure 11.1 is an innovative new method showing how to apply the PICO method when assessing qualitative research (Cooke et al 2012).

STUDENT CHALLENGE

Now let's think about a question from nursing. You observe that some of the patients you come across in the community from certain cultural groups tend to put honey on wounds (particularly burns) and swear that it helps heal them. You have heard honey has antibacterial properties and wonder if there could be some benefit in terms of wound healing. Using PICO, make this into a specific and searchable question.

- P:
- I:
- C:
- O:

PICO	SPIDER	JUSTIFICATION
P - Population/problem	S - Sample	Smaller groups of participants tend to be used in qualitative research than quantitative research, so this term was deemed more appropriate.
I - Intervention/exposure	PI – Phenomenon of Interest	Qualitative research aims to understand the how and why of certain behaviours, decisions, and individual experiences. Therefore, an intervention/exposure per se is not always evident in qualitative research questions.
C - Comparison	D - Design	The theoretical framework used in qualitative research will determine the research method that is used. As inferential statistics are not used in qualitative research, details of the study design will help to make decisions about the robustness of the study and analysis. In addition, this might increase the detection of qualitative studies in the databases in which titles and abstracts are unstructured.
O - Outcome	E - Evaluation	Qualitative research has the same end result as quantitative research methods: outcome measures. These differ depending on the research question and might contain more unobservable and subjective constructs when compared to quantitative research (e.g. attitudes and views and so forth), so evaluation was deemed more suitable.
	R - Research type	Three research types could be searched for: qualitative, quantitative, and mixed methods.

FIGURE 11.1
Beyond PICO: The SPIDER Tool for Qualitative Evidence Synthesis (Cooke et al 2012)

Conducting a literature review

Once you have a searchable question sorted out, you need to find out if someone else has already answered it. Doing a literature review will give you this answer and will also identify the gaps you may decide to address with your research. After completing the review you may need to change your question or you may simply confirm that your question is indeed important and still to be answered.

A literature review describes published materials that provide an examination of recent or current literature. Generally, a literature review involves some process for identifying materials for potential inclusion – whether or not requiring a formal literature search – for selecting included materials, for synthesising them in textual, tabular or graphical form and for making some analysis of their contribution or value. The purpose of doing a literature review is to identify what has been accomplished previously, build on previous work and avoid duplication by identifying omissions or gaps. There are risks, however; we may not pick up all of the literature we are looking for or we may only select literature that supports our preferred belief.

Searching the databases

As you have seen there are many databases out there that can be searched for literature. Generally when dealing with questions around health we focus on a few main ones. These include the Cochrane Library, MEDLINE, CINAHL and OVID (there are others as well). The Cochrane Library only covers intervention questions (e.g. testing treatments or technologies) and is often the first place people look for these. When searching the databases you need to use PICO (population/problem, intervention, comparator, outcomes) and any filters for the ideal study type. Remember, you can use Boolean operators that enable you to combine terms with 'or' or 'and' (see Chapter 2) and these may have a filter added such as meta-analyses so only meta-analysis (studies that combine the results of several studies) are included. So when we search for literature on perineal warm packs, for example, we need to use terms such as pregnancy, warm pack/warm compress, perineum, second stage, labour, pain and combine these in different ways (e.g. labour and compress). The process of searching the literature is described in more detail earlier in this book.

STUDENT CHALLENGE

Focusing Your Search

Think back to the question you designed to investigate the effects of applying honey to burns on wound healing. What terms would you use to search the databases? Think about the Boolean operators and filters you might also use.

Evaluating the literature

You know you need to appraise or review the literature critically, which means examining the existing literature on a particular topic, determining the weakness in the research or inconsistencies in the findings and understanding the strengths and limitations (Weaver & Olson 2006; Horsfall et al 2007) (Box 11.1). Refer back to Chapter 9. Remember, some basic guidelines for reading published research include:

Box 11.1
Checklist for appraising literature

1. Are the aims and objectives of the study clear?
2. Are the research questions and hypotheses (if appropriate) clear?
3. Is the research design/method adequately described?
4. Is the research method appropriate to answer the research question?
5. Are the tests used to determine reliability and validity of tools clearly described?
6. Is the source of the sample along with inclusion and exclusion criteria set out?
7. Was the statistical power used to detect or reject group differences discussed?
8. Are ethical concerns, including funding sources and author affiliations, covered?
9. Are the limitations of the methods and data analysis clearly spelt out?
10. Do the conclusions truly derive from the data without undue extrapolation?

Bowling (1997)

- Carefully read the abstract and skim read the body of the article to determine its relevance before you waste time printing out irrelevant information (Horsfall et al 2007).
- Don't be distracted by articles that are interesting but irrelevant or you will never finish the review (Asmundson et al 2002).
- More information is often not better, but more focused information is better in that it is time saving and relevant (Horsfall et al 2007).
- A literature review should be comprehensive and critical. It is important to read and understand the studies you have retrieved to refine your research question, give you up-to-date knowledge and assist with the detailed planning of your research plan (Horsfall et al 2007).

Being clear about what you are going to do

When you have done a literature review you need to be clear about what you are going to do in the study. When reviewing the literature on warm packs it was evident that, although much of it was anecdotal, both prevention of trauma and reduction of pain were advocated as potential benefits, so maternal comfort was incorporated as an important consideration. It was also the first observation Dahlen made on watching Lisa's reaction to the warm pack.

Women and midwives' evaluations of the warm packs were deemed to be as important as clinical outcome measures, as it seemed counterproductive to prove they work and then find women did not want to use them. It also seemed important to follow women up until 12 weeks following birth to determine possible long-term effects of warm packs, as we don't want to cause harm inadvertently. While this was time-consuming, it proved to be valuable, with some unexpected results.

So once you have a question and you have searched the literature and refined your question, you need to develop aims and objectives in order to be able to carry out the study.

Aims and objectives

You need to differentiate between the aims of your study and the objectives. Aims are the broad, conceptual general statements about what you hope to accomplish but usually aren't very measurable. The objectives are more specific and are operational or measurable. Objectives will often summarise and identify the variables or phenomena of interest in your research. Objectives can also be written in the form of a **hypothesis** to be tested or as research questions.

A common error is to describe the desired outcomes or potential benefits of the research rather than the aims of the research. Remember, there is a difference between the aims and objectives of your research and the benefits of the research. For example, a research project aims to test the outcomes of a particular intervention. The potential benefits of the research will be to improve the outcomes for clients.

Writing your aim

To write your aim, refer back to the overall problem or area of concern. Ask yourself: given the way we have described this problem and what we know about the obstacles, what are we trying to accomplish with the project?

The aim of the perineal warm pack trial was 'to evaluate the effect of applying warm packs to the perineum in the second stage of labour'.

Write an aim for your study on the use of honey on wound healing. Look back at your hypothesis to help you do this.

Write your objectives

We now need to write objectives to reflect what we are trying to achieve (don't describe how you will be doing your research: this is described in the methods section of your research proposal). Make your objectives realistic and pragmatic – it is useful to think 'small and possible'. It is OK to set out your objectives as a bullet-point list. List your specific objectives in no more than one or two sentences in approximate order of importance. Remember you can describe your research objectives in the form of a statement, hypothesis or research question. State your objectives, hypothesis or question in a way that can be evaluated or tested. That is, they must be measurable.

With the warm pack trial the objectives were:

1. To determine if applying warm packs to the perineum in the second stage of labour will reduce perineal trauma.
2. To determine if applying warm packs to the perineum in the second stage of labour will increase maternal comfort.

If you wrote this as a question rather than a statement it would look like this:

1. Will applying warm packs to the perineum in the second stage of labour reduce perineal trauma?
2. Will applying warm packs to the perineum in the second stage of labour increase maternal comfort?

Specifically, we wanted to know if there would be any differences in women's perineal outcomes and comfort when warm packs were applied to the perineum in the second stage of labour, compared with standard second-stage care that did not involve the use of warm packs.

Remember our question on the effect of honey on wound healing? Try writing the objectives of your study.

What is a hypothesis?

A hypothesis is a statement that predicts what you think you might find. For the warm pack trial the hypothesis would be:

- The application of warm packs to the perineum in the second stage of labour reduces perineal trauma and increases maternal comfort.

Sometimes this is phrased as a null hypothesis or a default position that states the opposite to what you might think you will find. Again, for the warm pack trial the null hypothesis would be:

- The application of warm packs to the perineum in the second stage of labour does not reduce perineal trauma or increase maternal comfort.

Now try and write a hypothesis and null hypothesis for the use of honey on wounds.

What are primary and secondary outcome measures?

In a quantitative study such as the warm pack trial we need to have outcome measures. How much of a difference in the incidence of perineal trauma and pain during the birth do I want to see before I say the warm pack makes a significant difference? The main thing we want to find out is called the primary outcome measure and it is what we use to work out how many people we need in a trial. In the warm pack trial our primary outcome measure was the proportion of women who required perineal suturing following birth. We thought that a 10% reduction in women needing to be sutured would be a good outcome and so, using a statistical package, we calculated we needed to recruit 694 women in the study, half of whom would be randomly allocated to receive the warm packs and the other half would have normal care that did not include the warm packs. Remember our question: will applying warm packs to the perineum in the second stage of labour reduce perineal trauma? If fewer women are sutured they are having less perineal trauma.

The secondary outcome measure or other thing we were interested in was women's comfort. Remember the other question was: will applying warm packs to the perineum in the second stage of labour increase maternal comfort? This was measured through pain scores at birth, days 1 and 2 following the birth, and at 6 and 12 weeks following the birth.

Again, reflect on the question about honey and wound healing. Can you think of a primary and secondary outcome measure you would be interested in finding out about?

Deciding on the most feasible study type to answer the question

Different questions will require different **research designs**. Because we wanted to ask an intervention question (if I apply a warm pack to the perineum, what will happen?) with the warm pack trial, a quantitative research study design was the most appropriate. A randomised controlled trial is the best way to answer intervention or treatment questions. If we had wanted to look at the perineal outcomes over a period of time, for example, 6 months, 12 months and 3 years after birth in a population of women, we would have undertaken a cohort study. If we had wanted to explore the experiences of women having warm packs then a qualitative method would have been used. Here is a quick revision of the two major research paradigms discussed in Chapters 5 and 6, just to reinforce the main differences.

Quantitative research designs

Quantitative research designs: describe the frequency of a variable in a **sample**/population; examine the relationships/correlation between variables in a sample/population; and are used to test theory and evaluate the effectiveness of interventions. The sample must be representative of the population you are studying to allow generalisation of the results. Quantitative research projects can describe, examine relationships and compare groups. **Data collection** tends to be more structured and the methods tightly defined and controlled in an attempt to decrease bias and ensure the sample is representative. The data collection may be via: survey, existing administrative datasets, medical records, physical measurements and tests. It is important the variables (factors, condition or trait) are measured using reliable and valid measurement tools and for this reason a description of how the variables are defined and measured is necessary. Statistical data analysis is carried out on quantitative data.

Qualitative research designs

Qualitative designs are generally used when little information is available or when an in-depth understanding of a process or experience is required. The strength of qualitative designs is that they can generate theory. Qualitative designs are not useful for testing hypotheses, nor are the results of this research necessarily applicable to a larger population, as they tend to use very small numbers of participants. Qualitative designs tend to use less structured forms of data collection such as interview, observation, focus groups or field notes. A combination of different data sources can be used. Variables are rarely defined at the initial phase of the research; rather, general areas of interest are identified. Analysis of the data can be carried out by various methods but most involve some form of thematic analysis such as grounded theory, ethnography and phenomenology.

It was decided during the early days of planning the warm pack trial that a randomised controlled trial methodology (quantitative) would be ideal. The randomised controlled trial methodology is widely accepted as the most rigorous way to test for the effect from a treatment or intervention. Random allocation to intervention and control groups ensures the groups being compared are on an equivalent footing at the outset of the study, thus eliminating selection and confounding biases (Schultz et al 2000). The randomised controlled trial is particularly effective in helping professionals and women choose between different forms of care. Randomised clinical trials were introduced into medicine in the 1950s as an objective way of determining the real effects of medical intervention, but the medical profession was slow to recognise their value (Enkin 2006). Other chapters have described different study designs in greater detail.

With your question about honey and wound healing, which research design might you use? Do you think a qualitative or quantitative design would be most appropriate?

Mixed methods

Mixed methods research involves the collection and integration of both qualitative and quantitative data within one study to gain a better understanding of the topic under investigation (Ivankova et al 2006; Tashakkori & Teddlie 2003). In health research this approach is becoming increasingly popular, as qualitative or quantitative methods on their own may not be sufficient to address the complex questions that arise in health care. By drawing on the strength of each approach we can gain a multifaceted perspective. An important part of mixed methods research is integrating the **data** and **findings** so there is one complete answer given to the research question. This is called integration and findings inform either the type of data collected in the next stage or questions asked and/or these findings are integrated to generate a deeper and often more useful answer to the overall study aim (Creswell 2008).

Helpful tips before you start your research

Organise a good working team

Doing research alone is very difficult. Collaborating with others gives you the advantage of different ideas, skills and orientations (Weaver and Olson 2006) (Box 11.2). When you start out undertaking research you generally do so on a small scale with a supervisor/supervisors to guide you. However, like clinical practice it is very hard and not advantageous in the long run to undertake research in isolation. If you include clinicians in your team, for example, it makes it more likely that practice will change (Horsfall et al 2007). Getting a multidisciplinary team together is also beneficial as it means each discipline will view the clinical situation from a different perspective (Horsfall et al 2007). Another advantage is that you can undertake the research in a few different clinical sites and therefore end up with a larger and more diverse sample size.

Box 11.2
Six characteristics of successful research collaborators

1. Being amenable to listen to and consider new ideas and other perspectives.
2. Open-mindedness and acceptance of challenges to your perspective and position.
3. Willingness and ability to negotiate and compromise so that some sort of consensus can be achieved throughout the project.
4. Being able to work both independently and interdependently at different stages of the research.
5. Well-developed and confident communication skills, essential to keep everybody adequately informed about each phase of the project – when the work is going well and when there are difficulties.
6. Personal and professional commitment to ethical research from all team members.

Stone (1999)

Identify a mentor or supervisor if doing a higher degree

Who is supporting your research and how they support you is important to successfully starting and completing a study. This is especially relevant if you are a novice researcher. You need to be able to show that the research you are interested in undertaking is feasible and will be carried out to a high standard whether you are doing it as part of your clinical role, applying for money to undertake research or undertaking a higher degree. Identifying a mentor, or supervisor if you are doing an Honours or higher degree, can help you with tasks that you may find difficult and they can read your proposal and provide critical feedback. Possible mentors may be experienced researchers who work in your organisation or nursing/midwifery academics from a nearby university. Asking other students who have been supervised by your potential supervisor can help you understand if the two of you might work well together.

Various forms of support may be available to you:

- experienced researchers
- managers
- methodological experts
- statistical/epidemiological experts
- topic area experts
- the combined support of a research group.

Read the literature around the topic

You may have already carried out a literature review for a university subject but it is important to refine, update and restructure the information. You have to persuade the reader about the importance and relevance of your research. For example, why is your topic important? What has been done before? What are the gaps in knowledge? You will require this information to describe the background of the research, to demonstrate how your research will address some of the gaps in knowledge around this topic and to identify why your research is important. This will also be important when you apply for ethics approval for your study, as your research should be making an important contribution to knowledge.

Look at how other authors describe their studies

In particular, read the literature on the specific methodologies you will be using, such as ethnography, phenomenology, grounded theory, randomisation/experimental or epidemiology. This will give you information about how best to describe your research design and the methods and procedures you will be using.

Find out if the research is feasible

Finding out if the research is feasible is essential before you embark on a study. For example, can you get access to patients, staff and/or patient records to collect the data you require for your research? Will you be able to collect enough data within the timeframe you have available to you? What is the most rigorous, ethical, efficient, easiest and non-intrusive way of recruiting participants (and, if relevant, doing an intervention) in the organisation in which your research is being conducted? Can you afford to do the study? This may influence the aim of the research and methods you will use. A variety of people may need to be approached depending on who is to be involved in the research and the type of organisation in which the research is taking place (e.g. directors of nursing, hospital data managers, nurse unit managers, medical records department or medical consultants). Feasibility planning for the research should allow you to build collaborations for the research within the organisation in which the research will be conducted. This will allow you to identify and prevent potential barriers to the research and to build consensus and commitment for the research within the organisation.

If your research is not feasible, you will need to review the design – sometimes this will require a change in research topic and you will need to start the process again. If your research is feasible then you need to consider the time and resources you will require to do the research and gather information on the cost of those resources.

Coming back to the question of whether honey helps wounds to heal, think about some of the obstacles you might face when trying to undertake this research. What strategies might you employ to overcome these?

A research proposal

What is a research proposal?

Carrying out research demands a thoughtful, careful, organised and sequential set of activities, rather than an enthusiastic, 'gung ho' approach (McGuire & Yeager 1999). Enthusiasm is of course needed but it does need to be organised enthusiasm. Whether you are undertaking an Honours, embarking on a higher degree or convincing your employer to support research you are interested in, you generally need to start with a research proposal plus supporting information that demonstrates you are eligible to conduct the research and you have approval and support from your employer and/or university.

The research proposal describes the blueprint or plan for the study and also must persuade the reader that the research:

- is important to nursing and midwifery practice
- has been informed by previous research
- has clear aims and objectives
- is scientifically reliable and valid; that is, rigorous
- is doable and you can do it (especially if applying to undertake a higher degree)
- is worthy of the degree of funding if this is requested.

It is important to have a well-developed plan before writing the research proposal. You should consider collecting information that will be required for your application. Managers and clinicians in the setting in which you are considering conducting the research should have input into the research plan to increase the feasibility of the project and to develop support for the project.

There are several steps you need to carry out while you are planning your project, which will assist you in writing your research proposal.

With the warm pack trial, once a literature review had been undertaken and the research aim and objectives were clear, a detailed document was written on how the study would be undertaken. The first author needed to be able to convince her research supervisors and other academics (necessary if you are doing a higher degree), clinical managers and ethics committees that the study was important, ethical, feasible and that she had the skills and support to complete it. Remember, the only good research is completed research! There are a lot of great ideas that are simply not feasible without significant funding and expertise.

The purpose of the research proposal

- To persuade the reader of the importance of the research (e.g. background, benefits to nursing/midwifery, dissemination).
- To describe how the research will be carried out (e.g. research plan, timeline).
- To describe the feasibility of the research (e.g. background, research plan, supervision and timeline, budget).
- To describe the scientific rigour and ethics of the research (e.g. background, research plan, ethics).
- To identify the value of the research (all the way through).

Some of the components which may need to be described in the methods section of the research proposal are:

- Research design (what?): the overall design or methodology that guides the research; for example, ethnography, grounded theory, experimental study (randomised controlled trial, cohort study).

- Sample (who?): a description of the participants/records from which data will be collected.
- Recruitment (how?): a description of how participants become involved in the research.
- Intervention (how?): a description of the treatment/education/system change being tested in the research project (only necessary for evaluation trials).
- Data collection/procedure (when? how?): a description of when, where and how and by whom data are collected. In the case of qualitative research this might include a description of the general topic areas of interest to the research field.
- Data collection/variables/tools/measures (how? what?): a description of the variables being measured and how they are being measured; that is, tests, measurement tools or scales, equipment used to measure variables (not usually necessary for qualitative research projects, although observational schedules may be used in some observational studies).
- Data analysis (how?): a description of the processes that will be used during the analysis of data.
- Ethical considerations: ethics approval is needed before the start of the study.

STUDENT CHALLENGE

Outlining Your Research Proposal

Using the components above that are needed in the methods section of a research proposal, describe what you would need to consider for the study on honey and wound healing. We are not expecting you to know all these answers but have a go.

Research design (methodology)

Sample

Recruitment

Intervention (we are assuming here you identified that a quantitative design would be best to test the effect of honey on wound healing)

Data collection

- Procedure
- Variables
- Tools
- Measures

Data analysis

Not all projects will have all of these components; for example, qualitative research projects rarely have an intervention to describe and do not usually describe variables or measurement tools. Different terms may also be appropriate; for example, qualitative researchers often describe participants rather than sample. Subheadings should be provided within the research plan to aid the reader. If both qualitative and quantitative methods are being used in the research or a variety of samples and methods of data collection are being used, it is important to be clear about what form of data collection is being used for each sample and how each type of data will be analysed.

Other important considerations

Ethics

You discovered in an earlier chapter on ethics how important an ethical approach is in research and we emphasise it again here. There can be no doubt that research conducted in clinical settings presents multiple ethical considerations and an ethical design to a research project is a moral requirement (Aita & Richer 2005). Principles of integrity, respect for persons, beneficence and justice need to be considered throughout the research process (Box 11.3). These concepts were first explored in the Nuremberg Code of 1947 and further developed and defined by the Belmont Report of 1979 (Aita & Richer 2005). The wellbeing of the participants in research must take precedence over data collection at all times (Thompson et al 2000). Making sure that participants have accurate information about the benefits and risks of participating and getting signed consent to be part of the study are core

Box 11.3
Six general ethical guidelines

1. Participants' welfare and rights take precedence over everything else.
2. They have the right to be clearly and adequately informed about the purpose of the study and its likely benefits.
3. They have the right to be clearly informed about the risks involved in participating, including the right to be informed about alternative treatment and approaches over and above those used in the study.
4. They have the right to refuse to participate without any impact on present or future treatment or other services.
5. They also retain the right to withdraw from the study at any time without any possible penalty in the present or the future.
6. Any information arising from their participation is to be kept confidential.

Asmundson et al (2002)

components of ethical research (Bowling 1997). It is also important that the participants feel they can say no or withdraw from the study without their care being compromised (Asmundson et al 2002; Thorpe & Anderson 2006). Being able to maintain the confidentiality of participants during research is another essential ethical consideration. There is also no point in performing research that does not have scientific merit and will not contribute to knowledge (Horsfall et al 2007). Planned submission of the research proposal to the Health Research Ethics Committee (HREC) is one way of demonstrating that ethical standards are being met. However, if there are ethical issues that are specific to your proposal, it is also important to demonstrate you are aware of these. For example, if the research participants come from a population of patients with dementia, what methods will be used to ensure that consent is obtained and no harm will come to participants? Get support the first time you go to submit an ethics application, as it is more complex than you may think.

How would you ensure that appropriate ethical considerations were in place for your honey and wound-healing study?

Timeline

The purpose of the timeline is to show the research is both realistic and feasible. The timeline will help you and others know how much time you have to allocate to the research given your other roles and responsibilities and whether the time anticipated for carrying out the study is realistic. The timeline needs to reflect these aspects and should indicate:

- when each component will commence and finish
- how long each of the components of the research will take you to carry out
- the duration of the project
- how many tasks will be occurring consecutively.

Some of the research components that may need to be accounted for in a timeline are ethical approval, staff training for research protocols, recruitment, data collection, intervention, data entry, data analysis, report writing and dissemination.

Budget

The budget outlines the costs of the research. What resources do you need and what will they cost you? (The human resource department may be useful for costs of personnel; the transport department may assist with transport costs.)

Examples of items under each heading are provided:

- Personnel: include positions, proposed date of employment/duration of employment, salary on cost and total amount; for example, research assistance, statistical assistance and data entry.

- Equipment: rental only; for example, digital recorders: duration of time required and costs.
- Maintenance and travel: type of car used and costs per kilometre travelled; photocopying/printing number of pages and cost, postage.

You may be lucky enough to get money from a funding source such as your university if you are a student or health service where you work to assist with the research. While gaining access to big grants will not happen until you are a more experienced researcher, any small amount of money should be kept track of in your curriculum vitae as it helps to convince people later on that they should fund your research.

Putting it all together

Now let's put all this information together. We began this story with the inception of the warm pack trial and the question that arose in the first author's mind during a birth. The question was, 'I wonder if warm packs reduce women's pain in the second stage of labour.' On reviewing the literature, much of it was anecdotal and there was also a suggestion that warm packs might reduce the incidence of perineal trauma. It became clear there was almost no scientific evidence to support or refute the belief that warm packs had an effect on perineal trauma or comfort during second stage. So the aim became 'to evaluate the effect of applying warm packs to the perineum in the second stage of labour'. The questions we asked were: will applying warm packs to the perineum in the second stage of labour reduce perineal trauma? Will applying warm packs to the perineum in the second stage of labour increase maternal comfort?

The perineal warm pack trial therefore was designed to investigate the effects of applying warm packs to the perineum during the late second stage of labour on perineal trauma and maternal comfort. Because this was asking an intervention question, then a randomised controlled trial (quantitative method) became the best way of evaluating the effectiveness of warm packs. In the late second stage of labour, first-time mothers ($n = 717$) giving birth were randomly allocated to having warm packs ($n = 360$) applied to their perineum or standard care ($n = 357$). The primary outcome measure was the requirement for perineal suturing and the secondary outcome measure was maternal comfort (remember the questions we asked).

There was no statistically significant difference in the number of women who required suturing following birth. Women in the warm pack group had significantly lower perineal pain scores when giving birth, on day 1 and on day 2 following the birth.

Warm packs were highly acceptable to both women and midwives as a means of relieving pain during the late second stage of labour. Almost the same number of women (79.7%) and midwives (80.4%) felt the warm packs reduced perineal pain during the birth. Both women and midwives were positive about using warm packs in the future. The majority of women (85.7%) said they would like to use perineal warm packs again for their next birth and similarly would recommend them to friends (86.1%). Likewise, 91% of midwives were positive about using the warm packs, with 92.6% considering using them in the future as part of care in the second stage of labour.

Several papers have now been published from this research (Dahlen et al 2007, 2009; Dahlen & Homer 2008, 2010) and in many hospitals it is common practice to use warm packs as a method of second-stage comfort. It all began, however, with a question and the research journey unfolded from there.

The story continues

In 2012 a group of authors published a Cochrane Systematic Review examining perineal techniques during the second stage of labour for reducing perineal trauma (Aasheim et al 2012). Amongst other things they looked at warm compresses to the perineum. They found two studies (one was undertaken by the first author) and putting them together were able to end up with a very big number of participants and do what is called a meta-analysis. They found finally that the use of warm compresses on the perineum was associated with a decreased occurrence of perineal trauma and that the procedure has shown to be acceptable to women and midwives and should be offered to women. So this now became Level 1 evidence, which is the highest level of scientific evidence available. What began as a simple observation and what I found was commonly used by midwives and had been for centuries (Dahlen, Homer, Leap, & Tracy 2011) now moved from the domain of 'tradition and custom' (remember the first chapter) ' to Level 1 evidence. When the Cochrane review was published in 2012 the first author was asked to write a critique of the review, which amused her no end (Dahlen 2012). It is now up to midwives themselves to transfer/ translate this knowledge to practise. You have been reminded of the importance of knowledge translation (KT) in the previous chapter. And so ends (but perhaps not) a journey of seeing, questioning, searching, doing finding and disseminating, which in essence, is what research is all about.

We hope you found this chapter helpful in strengthening and clarifying your understanding of many of the concepts presented in this book. Good luck with your research journey and remember to enjoy it!

STUDENT CHALLENGE

1. What steps might clinicians take to facilitate translation of this knowledge into their own practice?
2. Can you think of any barriers to integrating this research?
3. Will this evidence need reviewing at any stage?

You may want to read Chapter 12 and come back to this.

RESOURCES KIT

Librarians are your friends. Make time to talk to them and seek their help. They will make the library and searching for scientific journals much less daunting.

When you read research articles look for evidence of the research process – there should be a clear decision trail laid as to how the study was planned and conducted. Here are some useful websites to assist you in understanding the research process:

Foundation Center. Proposal writing short course. http://foundationcenter.org/getstarted/tutorials/shortcourse/index.html.

Ohio State University. Smart research strategies. http://liblearn.osu.edu/tutor/les6.

WikiEducator. How to get started on research. http://wikieducator.org/How_to_get_started_on_research.

See if you can find other useful resources on the web more generally or in electronic databases.

References

Aasheim V, Nilsen ABV, Lukasse M, et al: Perineal techniques during the second stage of labour for reducing perineal trauma, *Cochrane Database of Systematic Reviews* (2):Art. No.: CD006672, 2012. doi: 10.1002/14651858.CD006672.pub2.

Aita M, Richer C: Essentials of research ethics for health professionals, *Nursing and Health Sciences* 7:119–125, 2005.

Asmundson GJ, Norton GR, Stein MB: *Clinical research in mental health: a practical guide*, Thousand Oaks, California, 2002, SAGE Publications.

Bowling A: *Research methods in health. investigating health and health services*, Buckingham, 1997, Open University Press.

Cooke A, Smith D, Booth A: Beyond PICO: The SPIDER Tool for Qualitative Evidence Synthesis, *Qualitative Health Research* 22(10):1435–1443, 2012.

Creswell J: *Research design: qualitative, quantitative and mixed methods approaches*, London, 2008, Sage UK.

Dahlen H, Homer C: Perineal trauma and postpartum perineal morbidity in Asian and non-Asian primiparous women, *JOGNN – Journal of Obstetric, Gynecologic, & Neonatal Nursing* 37:455–463, 2008.

Dahlen H, Homer C: Infant feeding decisions in the first 12 weeks following birth: A comparison of the experiences of women from Asian and non-Asian backgrounds in Australia, *Women and Birth* 23:22–28, 2010.

Dahlen H, Homer CSE, Cooke M, et al: Perineal outcomes and maternal comfort related to the application of perineal warm packs in the second stage of labor. A randomized controlled trial, *Birth (Berkeley, Calif.)* 34:282–290, 2007.

Dahlen HG, Homer CSE, Cooke M, et al: 'Soothing the ring of fire'. Australian women and midwives' experience of using perineal warm packs in the second stage of labour, *Midwifery* 25:39–48, 2009.

Dahlen H: Systematic review: Perineal warm compress reduces risk of third and fourth degree tears and should be part of second stage care, *Evidence-Based Nursing* 15(4):103–104, 2012.

Dahlen H, Homer C, Leap N, et al: Social to surgical: Historic perspectives on perineal care during labour and birth, *Women and Birth* 24:105–111, 2011.

Dobratz M: Putting the pieces together: Teaching undergraduate research from a theoretical perspective, *Journal of Advanced Nursing* 41:383–392, 2003.

Enkin M: Beyond evidence: The complexity of maternity care, *Birth (Berkeley, Calif.)* 33:265–269, 2006.

Henderson S: *From Strength to Strength: an autobiography*, Melbourne, 1993, Sun Books.

Horsfall J, Cleary M, Walter G, et al: Conducting mental health research: Key steps, practicalities, and issues for the early career researcher, *International Journal of Mental Health Nursing* 16(Suppl 1):S1–S20, 2007.

Ivankova N, Creswell J, Stick S: Using mixed methods sequential explanatory design: From theory to practice, *Field Methods* 18(1):3–20, 2006.

McGuire D, Yeager K: Implementing the study. In Kirchhoff MMK, editor: *Using and conducting nursing research in the clinical setting*, Philadelphia, 1999, W.B. Saunders, pp 300–315.

Sackett D, Straus SE, Richardson WS, et al: *Evidence-based medicine: how to practice and teach EBM*, ed 2, Edinburgh, 2000, Churchill Livingstone.

Schultz KF, Chalmers I, Grimes DA, et al: Assessing the quality of randomization from reports of controlled trials published in obstetrics and gynaecology journals, *JAMA: The Journal of the American Medical Association* 272:125–128, 2000.

Stone K: Collaboration. In Kirchhoff MMK, editor: *Using and conducting nursing research in the clinical setting*, Philadelphia, 1999, W.B. Saunders, pp 182–190.

Tashakkori A, Teddlie C: *Handbook of mixed methods in social & behavioral research*, Thousand Oaks, California, 2003, SAGE Publications.

Thompson C, Cullum N, McCaughan D, et al: Nurses, information use, and clinical decision making – The real world potential for evidence-based decisions in nursing, *Evidence-Based Nursing* 7:68–72, 2004.

Thompson IE, Melia KM, Boyd KM: *Nursing ethics*, London, 2000, Churchill Livingstone.

Thorpe J, Anderson J: Supporting women in labour and birth. In Pairman S, Thorogood JPC, Tracy S, editors: *Midwifery preparation for practice*, Marrickville, 2006, Churchill Livingstone, pp 393–415.

Weaver K, Olson J: Understanding paradigms for nursing research, *Journal of Advanced Nursing* 53:459–469, 2006.

CHAPTER 12

RESEARCH AND KNOWLEDGE: WHAT DOES THE FUTURE HOLD FOR NURSING AND MIDWIFERY?

Anne Gardner

CHAPTER OUTLINE

KEY TERMS

accreditation
continuing professional development
Excellence in Research for Australia (ERA)
lifelong learning
midwifery research
nursing research
Performance-Based Research Fund (PBRF)
policy
research

LEARNING OBJECTIVES

After reading this chapter and following critical reflection the student will be able to:

1. Explore research priorities in various areas of clinical practice across the lifespan
2. Recognise clinical leadership that influences and progresses clinical care, policy and collaboration
3. Describe the current contribution of nursing and midwifery research in clinical practice and discuss its potential future contribution
4. Identify two important trends in health care at the local and strategic level that influence clinical nursing and midwifery practice
5. Discuss the application of research results in clinical practice.

STUDENT QUOTE

I'm just a new grad, how can I make a difference?

ABSTRACT

Nursing and midwifery are wonderful careers that can be both rewarding and challenging. High-quality healthcare practice needs continually to respond to the many changes that influence health outcomes in Australian and New Zealand society. These changes occur at both general and healthcare-specific levels. They include the increasingly aged society, the ageing of the health workforce, proposed new models of healthcare delivery and increased demands placed on nursing and midwifery clinicians, managers and academics to demonstrate accountability for their work. In order to respond to these changes, nurses and midwives need to be lifelong learners and consumers of research. Moreover, we must be prepared to assume leadership roles in the multidisciplinary team. We have to ask the question: how can I be a change agent and leader in doing and/or using research in my practice setting?

Lifelong learning

This chapter will draw together the ideas you have been reading about in your journey through this book. It is hoped that this last chapter will inspire you to become a consumer of **research** and a leader in research utilisation as soon as you receive your professional registration. You should expect to be continually learning as you progress in your career. In this chapter, you will read about recent trends that will affect you in your first few years as a graduate nurse or midwife. Beyond these first few years it is not possible to predict, because health care is such a dynamic and changing service, but we hope this book will help you to be ready for changes that we cannot currently imagine.

What does the phrase **lifelong learning** mean? The term draws on many concepts from learning theory, including the well-established notion of adult self-directed learning (Knowles 1980). The expression embodies the idea of learning as empowerment to take on the challenges of rapid technological and economic advances. Successful adult learning depends on motivation, choice and a personal responsibility for identifying learning goals and meeting these goals. Your university education should teach you how to learn, as well as providing you with information and knowledge. Books such as this one offer guidance about how to find and read research studies. In Chapter 9 you learnt how you can evaluate the quality of research. Actively appraising what you read is an important component of continuing to learn. When you read, try to imagine you are having a conversation with the writers.

As registered nurses and midwives, we should continue our professional development throughout our working lives. This has been emphasised in many parts of this book. We have a responsibility to ensure we maintain our competency as practitioners. In doing so, we facilitate improved quality of health care to the community as well as advancing the standing of our profession. The process of sustained learning is a joint responsibility of the individual nurse, the employer and the profession (National Review of Nursing Education 2002).

In New Zealand the requirement for practical demonstration of continued competence on annual registration has been in place for several years now. From July 2010 this has been a national requirement in Australia too. It is referred to as **continuing professional development** or CPD and is 'the means by which members of the profession maintain, improve and broaden their knowledge, expertise and competence, and develop the personal and professional qualities required throughout their professional lives' (www.nursingmidwiferyboard.gov.au/FAQ-and-Fact-Sheets.aspx). The CPD cycle involves reviewing practice, identifying learning needs, planning and participating in relevant learning activities and reflecting on the value of those activities (Australian Nursing and Midwifery Board 2009).

Models of integration of research into practice

As you discovered in your reading of Chapter 10, evidence-based practice is an integral part of current nursing and midwifery practice, however there have been problems in its integration. Let us examine some examples of best practice implementation models that have included a very clear planning stage. One model, developed in the UK, is called the Promoting Action on Research Implementation in Health Services or PARIHS (Helfrich et al 2010; Rycroft-Malone et al 2002). This model considers the evidence, providing an explanation of the nexus between research, clinical experience and patient experience. It then defines the context (or setting). Finally, it looks at the process of facilitation and identifies the skills required for effective facilitation.

The model described by Rycroft-Malone and others (2002), however, stops short of identifying the evaluation of successful strategies. Another model, which has now been tested in several settings, is the Ottawa model (Logan & Graham 1998). The Ottawa Model of Research Utilisation (OMRU) is a model that can be used to improve the efficiency and effectiveness of the transfer of research evidence into practice. Broadly conceived, the OMRU incorporates:

- assessment of current conditions (including the practice environment, the potential adopters and the evidence-based recommendations)
- monitoring the transfer of evidence-based research (including developing strategies and measuring the adoption of the research)
- evaluating the outcomes of the process.

The authors acknowledge that, although some details are provided on how to operationalise each element of the model, much work is still required to determine how research evidence may best be transferred into practice. Successful use of the Ottawa model to implement pressure injury prevention strategies has been described by Graham and Logan (2004). The authors demonstrated an association between the implementation of the prevention strategies and a reduction in prevalence of pressure injury although they were unable to demonstrate this was a causal link. The authors conclude their article by stating:

> *Adoption and use of evidence takes longer than anticipated. Experience has taught us that we tend to underestimate the time it takes to change practice in complex environments, particularly with large groups. Moreover, scanning the external environment for support or threats to implementation must be constant (Graham & Logan 2004).*

Despite this cautionary note, the article by Graham and Logan is a positive one. One of the strengths of their initiative was the clinical practice area in which they chose to test the model, that of skin care and prevention of pressure injury. Prevention of pressure injury is one of the better-researched areas of clinical practice and there were established guidelines for prediction, prevention and treatment of pressure injury that could be adapted for local use. There are now Pan Pacific guidelines (www.awma.com.au/publications/publications.php#pipm) and newly released world guidelines to which the Pan Pacific Pressure Injury Alliance have contributed (www.internationalguideline.com).

There are many instances where there is a gap in clinical research relevant to healthcare practice. As a clinician, you will constantly be identifying these areas of deficiency so let us look at this issue in relation to specific clinical groups.

Addressing clinical and research priorities

Keeping informed of the current clinical and research priorities in a given area can help direct and guide your practice with whatever target population you choose to work. Let us take mothers and infants for example; the overall goal in maternal–infant care is focused on improving outcomes for mothers and infants. Priority issues in maternal–infant care and research can be drawn from several sources. These sources include Australian-specific sources such as the National Health and Medical Research Council (NHMRC) strategic and priority-driven research objectives and the Commonwealth Department of Health and Ageing, as well as international and global sources such as the (US) National Institute of Nursing Research and the World Health Organization global nursing and **midwifery research** priorities (Box 12.1).

Research priorities assist in identifying areas of concern in practice as well as drawing attention to which areas of care receive funding priority for

Box 12.1
Organisations concerned with maternal–infant care

- Australian College of Midwives
- Perinatal Research Centre (Royal Women's Hospital Foundation and University of Queensland)
- New Zealand College of Midwives
- Karitane
- Australian Neonatal Nurses Association
- Women's and Children's Hospitals
- Australian Breastfeeding Association
- La Leche League
- Pregnancy and Newborn Services Network (NSW)

research. The NHMRC identifies research that focuses on pregnancy and maternal–infant care for Australia's indigenous people as a priority area and this is a response to poorer maternal–infant outcomes in indigenous communities than are seen in other Australian communities. Internationally, the American Association of Women's Health, Obstetrical and Neonatal Nurses has generated a list of clinically relevant areas that are deemed research priorities. These can be viewed by visiting its website (www.awhonn.org/awhonn/content.do?name=03_JournalsPubsResearch/3D_ResearchPriorities.htm) and have included research on preventing unintended pregnancy, cardiovascular health, weight management, cancer screening, women's health and stress management. Although many professional and consumer organisations do not have published research priorities, they all have some sort of clinical, educational or outcomes-based aims and these can provide insight into the types of research areas they would support.

STUDENT CHALLENGE

Checking Maternal-Infant Priorities

1. Go to the SIDS Australia website: www.sidsandkids.org. Have a look at the areas that have been researched to try to find the causes and the ways of preventing sudden infant death syndrome (SIDS). Can you identify any current priorities?
2. Look at the list of organisations in Box 12.1. Visit some of the websites and look for research priorities related to maternal-infant care.
3. Can you locate any other sources or organisations that list or discuss priorities in maternal-infant care or research?
4. Choose one of the priority areas you have discovered. Run a literature search for the years 2010 to the present and see what, if any, nursing or midwifery-related research has been conducted in your selected area. Did you find anything that might be applicable to the clinical area of maternal-infant care?
5. Now go to the website of the Royal Children's Hospital Clinical Practice Guidelines (see the Resources kit, below). These guidelines are freely available to health professionals and to the public. The guidelines are a good example of national or international principles of best practice being adapted for use locally.
6. Browse the site. You will see that there is an alphabetical list of guidelines and links to the guideline development process. Follow the link and review their process. Do they follow best practice in guideline development?

Now consider the care and research priorities relevant to an adult population. Health maintenance, promotion and restoration remain key goals in the care of adults, as is combating diseases that carry high morbidity and mortality rates. Many areas of adult health require current and rigorous research activity. A browse of key websites such as those of the National Heart Foundation, the Cancer Council or Diabetes Australia will highlight areas of current concern.

STUDENT CHALLENGE

Checking Adult Care Priorities

1. Australia's national research priorities include mental health, obesity and cancer control. Check out the Australian health priority areas on the Australian government's AIHW website (Australian Institute of Health and Welfare) (see the Resources kit, below). What is new or different about these objectives?
2. Locate the World Health Organization's research priorities and see how they compare with Australian government initiatives.
3. Locate the latest research priorities of at least two nursing or midwifery specialty areas of interest relevant to adult care. (Use MEDLINE or CINAHL and do a search from 2010 to the present.)
4. Choose one priority area from one of the specialty areas. Run a literature search for the years 2010 to the present and see what nursing or midwifery-specific research has been conducted in your selected area.

Clinical chairs

Once an area of research need has been identified, a research project can be designed and conducted. The establishment of clinical chairs in Australia over the last 20 years or so has been an important development in the academic maturity of the nursing and midwifery professions. The primary aims for these positions are to conduct research in conjunction with clinical nurses and midwives and to foster evidence-based practice. In the past, the potential for clinical nurses and midwives to contribute at an intellectual level to healthcare research was limited for many reasons. These reasons included limited potential for tertiary-level educational preparation and a lack of recognition on the part of other members of the multidisciplinary team. It is good to be able to say that both of these reasons are no longer valid.

Establishing a clinically based nursing or midwifery research unit, usually led by a professor or associate professor, is a long-term commitment that requires much planning.

The model of clinical chair works something like this. A healthcare facility and a university that has a nursing and midwifery department come together and, after a period of discussion, agree on a role description for a senior academic nurse or midwife. This role description should address some of the needs of both institutions. The healthcare facility can be a hospital, community health service or, more rarely, a long-term residential facility. Usually each facility funds half the salary and other costs of the position and staff contracts are for between two and five years. The incumbent is then accountable to both institutions in terms of performance during the period of the contract.

When these positions are successful, the university is rewarded by increased involvement in clinical research. The healthcare facility increases its capacity for best practice initiatives and the integration of evidence into practice. Both institutions aim for improved nursing and midwifery care leading to better health outcomes for patients or clients. However, changes in health outcomes are rarely the consequence of one professional group in isolation, so the clinical academic unit must function in close collaboration with other clinical units where these coexist.

However, these outcomes are all rather nebulous and have to be demonstrated through more tangible productivity measures (often called 'outputs'). For the university, these outputs are measured in terms of successful grant applications, completed research projects and subsequent high-quality research publications. For the healthcare facility, the outputs are often less easy to define but the rewards include internal reports providing high-quality analysis of hospital data, targeted literature reviews of current best practice and the development of local policies based on current research.

The close connection of healthcare facility with university departments increases clinician involvement in successful research to answer clinical nursing and midwifery problems and result in 'best practice-savvy' clinicians. There are now many examples of successful clinical nursing and midwifery collaborations between university and the health industry. These centres also employ research fellows and research assistants, often clinical nurses who have or are working towards postgraduate degrees, but also professionals from other healthcare disciplines such as psychologists and epidemiologists. These additional staff are primarily funded from research grant monies although, importantly, most centres also have some recurrent funding for research support positions.

Let me use my experience of working in such centres as an example. Over a ten-year period I was a senior academic in positions that were jointly funded by healthcare organisations and universities. I led teams that conducted research on topics that were important to the hospital, such as healthcare-associated infections and the prevention of pressure injury (Gardner et al 2009). I also participated in clinical forums where research input was important, such as policy and practice committees. I, and other senior research staff, collaborated with clinicians in conducting quality improvement projects that led to practice change and also publication of peer-reviewed papers (O'Connor et al 2009a;

Hartig & Smyth 2009). Some of these local-level projects evaluated the quality of current evidence (O'Connell et al 2006) or identified areas for future clinical research (Laffin & Smyth 2011; McArdle & Gardner 2009). Both the latter papers are literature reviews and both have resulted in prospective studies being conducted and published (Hughes et al 2011; Laffin et al 2014). Staff in the research centres also helped with presentation of information at local, national and international forums. Most of the presentations and publications were collaborative with authorship teams comprising both clinicians and researchers, as are all of the examples provided in this section. The most successful clinical academic nursing units are ones where the clinicians are valued for their expertise in equal measure with the academic input.

The reality of research in small healthcare facilities

It is to be hoped that these successful clinical academic units are the way of the future but we must also recognise that, in small healthcare facilities, it is still very difficult for clinical nurses and midwives to make research a reality without a formal support structure. If you work in a rural hospital, a residential aged-care facility in a small town or other small facility such as specialist minor day surgery centre you may feel that engagement in research is not possible. However, implementation of research is a good place to begin. Chapter 10 gives you some good advice about how knowledge translation can take place. For example, go to the annual or biennial conference of your specialty association, such as your state or national wound-care group, infection control association or orthopaedic nursing society. If it is a vibrant society there will be presentations of both clinical and research papers. Some presentations will discuss changes in policy and practice. If they are discussing a clinical problem you have also identified in your facility, speak to the presenters and ask if you can try their ideas in your hospital. Most nurses and midwives are very happy to collaborate and are pleased their ideas have applicability beyond their own hospital or community centre. You should make sure you acknowledge their support in any policy or practice change that you effect in your workplace and, who knows, you may establish a career-long collaborative relationship with interstate or overseas colleagues.

Other suggestions, mentioned throughout this book, include the following:

- In your workplace search out the more senior nurses and midwives who are undertaking further education; they are likely to be involved in research utilisation and have good critical appraisal skills.
- Make contact with a former lecturer who was passionate about the clinical application of research and ask if he or she is interested in collaborating in a practice change project.

- Make contact with the nearest university school of nursing and midwifery and ask the same question.
- Seek out clinical nurse consultants, a practice development nurse, nurse educator or a senior midwife in your organisation with a research responsibility in his or her job description and start a journal club (O'Connor et al 2009b).

Current email and web-based resources make contact with former lecturers or likeminded staff you have met at conferences so easy and fast that support and guidance can be gained from many sources. One example of such collaboration at a distance between nursing staff at a small hospital and a university academic is the evaluation of stroke guidelines in a rural setting – see McCann et al (2009).

Finally, Chapter 10 closes with a section on strategies to strengthen your utilisation potential. Go through this section, choose the strategies that will work best for you and become a 'research consumer'! However, remember that research utilisation and practice change take time and you should see these as long-term projects rather than quick processes. Start with modest aims and reward yourself and your colleagues when you achieve a small win. Once your colleagues start to use clinical research findings, there will be one or two who start to think about undertaking research themselves. The next section briefly considers your place as a new graduate in these processes.

Nurses and midwives as leaders and change agents

Let me begin this section by asking you to think about who you regard as current leaders in nursing and midwifery. As a new graduate, you may think that leadership is a concept you are not going to have to worry about for a while. You may recognise good leadership skills in others but not yet picture yourself as a leader. Leaders and managers are often seen as requiring the same skill sets and, while the required competencies for both do overlap, a good manager is not necessarily a good leader and vice versa. In particular, good leaders are not necessarily the ones with the most power or formal authority. Let us concentrate on leadership here. Good leaders want to take risks and try new ideas. They are able to motivate others because they have passion about their work. They also have good social skills and are able to understand others and respond appropriately. Does this sound like you?

The current skill mix of healthcare teams is such that you may well be quite senior as soon as you graduate. You will be leading and mentoring undergraduate students (both registered nurses or midwives and enrolled nursing students). You may also be supervising personal care attendants and orderlies. Perhaps your organisation will have medical and allied health students, too. The way you interact with these groups will influence how they see the place of nurses and midwives in the multidisciplinary team. You want to create the impression of the nursing and midwifery profession as one that works to get the best patient outcomes, draws on knowledge of research findings and applies best practice initiatives.

Let us return to the process of the integration translation of research into practice. As we have already mentioned, this topic has been discussed in some detail in Chapter 10 and is summarised again in this chapter using the Ottawa model (Logan & Graham 1998; Graham & Logan 2004). There is frequent reference to the length and complexity of the process of integrating research into clinical practice. The end-users are very influential in any change process and, as new graduates, you are end-users or consumers of research. Remember that change agents are people who are able to see an idea in its very early stages and work to move it through to completion (Crookes & Froggatt 2004; Middleton 2012). A director of nursing colleague of mine, in her welcoming speech, tells each cohort of new graduates that she expects every one of them to see themselves as leaders from the beginning of their employment.

Finally, I want to mention a very specific group of leaders. The development of the nurse practitioner role in Australia and New Zealand is an exciting trend. The title 'nurse practitioner' is now legally protected in both countries and there is mutual recognition of registration between the two countries. Standards were developed and accepted by both national registration boards (Gardner et al 2006a) and have recently been updated here in Australia (www.nursingmidwiferyboard.gov.au/Codes-Guidelines-Statements/Codes-Guidelines/nurse-practitioner-standards-of-practice.aspx). Clinical leadership is a core role for nurse practitioners because in Australia these positions are at the pinnacle of clinical nursing leadership. Nurse practitioners should be influential in clinical, professional and political forums (Gardner et al 2006b). Senior nurses have traditionally worked to achieve the latter two but have rarely been seen as clinical leaders. Australian and New Zealand nurse practitioners are already taking a leadership role in the clinical management of patients in their care. This is something for you to aspire to.

Societal trends

In the introduction to this chapter, I stated that health care is a dynamic and changing service. Let us turn to the place of nursing, midwifery and health care in society more broadly. In this section, I am going to summarise two very different trends that influence the circumstances under which the healthcare system functions. The first trend is the ageing of the population. As you are probably already aware, the demographic profile of Australia, New Zealand and most other industrialised societies is changing. The second trend I am going to discuss may be less familiar to you. It is the imperative for increased accountability that we encounter in many facets of our lives. This second trend is a function of the changing social and political milieu that has introduced an increasing focus on economic efficiency and system performance. First, let us consider the impact of demographic changes on healthcare delivery.

The ageing society

Increased average Australian life expectancy is the result of financial affluence that brings improved conditions of everyday living such as better nutrition and prompt access to health care. The increased life expectancy means more people are living beyond 65 years of age. 'The population aged 75 or more years is expected to rise by 4 million between 2012 and 2060, increasing from about 6.4 to 14.4 per cent of the population' (stated in An Ageing Australia: Preparing for the future, Productivity Commission 2013, p 2). However, increasing longevity is associated with higher prevalence of chronic illness that, in turn, can increase the demand on health services. For example, a younger person with no chronic illness who sustains a fractured femur in a road traffic accident is likely to have a much simpler recovery trajectory than an elderly person who sustains a similar injury in the same crash but who also has chronic health problems such as dementia and congestive cardiac failure.

The increasing proportion of aged persons, coupled with lower birth rates in societies such as Australia and New Zealand, affects not only the profile of healthcare consumers but also the healthcare workforce profile. Population ageing is not just an issue because there is an increased number of older people, but also because this change alters the ratio of younger to older people (Productivity Commission 2013). Amongst other consequences of the altered ratio is the change to the share of the population who are in the workforce. People who are under 55 years of age have significantly greater workforce participation. Consequently, as more people move into the older age groups, overall workforce participation rates will fall. In Australia, we anticipate that the proportion of people aged 65 years or over will increase from 13% in 2010 to 23% by June 2050. At the same time the proportion of working-age people is expected to fall by 7%. This means there will be relatively fewer people of working age to support the increasing number of older Australians (Productivity Commission 2013). Half of the nurses and midwives currently employed in Australia will retire in the next ten years (Palumbo et al 2009). To prevent a crisis in healthcare staffing, measures to improve participation in the healthcare workforce are needed.

Accountability for services

Next, let us consider two particular issues of accountability, one for the healthcare industry and one for the university sector. Safety and quality in health care have become issues that are very publicly debated both in our region (www.safetyandquality.gov.au) and internationally (e.g. in the USA, www.ahrq.gov). Sometimes patients are severely injured or die as a consequence of unsafe or adverse health care. We now understand that many adverse incidents are most usefully considered as consequences of imperfect systems, rather than simply being explained as the outcome of individual mistakes. Detailed analysis of the incident can help to identify system problems.

Accreditation

The first example of accountability is hospital **accreditation**. Healthcare organisations are required to demonstrate they are monitoring the quality of care so that problems can be identified promptly. They are obliged to report regularly the level of their performance against agreed measures (often known as 'indicators'). These reports go to funding bodies such as local and national health departments. In many countries, there is now formal accreditation of health services to evaluate quality of care against agreed standards of care. In Australia, one of the best-known accreditation processes can be found on the Australian Council on Healthcare Standards (ACHS) website (www.achs.org.au/Home). The ACHS is a national organisation that evaluates Australian healthcare organisations against agreed standards.

ACHS has released the fifth version of its hospital standards, the Evaluation and Quality Improvement Program, known by the acronym EQuIP – www.achs.org.au/achs-international/products-and-services/evaluation-and-quality-improvement-program-(equip), with a four-phase cycle:

1. Organisation wide survey
2. Self assessment
3. Periodic review
4. Self assessment.

For successful accreditation, the organisations must also demonstrate that, where a problem is identified, they are intervening to reduce risk and improve the quality of care. Try exploring the website to see what key indicators of care are measured within the clinical standard section.

The Excellence in Research for Australia Initiative

The second example of accountability affects the university system across the board, not just the part that delivers education to healthcare workers and conducts healthcare-related research. The Australian Commonwealth government introduced an initiative called the **Excellence in Research for Australia** (**ERA**) initiative. This initiative comes under the Department of Innovation, Industry, Science and Research. Information can be found by investigating the Australian Research Council's website (www.arc.gov.au/era/default.htm).

A similar initiative in New Zealand, known as the **Performance-Based Research Fund** (PBRF), has already resulted in changes:

> *Funding for research will no longer be allocated to institutions according to student enrolments. Instead, research funds will be allocated through the PBRF according to the quality of the research produced in each*

institution. The system will take into account the quality of researchers, research degree completions and external research income (www.otago.ac.nz/research/pbrf).

The main aim of the Australian initiative is to 'assess research quality within Australia's higher education institutions using a combination of indicators and expert review by committees comprising experienced, internationally recognised experts' (www.arc.gov.au/era/default.htm). In principle, an expert panel reviews the quality and impact of research outputs submitted by universities. The results influence the amount of research funding that Australian universities receive from the Commonwealth government. Similar exercises, undertaken in New Zealand and the UK as well as previously in Australia, have raised contentious issues for some disciplines, including those of nursing and midwifery. We can learn important lessons by understanding the way that the processes have played out previously and in other countries. Many academics are sceptical about these frameworks and see them as simply another bureaucratic layer. However, nursing and midwifery researchers will be disadvantaged if they do not actively participate in the process and the Council of Deans of Nursing and Midwifery (Australia and New Zealand) is engaged in several initiatives to ensure that nursing and midwifery are represented as advantageously as possible. In the most recent ERA, many nursing and midwifery research centres produced encouraging results.

While it receives less consideration at present in Australian national research assessment, one of the most important aspects for nursing and midwifery is the 'impact' measure. We need to be explicit about the influence our research has on healthcare policy and practice. The way in which evidence is translated into good clinical practice is complex but very important. The integration of research into practice is a thread that runs right through this book. Why is this important to you as a new graduate, you may ask? Well, you can play a part if you understand the full implications for the disciplines of nursing and midwifery. Let me give you an example of how it would work. To understand the example, we need to spend a little time considering the place of policies in health care.

Policy development in clinical practice

Most organisations have very specific statements for the guidance of their staff about the way the organisation is to function. These statements are often called policies and may relate to human resources, financial issues and, of course, clinical issues. Policy is a word that is used in many contexts. **Policy** can be defined as:

> ... a written plan of an organisation's official position, based on the organisation's purpose and goals, on a specific health situation, intended to guide and determine decisions for improving a specific health situation (Osborne & Webster 2010, p 60).

First, let us consider policies as they are used to guide our clinical practice. These are policies that help us to deliver patient care that:

- is based on best practice and appropriate evidence
- is safe for healthcare workers as well as for patients and their families
- complies with relevant legal and ethical frameworks.

Let us consider a practical example. Some years ago, a group of intensive care nurses examined the unit policy for the taping of endotracheal tubes in patients who were receiving artificial ventilation. They examined the published literature and were unable to find much useful clinical research. They approached me and elicited the assistance of our **nursing research** centre. We collaborated on a systematic review of methods of taping endotracheal tubes for adults receiving artificial ventilation and published the results (Gardner et al 2005). While this is a satisfactory outcome (or quality output) for the academic unit (i.e. a peer-reviewed publication) it does not, in itself, indicate any influence over practice. However, that publication is cited in clinical policies in several major hospitals in Australia and formed the basis for New South Wales state-wide standards (Rolls & Gardner 2007).

These policy documents are evidence of an uptake of research. You, as graduates who are active consumers of clinical research, can read, evaluate and report on research that is relevant to clinical problems in your specialty. This book has helped you to develop skills in using the internet efficiently, accessing and researching different research methods, appraising research reports and identifying findings that are pertinent to your practice. Your reports can influence changes in local policy. You can also argue for the policies to include reference to current research. (This can be particularly exciting when you are citing your own publications!)

Policy development at the national and international level

Finally, let us spend some time considering policy development at the national and international level. This may not seem relevant to you as a newly practising health professional who simply wants to deliver the best care possible to the patients and families in your care. Nonetheless, wider health policy does affect the way you practise. For example, governments formulate health policy to direct the way in which national funds are spent to deliver health care. Other national policies regulate the way components of differing health services articulate with each other.

If you develop your skills as a consumer of healthcare research, then you will be in a position to comment on draft national policies and guidelines. Exerting influence at this national level will help to ensure that the translation of healthcare policy at the local, practical level is workable, relevant and appropriate for our clients. When new national policies need to be developed, or there is a proposal for a major change in direction, a discussion paper or draft document may be circulated to relevant organisations (such as the Australian College of Nursing). You, as an active consumer of the research literature, may be able to identify strengths or weaknesses in these draft policies and guidelines. You can participate in the formulation of a response and can then contribute to debate at the national level.

The potential for involvement does not stop at national borders. International bodies such as the International Council of Nurses (ICN [2011]) and the International Confederation of Midwives (ICM [2011]) produce policy statements to provide guidance and promote consistency across the world. The mission statement on the ICN website includes the word 'policies':

> *The International Council of Nurses (ICN) is a federation of more than 130 national nurses' associations representing the millions of nurses worldwide. Operated by nurses and leading nurses internationally, ICN works to ensure quality nursing care for all, sound health policies globally, the advancement of nursing knowledge ... and a competent and satisfied nursing workforce (ICN 2011).*

An excellent example of the influence that bodies such as the ICN can have is the influence that nurses and midwives have had internationally to promote breastfeeding (ICN 2013). Breastfeeding is promoted strongly in Australia, through the Baby Friendly Health Initiative that is governed by the Australian College of Midwives (http://www.midwives.org.au/scripts/cgiip.exe/WService=MIDW/ccms.r?pageid=10218); (www.babyfriendly.org.au/what-is-baby-friendly/bfhi-australia).

STUDENT CHALLENGE

Exploring International Nursing and Midwifery Policies

1. Go to the ICN website (www.icn.ch) or ICM (www.internationalmidwives.org). Find the section on policies.
2. What topics are covered in the policies listed?
3. Given that the ICN mission statement refers to global health policies, find two policies that are applicable to the country where you are a practising nurse and see if they compare to the nursing code of practice in your country. Do a similar comparison for midwifery.

Even citation in policies is not the end of the process for policies only work if they are utilised. We have considered how policies based on the best available evidence can influence patient outcomes when we looked at models for the integration of research into practice earlier in this chapter as well as in previous chapters.

Conclusion

We have come to the end of the book. I hope you have developed a sense that nursing and midwifery are wonderful careers that can be both rewarding and challenging. Throughout the book you will have seen that research literacy assists in understanding and responding to the many changes that influence healthcare outcomes and ultimately health in the Australian and New Zealand context. To play your part successfully you need to be a lifelong learner and prepared to assume a leadership role when required in the multidisciplinary team. We hope that as beginners you now have a better understanding of the current and future contribution that research can make in clinical practice and that you understand the place of clinical leadership in this process. We wish you all the very best for your future careers in nursing or midwifery.

My vision for the future of research in nursing and midwifery

In a previous edition of this book, I finished with a gaze into the crystal ball and said that, in ten years' time, I hoped that:

- Nursing and midwifery practice will truly be steeped in research. This research will be wide-ranging in methodology and will also influence the practice of other healthcare disciplines.
- The nursing and midwifery component of the Australian and New Zealand healthcare workforce will include a very strong clinical practice structure with nurse practitioners at the apex.
- Senior nursing and midwifery clinicians, including nurse practitioners, will have academic positions in most large public healthcare organisations as well as many of the larger private healthcare facilities. Knowledge translation will be fully integrated.
- Nurses and midwives will account for 50% of the members in successful research teams obtaining healthcare-related nationally competitive research funding.
- The impact of nursing and midwifery research on practice will clearly be evidenced.

Several years later we are well on the road to achieving these aspirations. Nurses and midwives contribute actively to multidisciplinary national and international practice guidelines and have a much better record of success at major research grants but there is still much work to do. The future of the nursing and midwifery professions rests with you!

RESOURCES KIT

Websites

Agency for Healthcare Research and Quality: www.ahrq.gov.

Australian Commission on Safety and Quality in Health Care: www.safetyandquality.gov.au.

Australian Council on Healthcare Standards: www.achs.org.au/Home.

Australian Digital Theses Program: adt.caul.edu.au.

Australian evidence-based nursing – Joanna Briggs Institute: www.joannabriggs.org.

Australian Government. Australian Institute of Health and Welfare. National Health Priority: www.aihw.gov.au/national-health-priority-areas.

Australian Government. Australian Research Council – The Excellence in Research for Australia (ERA) initiative: www.arc.gov.au/era.

Australian Health Practitioner Regulation Agency: www.ahpra.gov.au.

Australian Nursing and Midwifery Accreditation Council: www.anmc.org.au.

Australian Wound Management Association publications: www.awma.com.au/publications/publications.php#pipm.

Centre for Reviews and Dissemination, University of York, UK: www.york.ac.uk/inst/crd.

Cochrane collaboration: www.cochrane.org.

International Confederation of Midwives (ICM): www.internationalmidwives.org.

International Council of Nurses (ICN): www.icn.ch/publications/position-statements.

Medical Research Council, UK: www.mrc.ac.uk.

MEDLINE: www.ncbi.nlm.nih.gov/entrez.

National Health and Medical Research Council: www.nhmrc.gov.au.

NHMRC/HREC joint webpage: www.nhmrc.gov.au/health-ethics.

National Health and Medical Research Council National Health Priority Areas: www.nhmrc.gov.au/grants-funding/research-funding-statistics-and-data/funding-statistics-grants-and-funding-data.

New Zealand Health and Disability Ethics: www.ethicscommittees.health.govt.nz.

New Zealand Standards and Performance Assessment Agency for Health and Disability Services. Telarc Quality Health – Te Taumata Hauora: www.telarc.co.nz.

Nursing and Midwifery Board of Australia: www.nursingmidwiferyboard.gov.au.

Nursing and Midwifery Board of Australia. CPD FAQ's for Nurses: www.nursingmidwiferyboard.gov.au/Codes-Guidelines-Statements/FAQ/CPD-FAQ-for-nurses-and-midwives.aspx.

Nursing and Midwifery Board of Australia. Nurse Practitioner standards for practice: www.nursingmidwiferyboard.gov.au/Codes-Guidelines-Statements/Codes-Guidelines/nurse-practitioner-standards-of-practice.aspx.

Prevention and Treatment of Pressure Ulcers. Clinical Practice Guideline: www.internationalguideline.com.

Productivity Commission report. An Ageing Australia – preparing for the future: www.pc.gov.au/research/completed/ageing-australia/ageing-australia-overview.pdf.

Royal Children's Hospital, Melbourne, Australia. Clinical Practice Guidelines: www.rch.org.au/clinicalguide/cpg.cfm.

University of Hong Kong Clinical Trials: www.hkclinicaltrials.com.

References

Australian Nursing and Midwifery Board: Online. Available: www.nursingmidwiferyboard.gov.au/FAQ-and-Fact-Sheets.aspx 27 May 2015.

Crookes PA, Froggatt T: Techniques and strategies for translating research findings into healthcare practices. In Crookes PA, Davies S, editors: *Research into practice. Essential skills for reading and applying research in nursing and healthcare*, ed 2, Sydney, 2004, Bailliere Tindall.

Gardner G, Carryer J, Dunn S, et al: Nurse practitioner competency standards: findings from collaborative Australian and New Zealand research, *International Journal of Nursing Studies* 43:601–610, 2006a.

Gardner G, Carryer J, Gardner A, et al: Competency and capability: imperative for nurse practitioner education, *Australian Journal of Advanced Nursing* 24:8–14, 2006b.

Gardner A, Hughes D, Cook R, et al: Best practice in stabilisation of oral endotracheal tubes: a systematic review, *Australian Critical Care* 18:158–165, 2005.

Gardner A, Millar L, Legg S, et al: Pressure injury prevalence in a private health service: Risks and recommendations, *Wound Practice & Research* 17(3):134–145, 2009.

Graham K, Logan J: Using the Ottawa model of research use to implement a skin care program, *Journal of Nursing Care Quality* 19:18–24, 2004.

Hartig V, Smyth W: 'Everyone should buttonhole': a novel technique for a regional Australian renal service, *Journal of Renal Care* 35:114–119, 2009.

Helfrich CD, Damschroder LJ, Hagedorn HJ, et al: A critical synthesis of literature on the promoting action on research implementation in the health services (PARIHS) framework. *Implementation Science* 5, 2010. Online. Available: www.biomedcentral.com/content/pdf/1748-5908-5-82.pdf 27 May 2015.

Hughes K, Gardner A, McArdle J: Audit of factors associated with the intactness of central venous catheter exit site dressings for northern Australian haemodialysis patients, *Renal Society of Australasia Journal* 7:108–114, 2011.

International Confederation of Midwives (ICM): 2011. Online. Available: http://www.internationalmidwives.org/ 27 May 2015.

International Council of Nurses (ICN): 2011. Online. Available: http://www.icn.ch/publications/position-statements/ 27 May 2015.

International Council of Nurses (ICN): 2013. Online. Available: http://www.icn.ch/images/stories/documents/publications/position_statements/A02_Breastfeeding.pdf 27 May 2015.

Knowles MS: *The modern practice of adult education: from pedagogy to androgogy*, New York, 1980, Cambridge University Press.

Laffin N, Smyth W: Prevention of radiation-induced moist desquamation in the tropics: A literature review of the non-prescription skin care products, *Wound Practice and Research* 19:136–144, 2011.

Laffin N, Smyth W, Heyer E, et al: Effectiveness and acceptability of a moisturizing cream and a barrier cream during radiation therapy for breast cancer in the tropics: A randomized controlled trial, *Cancer Nursing* 2014. doi: 10.1097/NCC.0000000000000161.

Logan J, Graham K: Towards a comprehensive interdisciplinary model of health care research use, *Science and Communication* 20:227–246, 1998.

McArdle J, Gardner A: A literature review of central venous catheter dressings: implications for haemodialysis in the tropics, *Healthcare Infection* 14:139–146, 2009.

McCann L, Groot P, Charnley C, et al: Excellence in regional stroke care: an evaluation of the implementation of a stroke care unit in regional Australia, *Australian Journal of Rural Health* 17:273–278, 2009.

Middleton S: An outcomes approach to stroke care: the importance of teamwork and evidence-based nursing care, *International Journal of Stroke* 7:224–226, 2012.

National Review of Nursing Education: *Our duty of care*, Canberra, 2002, Commonwealth of Australia.

O'Connell B, Duke M, Bennett P, et al: The trials and tribulations of team nursing, *Collegian (Royal College of Nursing, Australia)* 13:11–17, 2006.

O'Connor L, Bennett P, Gardner A, et al: Implementing a journal club in a palliative care setting: a link in the chain of evidence-based practice, *Collegian (Royal College of Nursing, Australia)* 16:147–152, 2009a.

O'Connor L, Gardner A, Millar L, et al: Absolutely fabulous – but are we? Carers' perspectives on satisfaction with a palliative homecare service, *Collegian (Royal College of Nursing, Australia)* 16:201–209, 2009b.

Osborne S, Webster J: Development and use of clinical guidelines. In Courtney M, McCutcheon H, editors: *Using evidence to guide nursing practice*, ed 2, Marrickville, 2010, Churchill Livingstone, pp 59–72.

Palumbo MV, McIntosh B, Rambur B, et al: Retaining an ageing nursing workforce: Perceptions of human resource practices, *Nursing Economics* 27:221–227, 2009.

Productivity Commission: *An Ageing Australia: Preparing for the future*. Research report. Melbourne: Productivity Commission, 2013, Online. Available: www.pc.gov.au/research/completed/ageing-australia/ageing-australia-overview.pdf 27 May 2015.

Rolls K, Gardner A: *The Rolls & Gardner guideline is now available on elitepdf.com which requires sign up*. Online. Available: http://elitepdf.com/stabilisation-of-an-endotracheal-tube-for-the-adult-intensive-care-patient.html, 2007.

Rycroft-Malone J, Harvey G, Kitson A, et al: Getting evidence into practice: ingredients for change, *Nursing Standard* 16:38–43, 2002.

GLOSSARY

Aboriginal and Torres Strait Islander peoples the First Nation peoples of Australia. Aboriginal peoples live and maintain the mainland continent now named Australia and Tasmania and its seas, oceans and sky-heavens. Torres Strait Islander peoples reside in and maintain the Torres Strait Islands and its seas and heavens

abstract 'a brief, objective summary of the essential content of a book, article, speech, report, dissertation, or other work that presents the main points in the same order as the original but has no independent literary value' (Reitz J: *Dictionary of Library and Information Science,* Westport, CT, 2004, Libraries Unlimited, p 3)

accreditation a system whereby a service is required to meet a set of accreditation standards set by a governing body

action research enquiry aimed at developing applied practical knowledge, and underpinned by collaborative and participatory social processes. This is a complex method for experienced researchers

appraisal tool a structured guide to undertaking a crucial appraisal

archival database 'an organised collection of records in digital format, containing information to be retained for an indefinite period of time, usually for future reference' (Reitz J: *Dictionary of Library and Information Science,* Westport, CT, 2004, Libraries Unlimited, p 37)

authority knowledge gleaned from the expertise of others

autonomy the philosophical principle of respecting a person's right to make their own decisions based on full and accurate information

barriers and facilitators 'barriers are defined as factors that would limit or restrict implementation of shared decision making in clinical practice. Facilitators are defined as factors that promote or help implement shared decision making in clinical practice' (Légaré F: Assessing barriers and facilitators to knowledge use. In Straus S, Tetroe J, Graham I, editors: *Knowledge Translation to Health Care: Moving from Evidence to Practice,* ed 2, 2009, Wiley Blackwell Publishing, p 85)

basic social process social or psychological process identified as enduring over time regardless of environmental conditions (e.g. stages of death and dying)

beneficence the philosophical principle of doing good and avoiding harm

blinding the process of keeping study participants and sometimes those involved in the conduct of a trial unaware of which treatment or intervention is being administered

blog see weblog

bookmark a way to mark and easily access a favourite or frequently used website (bookmarks are sometimes referred to as 'favourites')

bracketing a process used in some forms of phenomenology to identify and hold in abeyance or 'reduce' the personal beliefs that are held by a researcher about the phenomenon under study

browser a program that opens and displays pages on the world wide web

call number each book in the library has a unique call number. A call number is like an address – it identifies where the book is located in the library. Call numbers appear on the spine of books, bound periodicals, microfilm and other items. See: http://library.ucr.edu/?view=help/guides/callnumbers.html 9 February 2015

case study in-depth research study of an individual unit (e.g. a person, family, group or other identified social unit). A case study generally uses both qualitative and quantitative data

catalogue 'a list of books, maps, or other items, arranged in some definite order. It records, describes and indexes (usually completely) the resources of a collection, a library or a group of libraries' (Prytherch R: *Harrod's Librarians' Glossary and Reference Book,* ed 9, Aldershot, 2000, Ashgate, p 123)

citation 'a reference to a text or part of a text identifying the document in which it may be found' (Prytherch R: *Harrod's Librarians' Glossary and Reference Book,* ed 9, Aldershot, 2000, Ashgate, p 148)

citation database citation databases enable you to identify and search for references to previously published works cited by authors in their bibliographies. See http://www2.liu.edu/cwis/cwp/library/ref/isiwos.htm 9 February 2015

client a program that can request services from another computer, called a server

clinical significance determined through establishing how much benefit or harm results from a treatment or intervention

code of conduct guidelines to ensure researchers adhere to appropriate ethical standards when conducting research

coding one of the processes by which data may be categorised and conceptualised. It is most often seen in studies using a grounded theory approach

collective case study a series of case studies that examine similar patterns about identified phenomena

colonisation was a political and social strategy where European nations established control of land seized through imperial action by subjugating the Indigenous peoples. Colonisation continues through the imposition of dominant culture and knowledge systems, which marginalise Indigenous peoples and their ways of knowing

concept mental picture of an object or phenomenon. Concepts may be concrete or abstract

conceptual definition statement attaching a specified meaning to a word or concept (e.g. what the word means for a particular research study)

conceptual framework loosely related collection of concepts that have not yet been tested

conceptual utilisation adapting and using research findings to broaden or alter thinking and perspectives

concurrent mixed methods design design in which the qualitative and quantitative data are collected at the same time, but independently of each other. The final study results are based on the findings from both sets of data

constant characteristic that does not vary for a particular research study

constant comparative method method of analysis used in grounded theory in which categories of meaning are derived by comparing collected data incidents to one another until concepts emerge

continuing professional development (CPD) the means by which members of the profession maintain, improve and broaden their knowledge, expertise and competence and develop the personal and professional qualities required throughout their professional lives

control mechanisms used by the researcher to reduce the influence of extraneous variables

copyright 'a procedure whereby the originator of a piece of intellectual property (book, article, piece of music, etc.) acquires a series of rights over the work created, including copying, publishing, performing, broadcasting and adaptation' (Prytherch R: *Harrod's Librarians' Glossary and Reference Book,* ed 9, Aldershot, 2000, Ashgate, p 186)

credibility steps taken to make certain of accuracy, authenticity and validity of data

critical appraisal a structured process through which the strengths and limitations of research are evaluated and clinical relevance is established

critical approaches endeavours to produce research findings to generate change of some sort. When referring to this concept of change, authors often state that their research has transformative or emancipatory potential (i.e. the potential to be a catalyst for change)

critical reader a critical reader does not take what they read as fact but rather examines the evidence or arguments presented. They determine what, if any, influences and limitations may be involved and examine interpretations made by the author. Critical readers thus recognise not only what a text says, but also how that text portrays the subject matter

critical theory 'is an emancipatory methodological stance that challenges the status quo and seeks to bring about change. For example, critical theory has been used to call into question such social issues/norms as racism, sexism and colonialism' (Bohman J: *Critical Theory, the Stanford Encyclopedia of Philosophy*. Summer 2015 edition. Zalta EN (editor). Online. Available: http://plato.stanford.edu/archives/sum2015/entries/critical-theory/ 30 June 2015)

critique inquiry into a line of thought in order to understand it and determine its limitations. It is not the same as criticism
culturally competent refers to nurses' and midwives' having a comprehension of their own world views, sociocultural positioning and acting in respectful and responsive ways with Indigenous people
culture a 'form of production' that shapes people's thoughts and actions
data information collected for the purpose of analysis
database 'a large, regularly updated file of digitised information (bibliographic records, abstracts, full-text documents, directory entries, images, statistics, etc.) related to a specific subject or field, consisting of records of uniform format organised for ease and speed of search and retrieval and managed with the aid of database management system (DBMS) software' (Reitz J: *Dictionary of Library and Information Science,* Westport, CT, 2004, Libraries Unlimited, p 202)
data collection the gathering of information necessary to address the research problem
data immersion repeated engagement with primary data to become familiar with its content, feeling and tone. This can mean listening and relistening to digitally recorded data and reading and rereading text
deductive reasoning also called deduction; sets out with a general case from which specific instances are deduced
deep web (or invisible web or hidden web) pages on the world wide web that are not indexed by common search engines
dependent variable variable that is affected by the action of the independent variable
descriptive statistics statistics used to describe and summarise collected data
directional hypothesis statement that identifies the predicted direction of a relationship or difference between the independent and dependent variables within a given population
domain hierarchical scheme for indicating the logical and sometimes geographical venue of a web page from the network
electronic database database that is accessed for a search via computer, for example, CINAHL and MEDLINE
epistemology the study of knowledge; theorising about the nature and origin of knowledge
ERA Excellence in Research for Australia (see below)
ethical codes of conduct the foundation of research integrity is the code of conduct. Codes stipulate the standards of responsible and principled conduct demanded of everyone who is engaged in research. Codes compel researchers to be mindful of ethical guidelines governing research, and to observe organisational and regulatory requirements
ethics committee (human research) committee responsible for review of research proposals to ensure that human subjects are protected from harm
ethnography qualitative research design that focuses on the world view of an identified cultural group
evidence proof or findings that can be used as the basis for decisions
evidence-based practice (EBP) applying the best available evidence to care
Evidence-informed decision making (EIDM) decision making that is based on best available evidence
Excellence in Research for Australia (ERA) a federal government-led research assessment exercise in which university disciplines, including nursing and midwifery, are required to subject the research of their staff to internal self-assessment, international and/or national peer review
experimental research quantitative research in which one concept (independent variable) is manipulated to determine whether another concept (dependent variable) is affected
extraneous variable variable that interferes with the relationship of the independent and dependent variables in a specified study and therefore may provide misleading results
field natural setting in which investigation and data collection take place in a qualitative study
field notes written accounts of what a researcher sees, hears, experiences and thinks during the course of data collection in a qualitative study
findings results of the analysis of study data

fraud the deliberate falsification of research by researchers

generalisation the ability to apply study results from the sample to the population

grey literature documentary material that is not commercially published and is typically composed of technical reports, working papers, business documents and conference proceedings

grounded theory qualitative research that develops theoretical propositions about identified social/psychological processes from collected data

historical method qualitative analysis of historical events to draw additional insights or inferences about how past events affect the present

holism belief that, for any aspect of life to be fully understood, the associated factors and context must also be recognised and understood

host a computer that is directly connected to a network and provides services to many users. A host computer will run server software as a means of interacting with a number of clients

human rights rights inherent to everyone regardless of our nationality, where we live, sex, race, religion, language, or any other status. Everyone is equally entitled to his or her human rights without discrimination. See http://www.ohchr.org/EN/Issues/Pages/WhatareHumanRights.aspx 9 February 2015

hypertext enables links to other web pages or related websites. It is the 'active' area of text (sometimes underlined), presented as a graphic or button on which you can click to retrieve another document

hypertext markup language (HTML) the codes and instructions used to control the appearance and function of a website. It inserts links, graphics and other multimedia objects on the web page

hypertext transfer protocol (HTTP) the language used to transfer web pages over an internet connection. The first letters in a URL for a site on the world wide web

hypothesis statement of predicted relationship or difference between two or more variables within a specified population. A hypothesis contains at least one independent and one dependent variable. The goal of any statistical test is to determine whether or not the null hypothesis should be rejected, or not rejected

identifying bias identifying influence or subjectivity that reduces objectivity in a study

implication inference drawn about the results of a research study

independent variable variable that causes a change in the dependent variable

index 'an alphabetically arranged list of headings consisting of the personal names, places, and subjects treated in a written work, with page numbers to refer the reader to the point in the text at which information pertaining to the heading is found' (Reitz J: *Dictionary of Library and Information Science,* Westport, CT, 2004, Libraries Unlimited, p 353)

Indigenous peoples the First Nations peoples throughout the world who have been colonised. We use this term to acknowledge peoples locally and internationally who have struggled with dominant colonial regimes

inductive reasoning reasoning that moves from the particular to the general; a form of reasoning process in which a conclusion is drawn from particular cases, that is, from the particular to the general; as opposed to deductive reasoning

inferential statistics statistics that are used to study relationships or differences among variables in a sample and infer the results back to the population

information literate 'skill in finding the information one needs, including an understanding of how libraries are organised, familiarity with the resources they provide (including information formats and automated search tools), and knowledge of commonly used research techniques' (Reitz J: *Dictionary of Library and Information Science,* Westport, CT, 2004, Libraries Unlimited, pp 356–357)

information quality information quality is a subjective measure of the worth attributed to the information by the user of that information

informed consent an agreement by a research subject to participate voluntarily in a study after being fully informed about the study and the inherent risks and benefits of participation

instrument device or technique used to collect data in a research study (e.g. biophysical instruments such as glucometers, psychological instruments such as questionnaires or interviews, behavioural instruments such as observation)

interdisciplinary teamwork the practice, in both clinical and research settings, of professionals from different disciplines working together to achieve a common goal
interlibrary loan (document delivery) a library service that allows books and copies of journal articles to be obtained from other libraries
internet contraction of international networks; a global collection of interconnected networks that use the internet protocol (TCP/IP) as a means of linking computers
internet protocol number or address (IP number or IP address) a unique identifying number given to every machine on the internet. It consists of four parts separated by dots, for example, 131.234.245.7
internet service provider (ISP) company that provides a connection to the internet (e.g. Telstra BigPond, Ozemail)
intuition a 'gut feeling' or 'hunch' that comes from a place of personal experience and might not be explained or backed up easily by logic or facts; to have insight into the whole of a situation without possessing readily supportable or confirming data
journal (periodical or magazine) 'a periodical devoted to disseminating original research and commentary on current developments within a specific discipline, subdiscipline, or field of study' (Reitz J: *Dictionary of Library and Information Science,* Westport, CT, 2004, Libraries Unlimited, p 382)
knowledge a means of surviving by understanding; essential information about the world around us that allows us to function more effectively
knowledge translation (KT) the thought processes involved in reading, appraising and making a decision about using research findings in practice; a means of operating by understanding essential information about the world around us that allows us to function more effectively
language the primary mode of thinking and being for humanity
lifelong learning maintaining currency with a body or bodies of knowledge throughout the lifespan
listserver (listserv) electronic mailing list
literature review critical summary of available theoretical and research literature on the selected research topic. It places the research problem for a particular study in the context of what is currently known about the topic and supports the need for the study
manipulation intervention or treatment introduced by the researcher in an experimental study
Māori peoples the tangata whenua (Indigenous peoples of the land) of Aotearoa New Zealand. They are identified by their iwi (tribal groups) and hapū (sub-tribes) connected to various areas in New Zealand
measurement set of rules used to assign numbers to variables
method steps taken by the researcher to collect the data for a specific study (e.g. survey, interview or focus group)
methodology approach used by the researcher to guide the conduct of the study (for example, phenomenology, grounded theory or randomised control trial)
microform 'a generic term for a highly reduced photographic copy of text and/or images stored on a translucent medium (microfiche or microfilm)' (Reitz J: *Dictionary of Library and Information Science,* Westport, CT, 2004, Libraries Unlimited, p 453)
midwifery research research usually conducted by midwives to generate knowledge that informs and develops the discipline and practice of midwifery
mixed methods research use of both qualitative and quantitative methods of data collection in a single study. For example, combining qualitative interviews and quantitative survey data collection (see: Lee LYK, Holroyd E: Evaluating the effect of childbirth education class: a mixed-method study, *International Nursing Review* 56:361–368, 2009; Sands N: An exploration of clinical decision making in mental health triage, *Archives of Psychiatric Nursing* 23:298–308, 2009)
monograph 'a relatively short book or treatise on a single subject, complete in one physical piece, usually written by a specialist in the field' (Reitz J: *Dictionary of Library and Information Science,* Westport, CT, 2004, Libraries Unlimited, p 461)
multi methods research use of two or more data collection methods from the same research tradition. For example, participant observation and interviews (qualitative), or survey and

population census data (quantitative) (Teddlie C, Tashakkori A: *Foundations of Mixed Methods Research: Integrating quantitative and qualitative approaches in the social and behavioral sciences*, Thousand Oaks, California, 2009, SAGE Publications)

national broadband network (NBN) an Australian government infrastructure initiative aimed at creating a national network providing internet connectivity. Connection to this network will be via a range of technologies including fibre to the premise, fixed wireless and satellite technologies and will deliver download speeds in excess of 100 megabits per second

non-experimental research quantitative research in which concepts are not manipulated, but are examined as they occur naturally

non-probability sample sample selected using non-random techniques

null hypothesis a statement that predicts no relationship between the independent and dependent variables

nursing research research usually conducted by nurses to generate knowledge that informs and develops the discipline and practice of nursing

open source software software program developed by the IT community using a copyright licence that permits anyone to study, change and improve the software, and to redistribute it in modified or unmodified form. A sizeable proportion of this is freely available for download

operational definition specifies how a variable is to be measured

paradigm philosophical underpinnings from which specific research approaches stem (e.g. qualitative, quantitative) (Weaver K, Olson JK: Understanding paradigms for nursing research, *Journal of Advanced Nursing* 53:459–469, 2006)

performance-based research fund (PBRF) a scheme for New Zealand universities allocated according to the quality of the research produced in each institution. The system takes into account the quality of researchers, research degree completions and external research income

personal/lived experience knowledge derived from the cumulative experiences of living

phenomenology the study of lived experience. Its purpose is to understand and attribute meaning to the phenomenon of interest

podcast a means of distributing audio or video (multimedia) files over the internet for playback on mobile devices and personal computers

policy 'a written plan of an organisation's official position, based on the organisation's purpose and goals, on a specific health situation, intended to guide and determine decisions for improving a specific health situation' (Osborne S, Webster J: Development and use of clinical guidelines. In Courtney M, McCutcheon H, editors: *Using evidence to guide nursing practice*, ed 2, Marrickville, 2010, Churchill Livingstone, pp 59–72)

population all known subjects that possess a common characteristic of interest to a researcher

power analysis a calculation to estimate the sample size that is needed to test hypotheses adequately

predication the likelihood that a study will foresee outcomes

privacy the expectation that information about participants will be kept confidential

probability (random) sample sample selected using techniques to ensure that each subject in the population has an equal chance of being selected

problem statement interrogative or declarative statement that describes the purpose of a research study, identifies key concepts and sets study limits

protocol the rules two computers must follow to exchange messages

qualitative analysis a systematic search for meaning, which can include searching for patterns, categories and themes in the data findings

qualitative research incorporates a range of methods of inquiry that, in the main, seek to explore the behaviour, perspectives and experiences of people through a systematic process of listening to and/or observing them

quantitative research systematic process used to gather and statistically analyse information that has been measured by an instrument and converted to numerical data

randomised controlled trial form of experimental research where participants are randomly allocated into either a control or experimental group. Used to test new interventions or prevention programs

reasoning use of logical thought processes to solve problems. May be inductive or deductive in nature

recommendation statement derived from a research study to guide future research about a specified topic

reference collection 'books not meant to be read cover to cover, such as dictionaries, handbooks, and encyclopedias, shelved together by call number in a special section of the library' (Reitz J: *Dictionary of Library and Information Science,* Westport, CT, 2004, Libraries Unlimited, p 601)

reliability characteristic of a good instrument; the assessed degree of consistency and dependability

replication conduct of additional research studies on an identified problem to determine whether consistent results can be achieved by repeating the research methodology in a different setting

research systematic process using both inductive and deductive reasoning to confirm and refine existing knowledge and to build new knowledge

research design the overall plan for collecting data in a research study

research hypothesis expected relationship between the dependent and independent variables; also referred to as the alternative hypothesis

research literacy describes the process to develop skills and capacity to become 'evidence-based practitioners who are capable of making evidence-informed decisions to provide relevant care' (Halcomb EJ, Peters K: Nursing student feedback on undergraduate research education: Implications for teaching and learning, *Contemporary Nurse* 33(1):59–68, 2009)

research process the series of steps which make up research from the development of an idea to the completed research report or paper

research question use of an interrogative format to identify the variables to be studied and possible relationships or differences between those variables

research utilisation the process of translating and adapting research findings into practice. This process is sometimes called evidence-based practice (EBP)

researcher journal journal kept by a researcher in which thoughts, ideas, feelings and reflections are recorded. Field notes or observations may also be recorded

reserve collection 'material which is in great demand because of being placed on reading lists and set on one side for very short limited periods' (Prytherch R: *Harrod's Librarians' Glossary and Reference Book,* ed 9, Aldershot, 2000, Ashgate, p 628)

risks the potential to harm participants

sample subset of a population selected to participate in a research study

sampling the process used to select the sample

saturation point at which sampling and data collection are stopped in a grounded theory study because the information being collected is redundant and repetitive. Similar to the concept of theoretical redundancy

search engine tool for finding and retrieving specific information on the web (e.g. Google, Altavista, Ask, Metacrawler and Nursing Search Engine)

search strategy 'in information retrieval, a systematic plan for conducting a search' (Reitz J: *Dictionary of Library and Information Science,* Westport, CT, 2004, Libraries Unlimited, p 641)

sequential mixed methods design a design where the findings from one type of data collection method (e.g. interviews) provide a basis for the collection of a second set of data (e.g. survey). The final study results are based on the findings from both datasets

server (host) computer that offers an information service over the internet to a client

setting the physical location and conditions under which a research study takes place

social justice involves having fair and just social and political systems that ensures all people have equal opportunities and outcomes

social media media posted by the user. It takes many different forms – for example forums, message boards, blogs, wikis and podcasts. Social media applications include Google, Facebook and YouTube

socio-historical context refers to critical background information or setting the scene for Indigenous peoples. This includes the historical (and ongoing) experiences of colonisation and trauma and their current socioeconomic status that has impacted their health and wellbeing

statistical hypothesis also known as the null hypothesis, where there is no relationship between the dependent and independent variables

statistical significance significance determined through testing hypothesis and establishing probability

TCP/IP transmission control protocol/internet protocol. In combination, these protocols provide the method by which computers communicate over the internet. TCP/IP directs internet traffic through the internet

theoretical perspective/framework the theoretical foundation or frame of reference for a research study

theoretical sampling procedure used in grounded theory to gather additional data about emerging concepts

theory integrated and interrelated set of concepts used to explain some phenomenon

tradition the handing down of knowledge from one generation to the next

trial and error the process of trying a succession of alternative solutions before solving a problem

triangulation use of two or more data sources, investigators, methods or theories in the study of a phenomenon (Halcomb EJ, Andrew S: Triangulation as a method for contemporary nursing research, *Nurse Researcher* 13:71–82, 2005). This may or may not involve the combination of qualitative and quantitative methods of data collection in a single study

trustworthiness the rigour of qualitative research and encapsulates the concepts of credibility, transferability, confirmability and dependability

type 1 error occurs when the researcher rejects the null hypothesis when it's true. Also known as a 'false positive' or an α error

type 2 error occurs when the researcher fails to reject the null hypothesis when it's false. Also known as a 'false negative' or β error

uniform resource locator (URL) the address system used by the internet to assist in locating a web page or file

utilisation criteria criteria used to evaluate whether research findings can be adapted for use in the clinical arena

validity characteristic of a good instrument; the extent of an instrument's ability to measure what it purports to measure

values the beliefs that members of a group agree about in terms of what is imperative, has merit, is decent or is immoral

variable concept, characteristic or trait that varies (e.g. takes on measurably different values) within an identified population in a research study

voice over internet protocol (VOIP) the transmission of voice over IP-based networks

volume 'in the physical sense, all the written or printed matter contained in a single binding, portfolio, etc.' (Reitz J: *Dictionary of library and information science,* Westport, CT, 2004, Libraries Unlimited, p 763)

vulnerable groups people who have diminished capacity to give informed consent or are considered to be not completely free to give consent

web feed (RSS feed) a data format that can deliver updated content directly to you as soon as it is published online. The RSS feed allows content to be distributed to others

weblog (blog) a web page similar to a journal or diary. It is available through a website and it can be managed (organised, searched and categorised)

wi-fi the underlying technology of wireless local area networks. Wi-fi is developed to be used for mobile computing devices such as laptops. More recently it has been used for internet and VOIP phone access services, gaming and basic connectivity for consumer electronics

wiki Hawaiian word meaning 'quick'. A website that permits the creation and editing of hyperlinked web pages via a web browser using a markup language

wireless should not be confused with cordless. Refers to telecommunications systems that use some form of energy (e.g. radiofrequency, infrared light or laser light) to transfer information without the use of wires

wireless hotspots enable a person with a wi-fi device (computer, telephone, or personal digital assistant) to connect to the internet when in proximity of a wi-fi access point. Hotspots can range from a single room or access point to many square kilometres of overlapping hotspots, as in a municipal wireless network. Many universities and schools have wireless network access points around their campuses

world views are paradigms that guide how people live as cultural beings and make sense of the world, informed by their respective knowledge systems or ways of knowing related to their environment, cultures and experiences

world wide web (WWW) collection of computers on the internet that are interconnected by hypertext and store websites

INDEX

Page numbers followed by 'f' indicate figures, 't' indicate tables, and 'b' indicate boxes.